Complex Infectious Disease Issues in the Intensive Care Unit

Editors

NAOMI P. O'GRADY
SAMEER S. KADRI

INFECTIOUS DISEASE CLINICS OF NORTH AMERICA

www.id.theclinics.com

Consulting Editor
HELEN W. BOUCHER

September 2017 • Volume 31 • Number 3

ELSEVIER

1600 John F. Kennedy Boulevard • Suite 1800 • Philadelphia, Pennsylvania, 19103-2899.
http://www.theclinics.com

INFECTIOUS DISEASE CLINICS OF NORTH AMERICA Volume 31, Number 3
September 2017 ISSN 0891–5520, ISBN-13: 978-0-323-54556-3

Editor: Kerry Holland
Developmental Editor: Donald Mumford

Infectious Disease Clinics of North America (ISSN 0891–5520) is published in March, June, September, and December by Elsevier Inc., 360 Park Avenue South, New York, New York 10010-1710. Periodicals postage paid at New York, NY and additional mailing offices. Subscription prices are $301.00 per year for US individuals, $588.00 per year for US institutions, $100.00 per year for US students, $357.00 per year for Canadian individuals, $734.00 per year for Canadian institutions, $428.00 per year for international individuals, $734.00 per year for international institutions, and $200.00 per year for Canadian and international students. To receive student rate, orders must be accompanied by name of affiliated institution, date of term, and the *signature* of program/residency coordinator on institution letterhead. Orders will be billed at individual rate until proof of status is received. Foreign air speed delivery is included in all *Clinics* subscription prices. All prices are subject to change without notice. **POSTMASTER**: Send address changes to *Infectious Disease Clinics of North America,* Elsevier Health Sciences Division, Subcription Customer Service, 3251 Riverport Lane, Maryland Heights, MO 63043. **Customer Service: 1-800-654-2452 (US). From outside of the US and Canada, call 1-314-447-8871. Fax: 1-314-447-8029. E-mail: JournalsCustomerService-usa@elsevier.com (print support) or JournalsOnlineSupport-usa@elsevier.com (online support).**

Infectious Disease Clinics of North America is also published in Spanish by Editorial Inter-Médica, Junin 917, 1er A 1113, Buenos Aires, Argentina.

Reprints. For copies of 100 or more, of articles in this publication, please contact the Commercial Reprints Department, Elsevier Inc., 360 Park Avenue South, New York, New York 10010-1710. Tel. 212-633-3874, Fax: 212-633-3820, E-mail: reprints@elsevier.com.

Infectious Disease Clinics of North America is covered in *MEDLINE/PubMed (Index Medicus), Current Contents/Clinical Medicine, Science Citation Alert, SCISEARCH,* and *Research Alert.*

Contributors

CONSULTING EDITOR

HELEN W. BOUCHER, MD, FIDSA, FACP
Director, Infectious Diseases Fellowship Program, Division of Geographic Medicine and Infectious Diseases, Tufts Medical Center, Associate Professor of Medicine, Tufts University School of Medicine, Boston, Massachusetts

EDITORS

NAOMI P. O'GRADY, MD
Medical Director for Patient Safety and Clinical Quality, Critical Care Medicine Department, National Institutes of Health Clinical Center, Bethesda, Maryland

SAMEER S. KADRI, MD, MS
Head, Clinical Epidemiology Section, Critical Care Medicine Department, National Institutes of Health Clinical Center, Bethesda, Maryland

AUTHORS

MOHANAD AL-OBAIDI, MD
Infectious Disease Fellow, Division of Infectious Diseases, Department of Internal Medicine, University of Texas Health Science Center at Houston, Houston, Texas

JOHN G. BARTLETT, MD
Professor of Medicine Emeritus, Division of Infectious Diseases, The Johns Hopkins University School of Medicine, Baltimore, Maryland

TAISON BELL, MD
Department of Critical Care Medicine, National Institutes of Health Clinical Center, Bethesda, Maryland

STEPHANIE L. BONNE, MD, FACS
Division of Trauma and Critical Care, Assistant Professor, Department of Surgery, Rutgers New Jersey Medical School, Newark, New Jersey

HENRY F. CHAMBERS, MD
Professor, Division of Infectious Diseases, Department of Medicine, Zuckerberg San Francisco General Hospital and Trauma Center, University of California San Francisco, San Francisco, California

DANIEL S. CHERTOW, MD, MPH
Chief, Emerging Pathogens Section, Department of Critical Care Medicine, National Institutes of Health Clinical Center, Bethesda, Maryland

SARAH B. DOERNBERG, MD, MAS
Assistant Professor, Division of Infectious Diseases, Department of Medicine, University of California San Francisco, San Francisco, California

DIANA F. FLORESCU, MD
Associate Professor, Transplant Infectious Diseases Program, Division of Infectious Diseases, Department of Internal Medicine, University of Nebraska Medical Center, Omaha, Nebraska

BRIAN T. GARIBALDI, MD
Medical Director, Johns Hopkins Biocontainment Unit, Division of Pulmonary and Critical Care, The Johns Hopkins University School of Medicine, Baltimore, Maryland

DAVID N. GILBERT, MD
Chief, Infectious Diseases, Providence Portland Medical Center, Professor of Medicine, Oregon Health & Sciences University, Portland, Oregon

SAMEER S. KADRI, MD, MS
Head, Clinical Epidemiology Section, Critical Care Medicine Department, National Institutes of Health Clinical Center, Bethesda, Maryland

ANDRE C. KALIL, MD, MPH
Professor, Transplant Infectious Diseases Program, Division of Infectious Diseases, Department of Internal Medicine, University of Nebraska Medical Center, Omaha, Nebraska

MICHAEL KLOMPAS, MD, MPH
Associate Professor, Department of Population Medicine, Harvard Medical School, Harvard Pilgrim Health Care Institute, Department of Medicine, Brigham and Women's Hospital, Boston, Massachusetts

NAOMI P. O'GRADY, MD
Medical Director for Patient Safety and Clinical Quality, Critical Care Medicine Department, National Institutes of Health Clinical Center, Bethesda, Maryland

LUIS OSTROSKY-ZEICHNER, MD
Professor of Medicine and Epidemiology, Division of Infectious Diseases, Department of Internal Medicine, University of Texas Health Science Center at Houston, Houston, Texas

LUCY B. PALMER, MD
Pulmonary, Critical Care and Sleep Division, The State University of New York, Stony Brook, New York

TARA N. PALMORE, MD
Hospital Epidemiologist, National Institutes of Health Clinical Center, Bethesda, Maryland

CHANU RHEE, MD, MPH
Assistant Professor, Department of Population Medicine, Harvard Medical School, Harvard Pilgrim Health Care Institute, Department of Medicine, Brigham and Women's Hospital, Boston, Massachusetts

URIEL SANDKOVSKY, MD, MS
Associate Professor, Transplant Infectious Diseases Program, Division of Infectious Diseases, Department of Internal Medicine, University of Nebraska Medical Center, Omaha, Nebraska

JEFFREY R. STRICH, MD
Clinical Fellow, Department of Critical Care Medicine, National Institutes of Health Clinical Center, Bethesda, Maryland

JAMES M. WALTER, MD
Instructor of Medicine, Division of Pulmonary and Critical Care, Department of Medicine, Northwestern University Feinberg School of Medicine, Chicago, Illinois

RICHARD G. WUNDERINK, MD, FCCP
Professor of Medicine, Division of Pulmonary and Critical Care, Department of Medicine, Northwestern University Feinberg School of Medicine, Chicago, Illinois

Contents

New sepsis definitions shift emphasis from the systemic inflammatory response syndrome to organ dysfunction, quantified using the Sequential Organ Failure Assessment (SOFA) score. The new definitions also propose Quick SOFA criteria to rapidly identify potentially infected patients at risk for poor outcomes. The diagnosis of septic shock requires vasopressor dependence and increased lactate levels. Strengths of these definitions include their simplicity and clear association with adverse outcomes. However, their utility in identifying patients with serious infections before frank sepsis ensues remains to be seen. This article reviews challenges in defining sepsis, strengths and weaknesses of the new definitions, and unresolved issues.

In 2017, most intensive care units (ICUs) worldwide are admitting a growing population of immunosuppressed patients. The most common causes of pre-ICU immunosuppression are solid organ transplantation, hematopoietic stem cell transplantation, and infection due to human immunodeficiency virus. In this article, the authors review the most frequent infections that cause critical care illness in each of these 3 immunosuppressed patient populations.

The combination of molecular pathogen diagnostics and the biomarker procalcitonin (PCT) are changing the use of antimicrobials in patients admitted to critical care units with severe community-acquired pneumonia, possible septic shock, or other clinical syndromes. An elevated serum PCT level is good supportive evidence of a bacterial pneumonia, whereas a low serum PCT level virtually eliminates an etiologic role for bacteria even if the culture for a potential bacterial pathogen is positive. Serum PCT levels can be increased in any shocklike state; a low PCT level eliminates invasive bacterial infection as an etiology in more than 90% of patients.

Lower respiratory tract infection is a leading cause of death in the United States. Advances in diagnostic testing have improved our ability to detect pathogens. Viral pathogens are important causal pathogens in immuno-competent patients. As the number of elderly adults and those with chronic medical conditions increases, the burden of viral respiratory infections will increase. Clinicians must be familiar with the characteristics of rhinovirus, human adenoviruses, respiratory syncytial virus, and human metapneumovirus. Major challenges include distinguishing true infection from asymptomatic carriage and characterizing patients admitted with severe lower respiratory tract infection who do not have a causative pathogen identified.

Patients in the intensive care unit are exposed to multiple stressors that predispose them to invasive fungal infections (IFIs), which carry high morbidity and mortality. Getting acquainted with the diagnostic methods and therapies is imperative for patient safety and for providing high-quality health care. This article focuses on the most frequent IFIs: invasive candidiasis and invasive aspergillosis.

Clostridium difficile infection is a major health care challenge in terms of patient and economic consequences. For the patient, it is a morbid and sometimes a life-threatening iatrogenic complication of antibiotic treatment. In the United States, the provider's institution may face financial penalties, because the Centers for Disease Control and Prevention views this as an iatrogenic health care–associated complication that may not be reimbursable by the Centers for Medicare and Medicaid Services; this has resulted in substantial incentives for new approaches to prevention and treatment.

Despite advances in antibiotic and surgical management and supportive care for necrotizing soft tissue infections, morbidity and mortality remain substantial. Although there are clinical practice guidelines in place, there still remains much variability in choice and duration of antibiotic therapy, time to initial surgical debridement, and use of adjuvant medical therapies. This article offers an overview of necrotizing soft tissue infections with a focus on current diagnostic and treatment modalities.

Antimicrobial stewardship programs aim to monitor, improve, and measure responsible antibiotic use. The intensive care unit (ICU), with its critically ill patients and prevalence of multiple drug-resistant pathogens, presents unique challenges. This article reviews approaches to stewardship with application to the ICU, including the value of diagnostics, principles of empirical and definitive therapy, and measures of effectiveness. There is good evidence that antimicrobial stewardship results in more appropriate antimicrobial use, shorter therapy durations, and lower resistance rates. Data demonstrating hard clinical outcomes, such as adverse events and mortality, are more limited but encouraging; further studies are needed.

Infection control in the intensive care unit (ICU) has seen many advances, including rapid molecular screening tests for resistant organisms and chlorhexidine use in daily baths. Although these developments advance the cause of infection prevention, compliance with some of the basic measures remains elusive. Hand hygiene, antimicrobial stewardship, and reduction in device use remain the low-technology interventions that could have a major impact on nosocomial transmission of antimicrobial-resistant organisms. Although continued research is needed on new and old ways of preventing nosocomial infections, ICU staff must persevere in improving adherence with the measures that are known to be effective.

Central venous catheters (CVCs) are commonly used in critically ill patients and offer several advantages to peripheral intravenous access. However, indwelling CVCs have the potential to lead to bloodstream infections, with the risk increasing with an array of characteristics, such as catheter choice, catheter location, insertion technique, and catheter maintenance. Evidence-based guidelines have led to a significant reduction in the incidence of bloodstream infections associated with CVCs. The combination of guideline implementation and newer technologies has the potential to further reduce morbidity and mortality from infections related to CVCs.

The recent Ebola virus disease outbreak highlighted the need to build national and worldwide capacity to provide care for patients with highly infectious diseases. Specialized biocontainment units were successful in treating several critically ill patients with Ebola virus disease both in the United States and Europe. Several key principles underlie the care of critically ill patients in a high-containment environment. Environmental factors, staffing, equipment, training, laboratory testing, procedures, and waste management each present unique challenges. A multidisciplinary approach is key to developing effective systems and protocols to maintain the safety of patients, staff, and communities.

Multidrug-resistant organisms are creating a challenge for physicians treating the critically ill. As new antibiotics lag behind the emergence of worsening resistance, intensivists in countries with high rates of extensively drug-resistant bacteria are turning to inhaled antibiotics as adjunctive therapy. These drugs can provide high concentrations of drug in the lung that could not be achieved with intravenous antibiotics without significant systemic toxicity. This article summarizes current evidence describing the use of inhaled antibiotics for the treatment of bacterial ventilator-associated pneumonia and ventilator-associated tracheobronchitis. Preliminary data suggest aerosolized antimicrobials may effectively treat resistant pathogens with high minimum inhibitory concentrations.

INFECTIOUS DISEASE CLINICS
OF NORTH AMERICA

THE CLINICS ARE AVAILABLE ONLINE!
Access your subscription at:
www.theclinics.com

Preface

On the Interface of Infectious Diseases and Critical Care Medicine

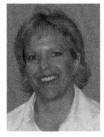 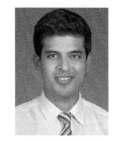

Naomi P. O'Grady, MD   Sameer S. Kadri, MD, MS
Editors

Infection occupies an overwhelming presence in the intensive care unit (ICU). Nearly half of the ICU patients worldwide are battling infection, and over two-thirds are pre-scribed antibiotics. Furthermore, this patient population we serve continues to grow in age, complexity, and vulnerability such that infection can easily tip the balance to-ward critical illness and death. Although outcomes from critical illness have improved over the years, patients with sepsis and septic shock continue to demonstrate unac-ceptably high mortality. The rise and fall of early goal-directed therapy for sepsis have renewed our realization of how important early recognition, prompt antibiotic de-livery, and source control are for a good outcome. Therefore, it is not surprising that infectious disease consultation has been shown to improve outcomes in a number of infections in the critically ill.

The last decade has witnessed increased activity on the interface of infectious dis-eases and critical care that has fostered combined training pathways in these two sub-specialties. This increased integration of specialties has contributed to dramatic decreases in central line–associated bloodstream infections, the expanding infrastruc-ture nationwide for extracorporeal membrane oxygenation in severe acute respiratory distress syndrome from influenza and bacterial pneumonia, resurrecting the antibiotic pipeline, prioritizing antibiotic stewardship, and bolstering emerging technology for rapid identification of pathogens. At the same time, both specialties have been hum-bled by the advent of pan-drug-resistant bacteria and serious outbreaks of emerging viruses such as severe acute respiratory syndrome coronavirus, Middle East respira-tory syndrome, and Ebola. We need a high degree of vigilance to detect, prepare for, and curb such epidemics, and we need to constantly appraise novel pathobiologic theories, biomarkers, and therapies as they emerge. Simply enhancing our repertoire

Infect Dis Clin N Am 31 (2017) xiii–xiv
http://dx.doi.org/10.1016/j.idc.2017.07.001
0891-5520/17/© 2017 Published by Elsevier Inc.

of intensive monitoring, resuscitation, and organ support for the critically ill will not be enough. It behooves us to stay abreast with local epidemiologic and susceptibility patterns, know which infections to anticipate with the increasing use of various novel immunomodulatory and biologic therapies for cancer and inflammatory diseases, recognize when adjunctive therapies are warranted, when enhanced isolation is indicated, when clinical judgment supersedes a biomarker test result, and when the risk of discordant antimicrobial therapy trumps the risk of selective pressure and *Clostridium difficile* infection.

The following issue of *Infectious Disease Clinics of North America* is a compilation of articles that combine current evidence with the opinion of experts in the fields of infectious diseases and critical care. We have attempted to cover nuanced epidemiologic and management issues on this interface of these two specialties. The information provided in this issue can benefit health care providers at all stages of training and practice, and it is hoped, patients and public health at large.

Naomi P. O'Grady, MD
Critical Care Medicine Department
National Institutes of Health Clinical Center
Bethesda, MD 20892, USA

Sameer S. Kadri, MD, MS
Clinical Epidemiology Section
Critical Care Medicine Department
National Institutes of Health Clinical Center
Bethesda, MD 20892, USA

E-mail addresses:
nogrady@mail.cc.nih.gov (N.P. O'Grady)
Sameer.kadri@nih.gov (S.S. Kadri)

New Sepsis and Septic Shock Definitions
Clinical Implications and Controversies

Chanu Rhee, MD, MPH[a,b],*, Michael Klompas, MD, MPH[a,b]

KEYWORDS

- Sepsis • Septic shock • Clinical diagnosis • SOFA • qSOFA • SIRS

KEY POINTS

- The new sepsis definitions shift emphasis from the systemic inflammatory response syndrome (SIRS) to organ dysfunction. They use the Sequential Organ Failure Assessment (SOFA) score as a simple, tested method of quantifying organ dysfunction, and require vasopressor-dependent hypotension and increased lactate levels in the absence of hypovolemia to diagnose septic shock.
- The new sepsis definitions also propose Quick SOFA (qSOFA) criteria (≥2 of hypotension, tachypnea, and/or altered mental status) for efficient bedside screening to identify potentially infected patients at risk for poor outcomes in out-of-hospital, emergency department, and general hospital ward settings.
- Although the new sepsis definitions have been endorsed by multiple professional societies, there have been concerns that their emphasis on organ dysfunction may lead to delays in identifying serious infections before they progress to organ dysfunction. Furthermore, the SOFA score has primarily been used as a research tool and is unfamiliar to many clinicians.
- Controversy also exists as to whether or not there is still a role for SIRS criteria, whether or not qSOFA is sufficiently sensitive as a screening tool for sepsis, and what the role of lactate testing is under the new sepsis definitions.
- Despite these controversies, the new definitions should not change the basics of sepsis management. The cornerstone remains early appropriate antibiotic therapy and source control for patients with serious infections, particularly those with signs of organ dysfunction, and rapid fluid resuscitation when hypotension is present.

[a] Department of Population Medicine, Harvard Medical School, Harvard Pilgrim Health Care Institute, 401 Park Drive, Suite 401, Boston, MA 02215, USA; [b] Department of Medicine, Brigham and Women's Hospital, 75 Francis Street, Boston, MA 02115, USA
* Corresponding author. Department of Population Medicine, Harvard Medical School, Harvard Pilgrim Health Care Institute, 401 Park Drive, Suite 401, Boston, MA 02215.
E-mail address: crhee@bwh.harvard.edu

Infect Dis Clin N Am 31 (2017) 397–413
http://dx.doi.org/10.1016/j.idc.2017.05.001
0891-5520/17/© 2017 Elsevier Inc. All rights reserved.

id.theclinics.com

INTRODUCTION

Sepsis is a major cause of death, disability, and cost to the health care system. However, despite its clinical significance, sepsis is difficult to define. For more than 2 decades, the sepsis classification framework has been based on identifying infection accompanied by the systemic inflammatory response syndrome (SIRS) (sepsis), and then looking for organ dysfunction (severe sepsis) or refractory hypotension (septic shock).[1] In 2016, the European Society of Intensive Care Medicine (ESICM) and Society of Critical Care Medicine (SCCM) released new consensus definitions (Sepsis-3) defining sepsis as "life-threatening organ dysfunction caused by a dysregulated host response to infection"[2] and eliminating SIRS criteria from the definition. The Sepsis-3 Task Force operationalized the new definition as infection associated with an increase in Sequential Organ Failure Assessment (SOFA) score by 2 or more points from baseline. In addition, a new set of simple clinical criteria were endorsed, called Quick SOFA (qSOFA), which can be easily calculated at the bedside to identify potentially infected patients at high risk for adverse outcomes who might merit additional care. The qSOFA score was also intended to prompt clinicians to consider the possibility of infection if not previously suspected.[3] In addition, septic shock is now defined as sepsis-induced hypotension requiring vasopressors and an increased lactate level in the absence of hypovolemia. Although the new definitions benefit from greater simplicity and clearer association with adverse outcomes, there are concerns that the emphasis on organ dysfunction and qSOFA may delay early identification and intervention in infected patients before they develop organ dysfunction. This article summarizes some of the challenges in defining sepsis, the history of sepsis definitions, the rationale and development of the new definitions, their strengths and weaknesses, and clinical controversies.

SEPSIS BURDEN AND NEW QUALITY MEASURES

Sepsis is the leading cause of death in noncoronary intensive care units (ICUs), the most expensive condition treated in hospitals, and a contributor in 30% to 50% of all hospital deaths.[4–6] Survivors are also at high risk for recurrent sepsis, readmissions, and long-term cognitive and functional impairment.[7,8] Reports based on administrative data have suggested an increase in sepsis cases over the past 2 decades,[9–11] although it is unclear whether this is caused by true increases in disease rates or greater recognition and more complete coding.[12,13] Nonetheless, increasing appreciation of the severe burden that sepsis imposes on society has prompted public education campaigns and quality improvement initiatives in hospitals around the world. In the United States, new regulatory requirements have been implemented, including the Centers for Medicare & Medicaid Services (CMS) SEP-1 measure, which compels hospitals to publicly report their compliance with 3-hour and 6-hour management bundles for patients diagnosed with sepsis.[14]

CHALLENGES IN DEFINING AND TRACKING SEPSIS

Sepsis is an elusive condition to define because it is a complex syndrome without a pathologic gold standard. It is often unclear whether a patient is infected or not, even when assessing the patient's clinical course in retrospect, and microbiological tests and cultures are often unrevealing.[15] Even positive microbiological tests do not always indicate active infection. Most clinicians would agree that a patient with bacteremia and hypotension or multiorgan dysfunction is septic, but blood cultures are positive in only a fraction of septic patients.[16] In addition, the line between normal organ function, chronic organ dysfunction, and acute organ dysfunction can be unclear, and attributing physiologic signs and organ dysfunction to infection versus a myriad of other potential causes is invariably subjective. Intensivists reviewing case vignettes of patients with suspected or documented infection and signs of organ dysfunction have high levels of disagreement about whether sepsis is present or not.[17]

Given these challenges, clinicians may wonder whether sepsis needs to be defined at all, or whether patients should simply be categorized according to their respective infectious syndromes, such as pneumonia or urinary tract infections. However, there is a compelling argument to define sepsis, above and beyond the underlying infection, because it carries important clinical implications for management. In particular, flagging sepsis helps clinicians identify the subset of patients who are at high risk of adverse outcomes and require immediate and aggressive resuscitation. Identifying sepsis may also help clinicians risk-stratify and prognosticate patients. In addition, defining sepsis is essential to understand the epidemiology of severe infections, track outcomes and quality of care, and set criteria for clinical studies.[18] These goals may be secondary priorities to practicing clinicians but they are vital for public health officials, researchers, administrators, and policy makers.

PRIOR SEPSIS DEFINITIONS

Sepsis has long been a confusing term to clinicians. Terms such as sepsis, septicemia, bacteremia, sepsis syndrome, and septic shock were used variably and sometimes interchangeably for many years. The first attempt to standardize sepsis terminology came with the American College of Chest Physicians/SCCM consensus conference in 1991.[1] At that time, sepsis was conceptually defined as the systemic inflammatory response to the presence of infection. SIRS criteria were proposed, consisting of 2 or more abnormalities in temperature, heart rate, respiratory rate, and white blood cell count, with severe sepsis referring to sepsis with organ dysfunction and septic shock referring to sepsis with refractory hypotension. This construct remained in place largely unchanged for the next 25 years. At the second consensus conference in 2001, the list of possible diagnostic criteria for sepsis was expanded but otherwise no significant change was made.[19] Importantly, no concrete definitions for organ dysfunction were offered with these first 2 sepsis definitions. The 2012 Surviving Sepsis Campaign guidelines, although not a sepsis definitions document, did offer a set of criteria for organ dysfunction, which have since been incorporated into the CMS SEP-1 measure.[20] However, use of these criteria is hampered by their lack of guidance on how to differentiate acute from preexisting organ dysfunction and the difficulty in knowing whether acute organ dysfunction was precipitated by infection or some other process.

WHY REVISE THE DEFINITION?

Since their inception, there has been ample recognition of the limitations of SIRS criteria.[21] SIRS is not specific for infection, and its usefulness as a screening tool for sepsis is limited by the high prevalence of these abnormalities in hospitalized patients. For example, one recent observational study showed that nearly half of all patients admitted to non-ICU wards met SIRS criteria at least once during their hospitalizations.[22] Equating SIRS with sepsis therefore risks promoting overuse of antibiotics and fluid resuscitation. At the same time, SIRS criteria still miss some patients with life-threatening infections. One large observational study showed that SIRS criteria were lacking in the first 24 hours of ICU admission in 1 out of 8 patients with infection and organ dysfunction, many of whom subsequently died in the hospital.[23] From a pathophysiologic standpoint, sepsis is now thought to represent a dysregulated host response to infection, whereas SIRS is a normal physiologic response to infection that may be adaptive. The Sepsis-3 Task Force consequently opted to deemphasize SIRS in defining sepsis and focused instead on organ dysfunction because this is the *sine qua non* of the complex pathobiology of sepsis that includes both proinflammatory and antiinflammatory responses. In addition, the term severe sepsis was thought to be confusing because most clinicians diagnose patients as septic when signs of hypotension or organ dysfunction are present. Septic shock was also thought to be more than just sepsis with refractory hypotension or cardiovascular dysfunction, requiring signs of cellular or metabolic abnormalities as well. In addition, the Sepsis-3 Task Force recognized the lack of uniformity in the thresholds for organ dysfunction and criteria for septic shock, which has confounded epidemiologic and clinical studies.[24]

SEPSIS-3: SEQUENTIAL ORGAN FAILURE ASSESSMENT, QUICK SEQUENTIAL ORGAN FAILURE ASSESSMENT, AND SEPTIC SHOCK

Sepsis was conceptually redefined as a "life-threatening organ dysfunction caused by a dysregulated host response to infection."[2] Operationally, the Sepsis-3 Task Force defined this as infection associated with an increase in the SOFA score by 2 or more points. The SOFA score, which describes organ failure across 6 systems, each from 0 to 4 points, was created by consensus opinion in 1996.[25] The new Sepsis-3 definitions and the SOFA score are summarized in **Table 1** and juxtaposed against the CMS SEP-1 definitions, which closely encompass the original sepsis definitions first proposed in 1991.

In contrast with the original consensus definition, which was created purely from expert opinion, the Sepsis-3 Task Force sought to use a data-driven approach to support their criteria. Specifically, a large electronic health record data set consisting of more than 1 million patient encounters at the University of Pittsburgh Medical System was used, from which approximately 150,000 patients were identified who had clinical evidence of suspected infection (imputed from clinicians' orders for clinical cultures and concurrent antibiotic administrations).[3] Among these patients, existing scores of inflammation (SIRS) or organ dysfunction (SOFA and the Logistic Organ Dysfunction System [LODS][26]) were compared for their ability to predict in-hospital mortality, prolonged ICU stay, or both. The discrimination for hospital mortality with SOFA and LODS was superior to that of SIRS. SOFA was chosen for operationalizing the definition rather than LODS because SOFA was thought to be simpler and more familiar within the critical care community.

In addition, a set of 21 bedside and laboratory criteria from Sepsis-2 that could be examined electronically were modeled in a multivariate analysis to derive parsimonious criteria with high predictive ability for the outcomes of mortality and/or prolonged ICU stay. This model led to the qSOFA criteria: systolic blood pressure less than or equal to 100 mm Hg, respiratory rate greater than or equal to 22 breaths/min, and altered mental status. Among ICU patients, SOFA and LODS were superior to qSOFA for discrimination of hospital mortality. Outside the ICU, greater than or equal to 2 qSOFA criteria had similar predictive ability as greater than or equal to 2 SOFA points and were superior to SIRS. Similar results were found on external validation of these criteria in 4 additional data sets. When comparing qSOFA with SIRS, qSOFA conferred a higher mortality risk at any baseline decile risk of in-hospital mortality. The task force thus proposed that the qSOFA score, which is simple, intuitive, and easy to apply at the bedside, can be used to rapidly identify patients with

Table 1
Sepsis-3 definitions versus the Centers for Medicare and Medicaid Services' SEP-1 definitions

Sepsis-3	CMS SEP-1 Definitions
Sepsis: documented/suspected infection and increase by ≥2 in SOFA score SOFA score: • Neurologic: Glasgow Coma Scale 13–14 = 1, 10–12 = 2, 6–9 = 3, <6 = 4 • Cardiovascular: MAP <70 mm Hg = 1, low-dose dopamine or dobutamine = 2, moderate-dose dopamine or low-dose epinephrine or norepinephrine = 3, high-dose dopamine or epinephrine or norepinephrine = 4 • Respiratory: Pao_2/Fio_2 ratio 300–399 = 1, 200–299 = 2, 100–199 + mechanical ventilation = 3, <100 + mechanical ventilation = 4 • Renal: creatinine 1.2–1.9 mg/dL = 1, 2.0–3.4 mg/dL = 2, 3.5–4.9 mg/dL or urine output <500 mL/d = 3, >5.0 mg/dL or urine output <200 mL/d = 4 • Hepatic: total bilirubin 1.2–1.9 mg/dL = 1, 2.0–5.9 mg/dL = 2, 6.0–11.9 mg/dL = 3, >12.0 mg/dL = 4 • Coagulation: platelet count 100–149 × $10^3/\mu L$ = 1, 50–99 = 2, 20–49 = 3, <20 = 4 Quick SOFA: (≥2 identifies patients at high risk for poor outcomes) • SBP ≤100 mm Hg • Respiratory rate ≥22 breaths/min • Altered mental status	Severe sepsis: documented/suspected infection and ≥2 SIRS criteria and ≥1 acute organ dysfunction SIRS: • Temperature >38.3°C or <36°C • Heart rate >90 beats/min • Respiratory rate >20 breaths/min or $Paco_2$ <32 mm Hg • WBC >12,000 cells/μL or <4000 cells/μL or >10% bands Organ dysfunction: • SBP <90 mm Hg or MAP <65 mm Hg or SBP decrease from baseline by >40 mm Hg • Lactate >2.0 mmol/L • Respiratory failure (need for noninvasive or invasive mechanical ventilation) • Creatinine >2.0 mg/dL or urine output <0.5 mL/kg/h × 2 h • Total bilirubin >2.0 mg/dL • Platelet count <100 × $10^3/\mu L$ • INR >1.5 or PTT >60 s
Septic shock: • Persistent hypotension after fluids, and • Requiring vasopressors, and • Lactate >2 mmol/L in the absence of hypovolemia	Septic shock: • Persistent hypotension after fluids (30 mL/kg), or • Initial lactate ≥4.0 mmol/L

Abbreviations: Fio_2, fraction of inspired oxygen; INR, International Normalized Ratio; MAP, mean arterial pressure; PTT, partial thromboplastin time; SBP, systolic blood pressure; WBC, white blood cell count.

suspected infection who are at high risk of poor outcomes in out-of-hospital, emergency department, or general hospital ward settings. SIRS was thought to be less useful because of its inferior predictive and discriminatory power compared with qSOFA.

Importantly, under the new definitions, greater than or equal to 2 qSOFA points associated with infection do not define sepsis. qSOFA is only intended to help clinicians identify patients who may have sepsis and who are at high risk for adverse outcomes. The qSOFA score was not formally incorporated into the sepsis definition because of the imperfect overlap between qSOFA and the full SOFA score. The qSOFA score misses some patients with 2-point increases in SOFA because it does not give points for all organ systems or variables accounted for in the SOFA score; namely, oxygenation, bilirubin, creatinine/urine output, and platelet counts. In contrast, some patients with greater than or equal to 2 qSOFA points might not have an increase in SOFA score by 2 because the qSOFA respiratory and blood pressure criteria are less severe than the SOFA thresholds for impaired oxygenation and circulatory function.[27]

Conceptually, septic shock was redefined as "a subset of sepsis in which particularly profound circulatory, cellular, and metabolic abnormalities are associated with a greater risk of mortality than with sepsis alone."[28] The clinical variables thought to represent these concepts were hypotension, vasopressor requirement, and increased lactate level.[28] Descriptive analyses within the Surviving Sepsis Campaign database showed that, among patients with different combinations of those variables, those with hypotension after fluids, a requirement for vasopressors, and lactate level greater than 2.0 mmol/L after volume resuscitation had higher mortalities (42.3%) than all other subsets. For example, infected patients with hypotension and a vasopressor requirement, but with a lactate level less than or equal to 2.0 mmol, had a mortality of 30.1%.

The conceptual differences in Sepsis-3 versus the prior sepsis definitions are shown in **Fig. 1**. Panel A shows the large overlap between SIRS and infection. Panel B shows the more modest overlap between organ dysfunction and infection. The size of the sepsis circle in panel B approximates the size of the severe sepsis circle in panel A, whereas the septic shock circle in panel B is smaller than septic shock circle in panel A (because of the more stringent definition of septic shock).

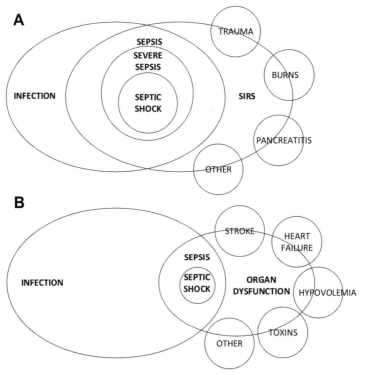

Fig. 1. Conceptual comparison of prior sepsis definitions (*A*) versus Sepsis-3 (*B*).

STRENGTHS OF SEPSIS-3

The new definitions have several strengths. First, the nomenclature better reflects clinicians' usual usage of the term sepsis. Clinicians rarely differentiated between sepsis and severe sepsis but instead used sepsis as an umbrella term for all patients with infection causing hypotension or organ dysfunction. The simpler terminology may, in the long run, decrease confusion among clinicians. Second, derivation of the new criteria was supported, in part, by robust analyses of electronic health record data sets rather than expert opinion alone. This support lends credibility and content validity because of the association of the new criteria with adverse outcomes. Old and new sepsis criteria have already been prospectively compared in an international cohort of patients presenting to emergency departments with suspected infection, and qSOFA was found to have higher prognostic accuracy for in-hospital mortality than both SIRS and severe sepsis.[29] External validation was also performed retrospectively in a large cohort study of patients admitted to ICUs in Australia and New Zealand with infection-related primary diagnoses, and an increase in SOFA by 2 or more points was found to have greater prognostic accuracy for in-hospital mortality than SIRS or qSOFA.[30] Both of these studies support the Sepsis-3 Task Force's recommendations of using qSOFA in non-ICU patients to efficiently identify potentially infected patients at high risk for adverse outcomes, but using the full SOFA score in ICU settings. Third, more standardized quantification of organ dysfunction (through SOFA) and septic shock criteria may allow better comparisons of sepsis cohorts across time and space. This possibility is important because interpreting trends in sepsis and septic shock incidence, severity, and mortality can be confounded by changes in the threshold to diagnose sepsis and organ dysfunction.[13,31,32]

For bedside clinical care, another benefit of the new definitions may be that they guide clinicians to pay more attention to organ dysfunction. The emphasis on organ dysfunction will ideally prompt clinicians to consider the possibility of undiagnosed infection when working up new organ dysfunction and to expedite resuscitation in infected patients with signs of organ dysfunction. Although most clinicians do not routinely calculate SOFA scores in their patients, the renewed emphasis on SOFA from Sepsis-3 could help clinicians better identify new organ dysfunction, and better prognosticate their patients. Furthermore, the qSOFA score is simple to calculate, clinically intuitive, and does not require any sophisticated equipment or laboratory testing. In addition, eliminating SIRS as a diagnostic criterion may potentially reduce inappropriate use of broad-spectrum antibiotics and fluid resuscitation.

POTENTIAL WEAKNESSES AND CRITICISMS OF SEPSIS-3

Despite the strength of the new definitions and the endorsements of multiple professional societies, they have not been universally embraced by the medical community. Several concerns about the new definitions are outlined here.

Using the New Sepsis Criteria Has Not Been Shown to Improve Clinical Outcomes

The use of large electronic health record data sets to develop definitions was a step forward from prior iterations, and some of the findings have already been prospectively validated.[29] However, showing that the new criteria are more strongly associated with adverse outcomes is different than showing that using these criteria can improve clinical care and outcomes. A prospective study comparing sepsis identification using the old versus the new methods and showing improved clinical outcomes with the new definitions would clearly lend the highest level of evidence to support Sepsis-3. Until rigorous real-world clinical testing is performed, the Sepsis-3 definitions will, in the eyes of many clinicians, remain provisional. Some have argued that the many successes of the Surviving Sepsis Campaign were specifically achieved under the rubric of SIRS and the old sepsis definitions and thus modifications to these definitions should require similar or better evidence of their capacity to improve outcomes before adoption.

Potential Delays in Early Identification and Treatment

Perhaps the most important concern is that eliminating SIRS and focusing on qSOFA/SOFA may delay early identification and treatment.[33,34] For example, under the new definition, infection with hypotension that does not require vasopressor support may not be classified as sepsis, but such patients clearly deserve prompt attention and therapy. Despite its faults, the SIRS/sepsis construct emphasized early recognition and halting the progression of infection to organ dysfunction. A good argument can be made that sacrificing specificity for the sake of sensitivity is appropriate for screening tools. Quality improvement efforts around the world have relied on the SIRS-as-sepsis framework for many years.[35–37] These efforts may have contributed to the observed decline in sepsis-related mortality over the past 2 decades.[32,38,39]

Along similar lines, it can be argued that the new septic shock criteria are not as clinically useful as the CMS definition. The CMS criteria (suspected infection with persistent hypotension after fluids, or initial lactate level ≥ 4.0 mmol/L) are essentially equivalent to the entry criteria into the early goal-directed therapy trials, and mandate urgent clinical interventions such as rapid fluid administration, antibiotics, and timely vasopressor administration.[40–44] Although the 3 most recent early goal-directed therapy trials showed no benefit compared with standard therapy, most of the patients in these trials were given fluids and antibiotics before enrollment.[45–47] Some experts have therefore concluded that the increasing emphasis over time on these basic, rapid interventions has been responsible for the significantly lower septic shock mortalities in recent trials compared with the original early goal-directed therapy trial.[48] Beyond portending a poor prognosis and suggesting a framework for thinking about sepsis, it is unclear whether the new Sepsis-3 septic shock definition is helpful to clinicians, because by the time patients meet these criteria they have already been fluid resuscitated and started on vasopressors.

Sequential Organ Failure Assessment Score: An Unfamiliar Clinical Tool Specific to the Intensive Care Unit

Another potential weakness of the new definitions is their reliance on the SOFA score. SOFA was created in 1996 primarily for research purposes in ICU settings. Scoring systems such as SOFA are generally not easy to memorize, which limits their everyday clinical utility. Many SOFA components are ICU specific, such as the Pao_2/Fio_2 (fraction of inspired oxygen) ratio or vasopressor requirements, or are not routinely measured in many patients, such as the Glasgow Coma Scale, which is problematic because most septic patients are initially managed in emergency rooms or on hospital wards rather than in an ICU.[49,50] Clinical practice changes in the past 2 decades also make the cardiovascular components of the SOFA score outdated, such as a deemphasis on dobutamine use after the negative early goal-directed therapy trials. Changes include less use of dopamine as a result of studies showing more adverse events compared with norepinephrine,[51] and greater use of vasopressin (which is not included in the score) in septic shock.[52] Furthermore, although using the SOFA score makes Sepsis-3's assessment of organ dysfunction more standardized than prior sepsis definitions, it does not address the clinical challenge of determining whether organ dysfunction is attributable to infection versus another cause.

Neither Sequential Organ Failure Assessment nor Quick Sequential Organ Failure Assessment Helps Identify Infection

The new definitions offer no guidance on identifying infection, but this is often the most important and challenging aspect to identifying sepsis. Every day, clinicians are faced with this deceptively simple question: is this patient infected or not? The Sepsis-3 Task Force did not tackle this question but reasoned that, functionally, the usual indication of severe infection is organ dysfunction and thus chose to emphasize the importance of detecting organ dysfunction with the hope that clinicians will then consider whether organ dysfunction may have been caused by infection. For the purposes of deriving and validating the new definitions, the Sepsis-3 Task Force chose to rely on clinicians' actions (culture orders and antibiotics) as proxies for suspected infection. Thus, clinicians should be cognizant that Sepsis-3 and qSOFA were derived in patients in whom infection was already suspected, and thus these scores do not help distinguish infected versus noninfected patients. Although the task force's reluctance to address the challenge of identifying infection is understandable, there have been major advances in the past decade in using biomarkers, such as procalcitonin, and molecular tests, including multiplex polymerase chain reaction, mass spectrometry, and array techniques, to help diagnose infection and guide antibiotic therapy.[53,54] These advances in infectious disease diagnostic tests could make a large difference in accurately and rapidly diagnosing sepsis, and in avoiding overprescription of antibiotics in noninfected patients. There is still much to be done to mature these technologies and define their roles in routine clinical practice. It is hoped that the science will sufficiently mature such that future sepsis definitions will embrace these new technologies and help guide clinicians in their appropriate use to identify and manage sepsis early.

Risk of Confusion with Concurrent Definitions

Although a transitional period is to be expected with the introduction of any new definition, sepsis terminology is particularly challenging because it has long been a source of confusion to clinicians and the public.[55] The new sepsis definitions risk making this problem even worse, at least in the short term.[14] It has taken decades of work to educate clinicians on the proper use of the prior sepsis definitions and to establish them in the medical lexicon. For example, although the first consensus definitions of sepsis, severe sepsis, and septic shock were published in 1992, it was not until 2002 that these terms were added to the International Classification of Diseases coding library. In the United States, the CMS SEP-1 measure still uses the old sepsis definitions and therefore compels hospitals to retain old terminology and definitions. Although CMS may eventually change their criteria to match the new definitions, they recently issued a statement that they have no immediate plans to do so pending further studies and field experience with the new definitions.[56]

PRESSING QUESTIONS AND CONTROVERSIES SURROUNDING SEPSIS-3 AND CLINICAL MANAGEMENT

The new definitions raise important practical questions about sepsis identification and clinical management, several of which are addressed below. Many of these questions cannot be adequately answered as of now in the absence of new data.

Is There Still a Role for Systemic Inflammatory Response Syndrome Criteria?

As discussed, one of the major criticisms of Sepsis-3 is the concern that deemphasizing SIRS will lead to delayed identification of patients with serious infections. However, the new definitions do not necessarily imply that SIRS criteria lack any clinical utility. In the analysis of electronic health record data sets by the Sepsis-3 Task Force, SIRS was moderately predictive of prolonged ICU stay and/or mortality. Other large observational studies have shown a stepwise increase in mortality with additional SIRS criteria,[23] and the mere presence of SIRS with infection carries a mortality of 7% or more.[57] Other studies have suggested that SIRS with infection progresses to sepsis with organ dysfunction in more than half of cases.[58] Thus, the continued use of SIRS as a screening tool for potentially infected patients is reasonable, so long as clinicians appreciate its imperfect sensitivity and pronounced lack of specificity. With these caveats in mind, many institutions may opt to continue using this approach to early sepsis identification.

Is Quick Sequential Organ Failure Assessment a Replacement for Systemic Inflammatory Response Syndrome?

The Sepsis-3 consensus definitions should not be interpreted as a call to replace SIRS with qSOFA. In the prior definitions, SIRS was a prerequisite to having sepsis, but this is not the case with qSOFA; qSOFA has merely been offered as an additional set of clinical criteria to identify patients with suspected infection who are at risk for poor outcomes and therefore merit increased vigilance and/or early intervention. In the Sepsis-3 derivation dataset, 75% of patients with suspected infection and 2 or more qSOFA points also had an increase of 2 or more SOFA points. However, the sensitivity of qSOFA for detecting the full range of organ dysfunction that can occur with sepsis seems to be poor. In a recent analysis of a prospective cohort of emergency department patients with suspected infection, qSOFA was specific (96.1%) but insensitive (29.7%) for organ dysfunction, whereas SIRS was less specific (61.1%) but more sensitive (72.3%).[59]

What Is the Best Screening Tool for Sepsis?

The poor sensitivity of qSOFA for organ dysfunction suggests that qSOFA alone is not an adequate screening tool for sepsis. The optimal screening tool remains a topic of debate. One recent study used a retrospective electronic health record data set to examine more than 30,000 patients with suspected infection in the emergency department or hospital ward and compared qSOFA and SIRS with the Modified Early Warning Score (MEWS) and the National Early Warning Score (NEWS), which are established scoring systems that identify patients who are clinically deteriorating.[60] The best discrimination for in-hospital mortality was with NEWS (area under the curve [AUC], 0.77), followed by MEWS (AUC, 0.73), qSOFA (AUC, 0.69), and SIRS (AUC, 0.65). SIRS was the most sensitive (91%), although it was nonspecific (13%) for predicting mortality or ICU transfer, versus 54% sensitivity and 67% specificity for qSOFA, 59% and 70% for MEWS greater than or equal to 5, and 67% and 66% for NEWS greater than or equal to 8. Furthermore, patients met SIRS criteria at an earlier time point before the combined outcome compared with qSOFA. This study suggests again that SIRS may have value in detecting potentially septic patients early, upstream from their eventual clinical deterioration, and that screening tools that are already in place in some health care systems may be superior to qSOFA. On the other hand, MEWS and NEWS may not be as simple and easy to memorize as qSOFA, and SIRS criteria may entail more risk of overtreatment of uninfected patients. Prospective trials comparing various strategies for early detection of sepsis (including qSOFA, SIRS, established early warning scores, and clinical vigilance alone), and their impact on clinical interventions and outcomes, are urgently needed to shed light on the optimal screening method.

What Is the Role of Lactate Testing with Sepsis-3?

Another controversial issue is the apparent diminished role of lactate testing in the Sepsis-3 definition. The Sepsis-3 Task Force did not include lactate as part of the qSOFA score because the addition of lactate did not improve predictive validity of the model for prolonged ICU stay and/or death. This finding is in contrast with the SEP-1 definition, in which increased lactate level is part of the severe sepsis criteria. The exclusion of lactate from Sepsis-3 should not downplay the clinical utility of lactate testing. The primary Sepsis-3 analysis assessed all events within 48 hours before to 24 hours following the onset of suspected infection. The analysis did not distinguish when within this period lactate was drawn and thus was insensitive to the possible clinical benefits of finding an increased lactate level before organ dysfunction occurs. Mortality rates were similar for patients with 1 qSOFA point and a lactate level of greater than 2 compared with those with 2 qSOFA points. Another recent study suggests that combining lactate level with qSOFA confers similar predictive utility for mortality compared with the full SOFA score.[61]

More notably, increased lactate level has been associated with mortality independent of other organ dysfunction, and several studies have shown that increased lactate levels can identify patients with suspected infection who have otherwise normal vital signs and no overt signs of organ dysfunction but have increased risk of death from sepsis.[62–64] Measuring lactate levels thus helps risk-stratify patients with suspected sepsis, prompts aggressive early treatment, and is central to monitoring the impact of therapy through serial testing.[65–70] Implementing bedside lactate measurements in the emergency department may improve the rapidity of fluid resuscitation in suspected sepsis and decrease rates of ICU admission and mortality.[71]

Thus, the available evidence suggests that lactate testing should still play a central role in sepsis identification and management. In support of this sentiment, the Surviving Sepsis Campaign issued interim recommendations after the publication of Sepsis-3 that continue to advise initiating the 3-hour and 6-hour bundles of care for sepsis with lactate level greater than 2.0 mmol/L (or other signs of organ dysfunction).[72]

Should Clinicians Routinely Measure Sequential Organ Failure Assessment Scores?

Sepsis-3 has increased the visibility of the SOFA score within the clinical community. Although SOFA was primarily created as a research tool, there is no particular reason why it could not be used as a clinical tool, especially because it tracks strongly with the risk of mortality. For example, in one large prospective study of ICU patients, a score of greater than 15 correlated with a 90% mortality.[73] Another prospective study found that an increase in SOFA score during the first 48 hours of ICU admission, independent of the initial score, predicted a mortality of greater than 50%, although a decrease in SOFA score was associated with a mortality of 27%.[74] In addition, the SOFA score has been validated and applied in diverse ICU patient groups, including medical, surgical, and cardiac patients, and those with burns.[75] It is simpler than many other ICU scoring systems, and it could be envisioned that, with the increasing sophistication of electronic health record systems, SOFA scores could be automatically calculated in real time and even function as an alert to clinicians for the possibility of sepsis. However, the clinical impact of routine SOFA score measurements by clinicians remains to be seen.

FINAL CAVEATS ON SEPSIS-3

Sepsis is inherently difficult to define because there is no true gold standard. As such, no single set of criteria can perfectly distinguish patients with sepsis from those without sepsis. Sepsis-3 merely represents the latest attempt to set clinical criteria to help clinicians speak the same language and to identify potentially infected patients who are at high risk for adverse outcomes. However, multiple competing approaches and terms may coexist when trying to define and measure sepsis, and there may be room for multiple definitions depending on whether the primary purpose is clinical care, research, surveillance, or audit.[18,76] For example, a sepsis definition meant to guide public health surveillance and benchmarking may favor objectivity, reproducibility, and ease of data capture, whereas a clinical definition may favor sensitivity, timeliness, and simplicity.[32,77] However, greater subjectivity and interrater variability is to be expected for a definition meant to guide clinical care, in which the timeliness of information is of great importance. A research definition meant for clinical trials may also emphasize timeliness and applicability at the bedside but allow for more complexity to enhance rigor. All these definitions may differ significantly from research definitions for animal models of sepsis pathobiology. Thus, clinicians should realize that different sepsis definitions may coexist, and their strengths, weaknesses, and differences must be interpreted in the context of their primary purpose.

SUMMARY

The ESICM/SCCM Sepsis-3 Task Force has redefined sepsis from the systemic inflammatory response to infection to life-threatening organ dysfunction secondary to a dysregulated host response to infection. From an operational standpoint, sepsis is now defined as infection leading to an increase in the SOFA score of 2 or more points, whereas septic shock is defined as infection leading to refractory hypotension requiring vasopressors and lactate level greater than 2 mmol/L in the absence of hypovolemia. The term severe sepsis has been discarded and SIRS criteria are no longer part of the sepsis definitions, although they may still be useful in helping identify patients with serious infections before they develop organ dysfunction. A set of simple bedside criteria consisting of 2 or more of systolic blood pressure less than or equal to 100 mm Hg, respiratory rate greater than or equal to 22 breaths/min, or altered mental status (qSOFA) have been suggested as an efficient screening method to identify patients at high risk of poor outcomes when infection is suspected in non-ICU settings.

The new definitions encompass the latest thinking in sepsis pathophysiology and are the result of a data-driven approach using large electronic health record data sets, but some clinicians have expressed concern that the shift in emphasis from SIRS to organ dysfunction may lead to delays in early identification and treatment of sepsis, and that the SOFA score is unfamiliar to many clinicians. Furthermore, the definitions offer no guidance on identifying infection, which is often the most challenging and important aspect of sepsis diagnosis for clinicians. They also risk causing confusion because they differ from definitions used for national quality measures in the United States and in global quality improvement initiatives. However, clinicians should remember that Sepsis-3 does not change the basics of sepsis management: the cornerstone remains early identification of infection, rapid treatment with antibiotics and source control when signs of organ dysfunction are present, and fluid resuscitation when hypotension is present. Further studies of sepsis are needed, including prospectively evaluating the impact of clinical care with the new versus the old criteria on patient outcomes, comparing the impact of different screening methods on patient outcomes, and identifying better measurements for organ dysfunction. Such studies will undoubtedly lead to improved future iterations of sepsis definitions.

REFERENCES

1. Bone RC, Balk RA, Cerra FB, et al. Definitions for sepsis and organ failure and guidelines for the use of innovative therapies in sepsis. The ACCP/SCCM Consensus Conference Committee. American College of Chest Physicians/Society of Critical Care Medicine. Chest 1992;101(6):1644–55.
2. Singer M, Deutschman CS, Seymour CW, et al. The third international consensus definitions for sepsis and septic shock (Sepsis-3). JAMA 2016;315(8):801–10.
3. Seymour CW, Liu VX, Iwashyna TJ, et al. Assessment of clinical criteria for sepsis: for the third international consensus definitions for sepsis and septic shock (Sepsis-3). JAMA 2016;315(8):762–74.
4. Minino AM, Murphy SL. Death in the United States, 2010. NCHS Data Brief 2012;(99):1–8.
5. Torio CM, Andrews RM. National inpatient hospital costs: the most expensive conditions by payer, 2011: statistical brief #160. Rockville (MD): Healthcare Cost and Utilization Project (HCUP) Statistical Briefs; 2006.
6. Liu V, Escobar GJ, Greene JD, et al. Hospital deaths in patients with sepsis from 2 independent cohorts. JAMA 2014;312(1):90–2.
7. Winters BD, Eberlein M, Leung J, et al. Long-term mortality and quality of life in sepsis: a systematic review. Crit Care Med 2010;38(5):1276–83.
8. Nesseler N, Defontaine A, Launey Y, et al. Long-term mortality and quality of life after septic shock: a follow-up observational study. Intensive Care Med 2013; 39(5):881–8.
9. Gaieski DF, Edwards JM, Kallan MJ, et al. Benchmarking the incidence and mortality of severe sepsis in the United States. Crit Care Med 2013;41(5):1167–74.
10. Martin GS, Mannino DM, Eaton S, et al. The epidemiology of sepsis in the United States from 1979 through 2000. N Engl J Med 2003;348(16):1546–54.
11. Dombrovskiy VY, Martin AA, Sunderram J, et al. Rapid increase in hospitalization and mortality rates for severe sepsis in the United States: a trend analysis from 1993 to 2003. Crit Care Med 2007;35(5):1244–50.
12. Rhee C, Gohil S, Klompas M. Regulatory mandates for sepsis care–reasons for caution. N Engl J Med 2014;370(18):1673–6.
13. Rhee C, Murphy MV, Li L, et al, for the Centers for Disease Control and Prevention Epicenters Program. Comparison of trends in sepsis incidence and coding using administrative claims versus objective clinical data. Clin Infect Dis 2015;60(1): 88–95.
14. Klompas M, Rhee C. The CMS sepsis mandate: right disease, wrong measure. Ann Intern Med 2016;165(7):517–8.
15. Phua J, Ngerng W, See K, et al. Characteristics and outcomes of culture-negative versus culture-positive severe sepsis. Crit Care 2013;17(5):R202.
16. Sands KE, Bates DW, Lanken PN, et al, Academic Medical Center Consortium Sepsis Project Working Group. Epidemiology of sepsis syndrome in 8 academic medical centers. JAMA 1997;278(3):234–40.
17. Rhee C, Kadri SS, Danner RL, et al. Diagnosing sepsis is subjective and highly variable: a survey of intensivists using case vignettes. Crit Care 2016;20:89.
18. Angus DC, Seymour CW, Coopersmith CM, et al. A framework for the development and interpretation of different sepsis definitions and clinical criteria. Crit Care Med 2016;44(3):e113–21.
19. Levy MM, Fink MP, Marshall JC, et al, SCCM/ESICM/ACCP/ATS/SIS. 2001 SCCM/ESICM/ACCP/ATS/SIS international sepsis definitions conference. Crit Care Med 2003;31(4):1250–6.

20. Dellinger RP, Levy MM, Rhodes A, et al, Surviving Sepsis Campaign Guidelines Committee Including the Pediatric Subgroup. Surviving Sepsis Campaign: international guidelines for management of severe sepsis and septic shock: 2012. Crit Care Med 2013;41(2):580–637.

21. Vincent JL. Dear SIRS, I'm sorry to say that I don't like you. Crit Care Med 1997; 25(2):372–4.

22. Churpek MM, Zadravecz FJ, Winslow C, et al. Incidence and prognostic value of the systemic inflammatory response syndrome and organ dysfunctions in ward patients. Am J Respir Crit Care Med 2015;192(8):958–64.

23. Kaukonen KM, Bailey M, Pilcher D, et al. Systemic inflammatory response syndrome criteria in defining severe sepsis. N Engl J Med 2015;372(17):1629–38.

24. Shankar-Hari M, Deutschman CS, Singer M. Do we need a new definition of sepsis? Intensive Care Med 2015;41(5):909–11.

25. Vincent JL, Moreno R, Takala J, et al. The SOFA (Sepsis-related Organ Failure Assessment) score to describe organ dysfunction/failure. On behalf of the Working Group on Sepsis-related Problems of the European Society of Intensive Care Medicine. Intensive Care Med 1996;22(7):707–10.

26. Le Gall JR, Klar J, Lemeshow S, et al. The logistic organ dysfunction system. A new way to assess organ dysfunction in the intensive care unit. ICU Scoring Group. JAMA 1996;276(10):802–10.

27. Vincent JL, Martin GS, Levy MM. qSOFA does not replace SIRS in the definition of sepsis. Crit Care 2016;20(1):210.

28. Shankar-Hari M, Phillips GS, Levy ML, et al, Sepsis Definitions Task Force. Developing a new definition and assessing new clinical criteria for septic shock: for the third international consensus definitions for sepsis and septic shock (Sepsis-3). JAMA 2016;315(8):775–87.

29. Freund Y, Lemachatti N, Krastinova E, et al, for the French Society of Emergency Medicine Collaborators Group. Prognostic accuracy of Sepsis-3 criteria for in-hospital mortality among patients with suspected infection presenting to the emergency department. JAMA 2017;317(3):301–8.

30. Raith EP, Udy AA, Bailey M, et al, for the Australian and New Zealand Intensive Care Society (ANZICS) Centre for Outcomes and Resource Evaluation (CORE). Prognostic accuracy of the SOFA score, SIRS criteria, and qSOFA score for in-hospital mortality among adults with suspected infection admitted to the Intensive Care Unit. JAMA 2017;317(3):290–300.

31. Rhee C, Murphy MV, Li L, et al, Centers for Disease Control and Prevention Epicenters Program. Improving documentation and coding for acute organ dysfunction biases estimates of changing sepsis severity and burden: a retrospective study. Crit Care 2015;19:338.

32. Kadri SS, Rhee C, Strich JR, et al. Estimating ten-year trends in septic shock incidence and mortality in united states academic medical centers using clinical data. Chest 2017;151(2):278–85.

33. Simpson SQ. New sepsis criteria: a change we should not make. Chest 2016; 149(5):1117–8.

34. Cortes-Puch I, Hartog CS. Opening the debate on the new sepsis definition change is not necessarily progress: revision of the sepsis definition should be based on new scientific insights. Am J Respir Crit Care Med 2016;194(1):16–8.

35. Levy MM, Rhodes A, Phillips GS, et al. Surviving Sepsis Campaign: association between performance metrics and outcomes in a 7.5-year study. Crit Care Med 2015;43(1):3–12.

36. Ferrer R, Artigas A, Levy MM, et al. Improvement in process of care and outcome after a multicenter severe sepsis educational program in Spain. JAMA 2008; 299(19):2294–303.

37. Miller RR 3rd, Dong L, Nelson NC, et al, Intermountain Healthcare Intensive Medicine Clinical Program. Multicenter implementation of a severe sepsis and septic shock treatment bundle. Am J Respir Crit Care Med 2013;188(1):77–82.

38. Stevenson EK, Rubenstein AR, Radin GT, et al. Two decades of mortality trends among patients with severe sepsis: a comparative meta-analysis*. Crit Care Med 2014;42(3):625–31.

39. Kaukonen KM, Bailey M, Suzuki S, et al. Mortality related to severe sepsis and septic shock among critically ill patients in Australia and New Zealand, 2000-2012. JAMA 2014;311(13):1308–16.

40. Kumar A, Roberts D, Wood KE, et al. Duration of hypotension before initiation of effective antimicrobial therapy is the critical determinant of survival in human septic shock. Crit Care Med 2006;34(6):1589–96.

41. Gaieski DF, Mikkelsen ME, Band RA, et al. Impact of time to antibiotics on survival in patients with severe sepsis or septic shock in whom early goal-directed therapy was initiated in the emergency department. Crit Care Med 2010;38(4): 1045–53.

42. Beck V, Chateau D, Bryson GL, et al, Cooperative Antimicrobial Therapy of Septic Shock Database Research Group. Timing of vasopressor initiation and mortality in septic shock: a cohort study. Crit Care 2014;18(3):R97.

43. Waechter J, Kumar A, Lapinsky SE, et al, Cooperative Antimicrobial Therapy of Septic Shock Database Research Group. Interaction between fluids and vasoactive agents on mortality in septic shock: a multicenter, observational study. Crit Care Med 2014;42(10):2158–68.

44. Bai X, Yu W, Ji W, et al. Early versus delayed administration of norepinephrine in patients with septic shock. Crit Care 2014;18(5):532.

45. Pro CI, Yealy DM, Kellum JA, et al. A randomized trial of protocol-based care for early septic shock. N Engl J Med 2014;370(18):1683–93.

46. ARISE Investigators, ANZICS Clinical Trials Group, Peake SL, Delaney A, Bailey M, et al. Goal-directed resuscitation for patients with early septic shock. N Engl J Med 2014;371(16):1496–506.

47. Mouncey PR, Osborn TM, Power GS, et al. Trial of early, goal-directed resuscitation for septic shock. N Engl J Med 2015;372(14):1301–11.

48. Lilly CM. The ProCESS trial–a new era of sepsis management. N Engl J Med 2014;370(18):1750–1.

49. Levy MM, Dellinger RP, Townsend SR, et al. The Surviving Sepsis campaign: results of an international guideline-based performance improvement program targeting severe sepsis. Intensive Care Med 2010;36(2):222–31.

50. Rohde JM, Odden AJ, Bonham C, et al. The epidemiology of acute organ system dysfunction from severe sepsis outside of the intensive care unit. J Hosp Med 2013;8(5):243–7.

51. De Backer D, Biston P, Devriendt J, et al. Comparison of dopamine and norepinephrine in the treatment of shock. N Engl J Med 2010;362(9):779–89.

52. Vail EA, Gershengorn HB, Hua M, et al. Epidemiology of vasopressin use for adults with septic shock. Ann Am Thorac Soc 2016;13(10):1760–7.

53. Rhee C. Using procalcitonin to guide antibiotic therapy. Open Forum Infect Dis 2016;4(1):ofw249.

54. Liesenfeld O, Lehman L, Hunfeld KP, et al. Molecular diagnosis of sepsis: new aspects and recent developments. Eur J Microbiol Immunol (Bp) 2014;4(1):1–25.

55. Poeze M, Ramsay G, Gerlach H, et al. An international sepsis survey: a study of doctors' knowledge and perception about sepsis. Crit Care 2004;8(6):R409–13.

56. Townsend SR, Rivers E, Tefera L. Definitions for sepsis and septic shock. JAMA 2016;316(4):457–8.

57. Rangel-Frausto MS, Pittet D, Costigan M, et al. The natural history of the systemic inflammatory response syndrome (SIRS). A prospective study. JAMA 1995; 273(2):117–23.

58. Brun-Buisson C. The epidemiology of the systemic inflammatory response. Intensive Care Med 2000;26(Suppl 1):S64–74.

59. Williams JM, Greenslade JH, McKenzie JV, et al. Systemic inflammatory response syndrome, quick sequential organ function assessment, and organ dysfunction: insights from a prospective database of ED patients with infection. Chest 2017; 151(3):586–96.

60. Churpek MM, Snyder A, Han X, et al. Quick sepsis-related organ failure assessment, systemic inflammatory response syndrome, and early warning scores for detecting clinical deterioration in infected patients outside the intensive care unit. Am J Respir Crit Care Med 2017;195(7):906–11.

61. Ho KM, Lan NS. Combining quick sequential organ failure assessment with plasma lactate concentration is comparable to standard sequential organ failure assessment score in predicting mortality of patients with and without suspected infection. J Crit Care 2016;38:1–5.

62. Howell MD, Donnino M, Clardy P, et al. Occult hypoperfusion and mortality in patients with suspected infection. Intensive Care Med 2007;33(11):1892–9.

63. Lokhandwala S, Moskowitz A, Lawniczak R, et al. Disease heterogeneity and risk stratification in sepsis-related occult hypoperfusion: a retrospective cohort study. J Crit Care 2015;30(3):531–6.

64. Mikkelsen ME, Miltiades AN, Gaieski DF, et al. Serum lactate is associated with mortality in severe sepsis independent of organ failure and shock. Crit Care Med 2009;37(5):1670–7.

65. Jones AE, Puskarich MA. Is lactate the "Holy Grail" of biomarkers for sepsis prognosis? Crit Care Med 2009;37(5):1812–3.

66. Nguyen HB, Rivers EP, Knoblich BP, et al. Early lactate clearance is associated with improved outcome in severe sepsis and septic shock. Crit Care Med 2004;32(8):1637–42.

67. Trzeciak S, Dellinger RP, Chansky ME, et al. Serum lactate as a predictor of mortality in patients with infection. Intensive Care Med 2007;33(6):970–7.

68. Shapiro NI, Howell MD, Talmor D, et al. Serum lactate as a predictor of mortality in emergency department patients with infection. Ann Emerg Med 2005;45(5): 524–8.

69. Jansen TC, van Bommel J, Schoonderbeek FJ, et al, LACTATE Study Group. Early lactate-guided therapy in intensive care unit patients: a multicenter, open-label, randomized controlled trial. Am J Respir Crit Care Med 2010;182(6): 752–61.

70. Jones AE, Shapiro NI, Trzeciak S, et al, Emergency Medicine Shock Research Network Investigators. Lactate clearance vs central venous oxygen saturation as goals of early sepsis therapy: a randomized clinical trial. JAMA 2010;303(8): 739–46.

71. Singer AJ, Taylor M, LeBlanc D, et al. ED bedside point-of-care lactate in patients with suspected sepsis is associated with reduced time to IV fluids and mortality. Am J Emerg Med 2014;32(9):1120–4.

72. Surviving Sepsis Campaign. The Surviving Sepsis Campaign responds to Sepsis-3. 2016. Available at: http://www.survivingsepsis.org/SiteCollectionDocuments/SSC-Statements-Sepsis-Definitions-3-2016.pdf. Accessed December 4, 2016.

73. Vincent JL, de Mendonca A, Cantraine F, et al. Use of the SOFA score to assess the incidence of organ dysfunction/failure in intensive care units: results of a multicenter, prospective study. Working Group on "Sepsis-related Problems" of the European Society of Intensive Care Medicine. Crit Care Med 1998;26(11): 1793–800.

74. Ferreira FL, Bota DP, Bross A, et al. Serial evaluation of the SOFA score to predict outcome in critically ill patients. JAMA 2001;286(14):1754–8.

75. Vincent JL, Moreno R. Clinical review: scoring systems in the critically ill. Crit Care 2010;14(2):207.

76. Seymour CW, Coopersmith CM, Deutschman CS, et al. Application of a framework to assess the usefulness of alternative sepsis criteria. Crit Care Med 2016;44(3):e122–30.

77. Rhee C, Kadri S, Huang SS, et al. Objective sepsis surveillance using electronic clinical data. Infect Control Hosp Epidemiol 2016;37(2):163–71.

Sepsis and Challenging Infections in the Immunosuppressed Patient in the Intensive Care Unit

Diana F. Florescu, MD, Uriel Sandkovsky, MD, MS,
Andre C. Kalil, MD, MPH*

KEYWORDS

- Sepsis • Infection • Critically ill • Immunosuppressed

KEY POINTS

- The clinical approach to both diagnosis and treatment of infections in the critically ill immunosuppressed patient is highly dependent on the specific cause of the immunosuppression.
- The opportunistic infections affecting patients with human immunodeficiency virus (HIV) are different from those affecting patients with solid organ transplantation, which in turn are also different from those affecting patients with hematopoietic stem cell transplantation.
- Furthermore, important epidemiologic questions, such as how advanced the HIV disease is, how far the patient with solid organ transplantation is from the surgical procedure, and what type of stem cell transplant was performed, are all important to guide the clinician toward the most probable infection etiology that could be causing the critically ill status.
- The general treatment approach is dependent on the precision of the diagnostic approach and consists of rapid initiation of antimicrobials, source control, and minimization of immunosuppression by either reducing immunosuppressive drugs, or reconstituting the immune system with antiretroviral drugs for patients with HIV.

INTRODUCTION

Sepsis remains a major public health problem, one of the top causes of death among immunosuppressed critically ill patients who have undergone solid organ transplantation (SOT) and hematopoietic stem cell transplantation (HSCT).[1,2] These are small but unique and growing populations that are often excluded from randomized controlled trials evaluating therapies for sepsis and infection.[3] The incidence of sepsis is 20% to

Transplant Infectious Diseases Program, Division of Infectious Diseases, Department of Internal Medicine, University of Nebraska Medical Center, 985400 Nebraska Medical Center, Omaha, NE 68198-5400, USA
* Corresponding author.
E-mail address: akalil@unmc.edu

Infect Dis Clin N Am 31 (2017) 415–434
http://dx.doi.org/10.1016/j.idc.2017.05.009
0891-5520/17/© 2017 Elsevier Inc. All rights reserved.

id.theclinics.com

60% of all SOT recipients, with an in-hospital mortality of 5% to 40%.[4,5] Severe sepsis in HSCT recipients is approximately 5 times more frequent when compared with the nonimmunocompromised population, with a twofold higher mortality for allogeneic HSCT recipients than autologous recipients; reported in-hospital mortality is 55% to 70% for allogeneic and 30% to 58% for autologous HSCT recipients.[6] Most infections and sepsis in patients with HSCT are related to neutropenia (neutrophil count $\leq$500/mm^3 or $\leq$1000/mm^3 with a predicted decrease to $\leq$500/mm^3) and mucositis induced by cytoablative chemotherapy, or delayed engraftment following HSCT.[7] Patients with solid tumors usually undergo less intense chemotherapy and rarely become neutropenic.

Detailed epidemiologic information and clinical history are vital to understand the risk of different infections in immunocompromised patients. Exposures to contacts with respiratory illness would suggest influenza, parainfluenza, respiratory syncytial virus (RSV), and adenovirus infections; exposure to construction sites or environmental sources would make us suspect *Histoplasma*, *Aspergillus*, or *Nocardia* infections; exposure to water sources can be followed by *Legionella* or atypical mycobacterium infections; travel to certain areas might raise suspicion for endemic fungal infections (histoplasmosis, cryptococcosis, coccidioidomycosis).[8,9] The risk for certain opportunistic infections (invasive aspergillosis, cryptococcosis, nocardiosis, *Pneumocystis* pneumonia, cytomegalovirus [CMV] disease) depends on the net state of immunosuppression, a direct reflection of previous use of T-cell depleting antibodies for induction or rejection, myeloablative regimens, and the chronic immunosuppression.[10,11] SOT and HSCT recipients with infections and sepsis frequently are afebrile, but tend to have more thrombocytopenia and develop organ failure.[12]

CLINICAL SYNDROMES
Vascular Access Device–Related Infections

Please refer to the article by Taison Bell and Naomi O'Grady, "Prevention of Central Line-Associated Bloodstream Infections," in this issue.

Prolonged vascular access may be needed for longer periods for renal replacement therapy, total parenteral nutrition, treatment of acute rejection, or graft-versus-host disease (GVHD).[13–15] Vascular access device (VAD) infections can originate from the skin flora or from severe gastrointestinal mucositis (due to chemotherapy or bowel ischemia).[13–15] To determine the role of VAD in the etiology of bloodstream infections, the time-to-positivity between peripherally and centrally drawn blood cultures should be compared; a centrally drawn blood culture that is positive at least 120 minutes earlier than a peripherally drawn blood culture is highly sensitive and specific for VAD-related infection. Most VAD exit site infections can be treated with anti-infective therapy without line removal. However, VADs should be immediately removed in patients with septic shock, septic phlebitis, and tunnel or port pocket infection. VAD should be removed in patients with infections caused by *Staphylococcus aureus*, *Bacillus* spp, *Acinetobacter*, *Pseudomonas aeruginosa*, *Stenotrophomonas maltophilia*, *Corynebacterium jeikeium*, nontuberculous mycobacteria, yeasts, and molds. Management of VAD should follow the published guideline.[15,16]

Pneumonia

The respiratory tract remains one of the most frequent portals of entry for community-acquired, nosocomial, or opportunistic pathogens. In SOT, during the first month after transplantation, nosocomial infections, including hospital-acquired or ventilator-associated pneumonia are common, whereas pulmonary aspergillosis and viral infections are not frequently seen.[11,17] Between 1 and 6 months, nosocomial pathogens are still responsible for a significant number of infections; community-acquired pathogens are more frequently seen along with opportunistic infections (CMV, aspergillosis, cryptococcosis, histoplasmosis, coccidioidomycosis, and nocardiosis).[10,11] After 6 months, in most of the transplants, community-acquired infections (with *Streptococcus pneumoniae*, *Legionella* spp, *Haemophilus* spp) are predominant, whereas the risk of opportunistic infections diminishes.[10,11] Lung transplant recipients are at particularly high risk of developing pneumonia, empyema, or lung abscesses after transplantation, multidrug-resistant organisms being usually isolated in conjunction with colonization before surgery.[18,19] In HSCT recipients, during the pre-engraftment period (<30 days after transplantation), nosocomial pathogens and respiratory viruses are common causes of pneumonia and sepsis.[20,21] Invasive aspergillosis is usually seen with prolonged neutropenia.[21–23] Early after engraftment (30–100 days posttransplantation), pneumonia is usually caused by respiratory viruses, CMV, *Pneumocystis*, and *Aspergillus*. During the later period postengraftment (>100 days posttransplantation), the risk for CMV and *Aspergillus* infections remains high, with increased risk for community-acquired pneumonia (respiratory viruses and encapsulated bacteria).[21]

Community-acquired pneumonia remains a common problem, even months or years after transplantation, with a higher incidence in HSCT and SOT recipients when compared with the general population.[21,24] Pneumonia should be suspected in patients with fever, respiratory distress, and increased oxygen requirements. Ideally, sputum and blood cultures should be obtained before treatment is started. Urine *S pneumoniae* antigen, *Legionella* antigen tests, and respiratory multiplex polymerase chain reaction (PCR) panels may allow rapid diagnosis.[25–28] The threshold to perform bronchoscopy with bronchoalveolar lavage (BAL),[29] or lung biopsy should be lower for SOT or HSCT recipients.[30] The specimens obtained should be sent for bacterial, fungal, and mycobacterial cultures, and PCR for respiratory viruses, *Aspergillus* galactomannan, *Histoplasma* antigen, and cytology. Chest radiograph (CXR) is useful for detecting pulmonary infiltrates, but in hospitalized patients, underlying atelectasis, concomitant edema, or pleural effusions make the diagnosis more difficult.[31,32] Computed tomography (CT) scans are more sensitive to delineate pulmonary infiltrates, lung necrosis, cavitary lesions, lung abscesses, lymphadenopathy, and empyema.[32,33] Findings suggestive of invasive fungal infections ("halo sign" or "crescent sign") are more likely to be seen on CT scans.[33,34] Antimicrobial therapy for pneumonia depends on previous use of antibiotics, colonization with multidrug-resistant organisms, local antibiogram, and should follow the published guidelines[15,35,36]

Mediastinitis

Mediastinitis is usually a complication from esophageal perforation, progressive retropharyngeal infections, or after cardiothoracic surgery (left ventricular assist device [LVAD] or total artificial heart implantation, heart and/or lung transplantation). Several factors for mediastinitis have been reported: diabetes, obesity, immunosuppressed status, reintervention for bleeding, prior methicillin-resistant *S aureus* colonization, and previous LVAD infections.[37–39] Clinical presentation can be fulminant or subacute; most patients will present with fever, purulent drainage or dehiscence of the wound, or leukocytosis.[37,38] CT scan of the chest usually shows fluid collections or hematomas, common findings in the early postoperative period.[37,40,41] Aspiration of fluid collections or culture of the fluid during the surgical procedure is essential to guide antibiotic treatment.[42,43] Most commonly, gram-positive organisms (*S aureus*, coagulase-negative *Staphylococci*, and *Streptococci*) are isolated.[44] Empiric antimicrobial therapy should include piperacillin/tazobactam or cephalosporins with activity against non–lactose-fermenting gram-negatives, along with vancomycin; once the results of the cultures become available, more targeted treatment would be indicated.

Acute Abdomen

Abdominal pain is a common complaint in patients with mucositis after chemotherapy, GVHD, and after SOT. Most of the complications in the early posttransplantation period (cholangitis, peritonitis, intrahepatic and extrahepatic abscesses, surgical wound infections, biliary leak) are related to surgical procedures and may have more subtle clinical presentation due to the anti-inflammatory effects of steroids and other immunosuppressive drugs; sepsis is not uncommon, especially in liver and small bowel transplant recipients.[12–14,45] If peritonitis is diagnosed in the early postoperative period, it is usually due to dehiscence of anastomosis (ie, biliary, ureteral, ostomy), biliary leak, intestinal perforation, or bacterial translocation if there is bowel necrosis. Development of hepatic abscesses might suggest hepatic artery thrombosis, whereas intra-abdominal abscesses would suggest intestinal ischemia, anastomosis dehiscence, or development of fistulas.[14] Biliary strictures can complicate with recurrent cholangitis, liver abscesses, and sepsis, especially after retrograde cholangiography and t–tube cholangiography manipulation.[2] Acute abdomen that might require further intervention is indicated by unstable vital signs, abdominal tenderness on palpation, and rebound tenderness. Usually Enterococci, gram-negative organisms, aerobes and anaerobes are isolated. Abdominal ultrasound, CT scan with contrast, and MRI with contrast of the abdomen and pelvis can guide if further surgical intervention is needed.

Life-threatening enterocolitis or typhlitis are commonly described in neutropenic patients after chemotherapy for hematologic malignancies and in patients with breakdown of the intestinal mucosal integrity.[15] Patients typically present with fever, vomiting, nausea, diarrhea, abdominal pain, abdominal distension, or hematochezia; presence of peritoneal signs should raise the suspicion for perforation[15,46–49] Clostridium difficile infection, GVHD, CMV enteritis, or colitis should be considered in the differential diagnosis.[15] These infections are usually polymicrobial, including C difficile, aerobic and anaerobic, gram-negative, and gram-positive organisms.[15] Abdomen radiographs are suboptimal, sometimes showing fluid-filled distended cecum with dilated adjacent small bowel loops or thumb printing; in patients with complications, pneumatosis intestinalis or intraperitoneal free air can be seen.[49] CT scan is the preferred diagnostic test; the findings, occasionally limited to the right colon or to the cecum are bowel wall thickening, mesenteric stranding, and bowel loop dilation.[15,50] Initial treatment should be conservative: nasogastric suction, bowel rest, total parenteral nutrition, and broad-spectrum antibiotics.[15] Surgical intervention is required in up to 5% of patients who develop complication (perforation, intractable bleeding, refractory sepsis).[15]

Sepsis and Neutropenic Fever

The initial empiric regimen for the unstable neutropenic patient should be based on the local antibiogram, colonization with multidrug-resistant organisms, and recent antibiotic exposure; it should include a broad-spectrum beta-lactam, an aminoglycoside, vancomycin, and echinocandin (if the patient is not already on an antifungal agent).[15] Subsequently, the regimen should be tailored based on the culture results and radiologic data. In patients with persistent fever, the following should be considered: viral or mold infection, atypical mycobacterial infection, undrained closed space infection, deep venous thrombosis or pulmonary embolism, adrenal insufficiency, and drug-induced fever.[15] It is also important to consider breakthrough infections in patients who are already on antibiotics; that is, extended-spectrum lactamase-producing bacteria in patients on cephalosporins, or *S maltophilia* in patients on carbapenems.[15]

Urinary Tract Infections

Infections of the urinary tract (UTIs) are common causes of sepsis in immunosuppressed patients. In kidney transplant recipients, UTIs can be diagnosed any time after transplantation, with the highest incidence in the first 3 to 6 months.[51] There are several known risk factors for complicated UTIs: female gender, anatomic (stones, tumors, urinary tract stenosis, anastomotic leaks, and lymphoceles), presence of indwelling catheter, and comorbidities (diabetes, neurogenic bladder, urinary reflux especially before kidney transplantation, increased immunosuppression, malnutrition).[2,51–53] Patients with complicated UTI or pyelonephritis can present with fever, chills, dysuria, urgency, frequency, or suprapubic, flank or allograft pain; some patients can present without urinary tract symptoms or nonspecific sepsis syndrome.[51] In kidney transplant recipients, as in any other immunocompromised hosts, gram-negative bacteria account for most infections, with *Escherichia coli* being the most frequently isolated pathogen.[51] The diagnosis of complicated UTI relies on blood cultures and quantitative count of bacteria in the urine culture. Approximately two-thirds of the patients with pyelonephritis have positive urine cultures, and one-third are bacteremic.[51] Both kidney allograft rejection and pyelonephritis can lead to loss of renal function, but rejection shows urine analysis and cultures negative for acute infection. Complicated UTIs after kidney transplantation can originate from the native kidney or from the allograft.[51] Abdominal ultrasounds should be performed in patients with renal failure and/or sepsis of urinary tract origin to evaluate for ureteral obstruction, abscesses, or dilatation of the collecting system.[2] CT of the abdomen and pelvis, and cystoscopy might be necessary for further diagnostic purposes and stent removal for source control. Empiric antimicrobial treatment depends on the severity of illness, hospital epidemiology, and patients with multidrug-resistant organisms, following published guidelines.[51] Treatment should be tailored based on the culture results. Renal transplant recipients with recurrent UTIs require evaluation for anatomic and functional abnormalities with ultrasound, CT scan, urodynamic studies, and cystourethrogram; they also may require prolonged courses of antibiotics and reevaluation of anatomic and/or functional abnormalities.[51] Although BK virus may lead to nephritis and rarely to hemorrhagic cystitis in SOT, adenovirus is a more common cause of hemorrhagic cystitis in patients with HSCT.

Organisms of Special Interest

Clostridium difficile

Please refer to the article by John G. Bartlett, "*C difficile* infection," in this issue.

C difficile infections (CDIs) occur in 20% of HSCT and 10% of SOT recipients (with the highest rate in lung, heart, and intestine allograft recipients), with a recurrence rate up to 30%.[54–56] A higher frequency of CDI is described during the first months after HSCT and SOT, when the patients are exposed to health care and receive more intense immunosuppression and antibiotics.[54,57,58] History is important to identify risk factors for CDI, such as age older than 65, antimicrobial exposure, medication to suppress gastric acid production, uremia, hypogammaglobulinemia, and prolonged hospitalization. Certain risk factors are more specific for SOT recipients (recent gastrointestinal surgery, presence of nasogastric or endotracheal tube), whereas other risk factors are more specific for HSCT recipients (gut GVHD, total body radiation, and cord blood use).[54,59–63] Severe CDI and life-threatening complications of CDI (ie, toxic megacolon, multiorgan failure) have been linked to older age and hypoalbuminemia.[62] Cessation of the antimicrobial agent or changing to a more narrow-spectrum regimen if the antimicrobial treatment needs to be continued should be the first intervention.[62] Fulminant colitis can develop in SOT and HSCT recipients, colectomy, diverting ileostomy, or colostomy may be required in patients who fail to respond within the first 48 hours to medical therapy, or have toxic megacolon, bowel perforation, or multiorgan failure.[15,58] The antimicrobial therapy depends on the severity of the illness and recurrence of the infections as described in the published algorithms.[15,62]

Nocardiosis

Nocardiosis, a rare opportunistic infection, is diagnosed in up to 4% of the SOT and HSCT patients, with the highest reported incidence in lung transplant recipients.[64] Nocardiosis is diagnosed at 8 to 30 months after SOT and 6 to 10 months after HSCT, mainly in patients on an intense immunosuppressive regimen (high-dose steroids and high calcineurin inhibitor levels) and with previous CMV infection.[64] Invasive nocardiosis (pulmonary, central nervous system [CNS], or disseminated infections) account for most cases. The CNS is the most common extrapulmonary site affected; patients present with signs of increased intracranial pressure, focal neurologic deficits, or coma.[64] Cutaneous nodules, pustules, and abscesses can be found on physical examination and might represent the portal of entry for *Nocardia* or might be part of a disseminated process.[64] Diagnosis relies on isolation and identification of the organism from a clinical sample: BAL specimen, transbronchial or transthoracic lung biopsy, fine-needle aspiration of an abscess, or stereotactic brain biopsy.[64] CXR and CT scan of the chest commonly show nodular or cavitary lesions, whereas lobar consolidations and ground-glass opacities are less frequently seen.[64] Imaging of the CNS with CT scan or MRI is vital in any patient with invasive disease, the need for lumbar puncture or drainage, and to determine the length of therapy. Imaging of the brain usually shows single or multiple abscesses with surrounding edema.[64] Coinfections have been reported in a high percentage of SOT recipients.[64] Antimicrobial therapy should be initiated based on clinical and radiological suspicion and should take into account the site of involvement, the severity of the disease, and drug interactions.[9,15] For patients with severe disease, a combination of imipenem/cilastatin and trimethoprim/sulfamethoxazole (TMP-SMX) or amikacin is recommended.[9,15]

Pneumocystis jirovecii infections

Pneumocystis pneumonia has been recognized as a severe life-threatening infection; it is usually diagnosed within the first 2 months after HSCT, mainly in patients who are not compliant with TMP-SMX prophylaxis[65]; SOT recipients, due to longer prophylaxis with TMP-SMX, tend to present much later.[66,67] The incidence of *Pneumocystis* pneumonia seems to be highest in lung and lung-heart transplant recipients.[67] Several risk factors have been associated with this infection: high doses of corticosteroids for prolonged periods of time, antilymphocyte therapy, prior CMV infection, allograft rejection, lymphopenia, and especially low CD4 cell count, neutropenia, agammaglobulinemia, and anti–tumor necrosis factor antibody treatment.[67,68] Patients usually have a rapid clinical deterioration that starts with fever, cough, and progressive shortness of breath; they become hypoxemic, and if not treated promptly, they progress to acute respiratory failure.[67,68] Coinfections with other respiratory viruses or CMV are not uncommon.[67] Bronchoscopy with BAL (and detection with immunofluorescent antibody stain, Gomori methenamine-silver, Giemsa and Wrights stains) remain the gold standard diagnostic approach.[67,68] Transbronchial biopsy might increase the diagnostic yield.[67] As an adjunctive diagnostic tool, $(1\rightarrow3)$-β-d-Glucan assay has been used, but it can be positive with other fungal infection and has a low specificity for *P jirovecii* pneumonia.[67] CT scan of the lung is a more reliable diagnostic tool compared with CXR, detecting usually ground-glass infiltrates, consolidation, linear and/or reticular opacities, cystic changes, and nodular lesions.[67,69] First line of therapy regardless of disease severity should be TMP-SMX, with the exception of patients with history of immediate hypersensitivity to sulfa, Stevens Johnson syndrome, or toxic epidermal necrolysis.[67,69] Second-line therapy should be used as per available guidelines.[67,69] In cases with severe hypoxemia (Pao_2 <70 mm Hg on room air) adjunctive corticoids should be administrated.[67,69]

Aspergillosis

Please refer to the article by Luis Ostrosky-Zeichner and Mohanad Al-Obaidi, "Invasive Fungal Infections in the Intensive Care Unit," in this issue.

Aspergillus is the most common invasive fungal infection after HSCT. In this population, prolonged neutropenia, GVHD, CMV infection, and augmented immunosuppression have been described as risk factors for invasive disease.[70] The incidence in SOT varies according to the transplanted organ, with the highest incidence in heart and lung transplant recipients.[71] Risk factors depend on the allograft and include the intensity of immunosuppression, retransplantation, reoperation, treatment for rejection, colonization of the airways with *Aspergillus*, severe hypogammaglobulinemia, renal failure requiring renal replacement therapy, and CMV infection.[71] Clinical presentation depends on the site of involvement and includes fever, cough, or hemoptysis in patients with pulmonary aspergillosis, and focal neurologic signs and confusion in patients with CNS aspergillosis. Sputum culture has low sensitivity, and detection of *Aspergillus* does not always correlate with presence of invasive disease, but it has a high positive predictive value for subsequent development of disease.[71] BAL fluid and tissue biopsies should be submitted for both culture and histopathological examination.[70] Serum and BAL *Aspergillus galactomannan* are recommended adjunctive tests for invasive aspergillosis (IA) in patients who are not on antifungal prophylaxis, with probable greater utility in HSCT than in SOT recipients.[70,71] The $(1 \rightarrow 3)$-β-d-Glucan assay nonspecific test for IA can be used as an adjunctive diagnostic tool in high-risk HSCT recipients.[70] CT scan is the preferred imaging in patients with suspected IA.[70] Early initiation of treatment with voriconazole is recommended for CNS aspergillosis if IA is suspected; lipid formulations of amphotericin B are considered alternative treatment options.[70,71] Combination therapy (voriconazole and an echinocandin) can be used in severe infections, but its role remains to be defined.[70,71] Voriconazole is a potent inhibitor of CYP34A and the doses of calcineurin inhibitors and sirolimus should be adjusted and the levels monitored.[71] Overall immunosuppression should be reduced if possible. In neutropenic patients, colony-stimulating factors can be considered, or in HSCT recipients with refractory IA, granulocyte transfusions can be used.[70]

Cytomegalovirus

CMV reactivates in up to 30% of HSCT and up to 55% of SOT recipients.[72–74] The risk for CMV infection in HSCT is higher in CMV-seropositive recipients, and patients undergoing allogeneic HSCT, receiving alemtuzumab, with GVHD.[15] In SOT, the risk factors are CMV serostatus D+/R−, allograft type (highest rate in intestine and lung transplant recipients), use of lymphocyte-depleting agents, increased immunosuppression for treatment of rejection, coinfection with human herpesvirus (HHV)-6 or HHV-7.[75] Late CMV disease remains a persistent problem in SOT and HSCT recipients, even with prophylaxis and preemptive therapy.[15,75] For example, in SOT, because of ganciclovir or valganciclovir prophylaxis, the disease usually presents 1 to 3 months after drug discontinuation and sometimes later, in conjunction with treatment for rejection. Fever, generalized weakness, malaise along with cough, shortness of breath, and hypoxemia are common findings in patients with CMV pneumonia.[75,76]

CMV can affect the gastrointestinal tract anywhere from the oral cavity to the rectum. Patients usually present with fever, malaise, nausea, vomiting, abdominal pain, and diarrhea. Severe cases of CMV enteritis and colitis can present with significant anemia, dehydration, renal failure, hypotension, or even shock secondary to gastrointestinal bleeding or perforation.[77–79] The gastrointestinal tract is more susceptible to viral infections due to graft-versus-host reaction (especially in HSCT recipients) and aberrant immune response within the allograft (mainly in liver and intestinal transplant recipients).[80–82] The diagnosis and treatment of CMV infection might be complicated in cases with GVHD or allograft rejection of the gastrointestinal tract.[83]

The diagnosis of active CMV infection is based on CMV antigenemia, quantitative nucleic acid testing (QNAT), and histopathology.[15,75,84–86] CMV pp65 antigenemia, a semiquantitative test, is cheap and easy to perform, but the test is not standardized and results are influenced by neutropenia.[86] CMV QNAT is expensive but the test is more sensitive, has been standardized, and can be used in other body fluids and tissue.[86] CMV viremia may be low or negative in patients with significant gastrointestinal or lung involvement.[86] Early colonoscopy can be beneficial for the early diagnosis and management of CMV colitis in transplant recipients, especially in cases with negative blood CMV QNAT.[87] Immunohistochemistry for CMV should be performed on all biopsy and BAL specimens, looking for inclusion bodies.[86] CT scan of the abdomen and pelvis would demonstrate circumferential wall thickening, focal or diffuse bowel dilatation, pericolonic fat stranding, lymphadenopathy, or pneumatosis coli.[88] CMV pneumonia may present with bilateral infiltrates, ground-glass opacities, consolidations, or nodular lesions seen on radiograph or CT scan of the chest.[32]

Initial treatment consists of intravenous ganciclovir or oral valganciclovir, reduction of immunosuppression, and CMV-specific immunoglobulin or intravenous immunoglobulin in selected patients (pneumonia, refractory or resistant infections).[75] In patients with severe CMV disease, in patients intolerant to oral treatment or with significant diarrhea, intravenous ganciclovir remains the preferred drug.[75,86] Foscarnet and cidofovir are reserved for treatment of ganciclovir-resistant CMV infection.[75] Viremia should be tested weekly while on therapy, and the treatment can be discontinued after 2 negative weekly assays.[75,86] The length of therapy depends on the site of infection, resolution of symptoms, and clearance of viremia.[75,89] Patients with severe CMV disease, high initial CMV viral loads, clinically refractory disease, and leukopenia or neutropenia should have immunosuppression decreased.[86]

Respiratory viruses

Please refer to the article by James M. Walter and Richard G. Wunderink, "Severe Respiratory Viral Infections: New Evidence and Changing Paradigms," in this issue.

Influenza, parainfluenza, RSV, metapneumovirus, and adenoviruses may all cause severe respiratory infections in immunocompromised patients.[90,91] Most immunosuppressed patients have mild upper respiratory tract infections manifested as rhinorrhea, nasal congestion, cough, fever, headache, sore throat, fatigue, malaise, and myalgia; some recipients may develop lower respiratory tract infections and present with shortness of breath, cough, and progressive hypoxemia.[92] Immunocompromised patients also may shed the viruses for prolonged periods, an important aspect when considering isolations.[90,91,93,94] The risk for progression of RSV, influenza, or parainfluenza infections to the lower respiratory tract is higher in older patients, those with smoking history, neutropenic or lymphocytopenic recipients, allogeneic HSCT or lung transplant recipients, mismatched or unrelated HSCT, marrow or cord blood HSCT, patients who received myeloablative regimens or antilymphocyte globulins, or patients with GVHD, systemic corticosteroid use, and pulmonary coinfections.[91,92] Complications after influenza infections are not uncommon: bronchiolitis obliterans, bacterial pneumonia, myocarditis, and encephalopathy.[90] Because the clinical signs and symptoms are similar for all the respiratory viruses, antigen detection and multiplex PCR assay (with high sensitivity and specificity) in the nasopharyngeal swab or wash should be used for fast.[91,92] If lower airways involvement is suspected, BAL should be performed.[91]

Treatment of influenza with neuraminidase inhibitors, such as oseltamivir or zanamivir, for an extended time may be used due to the risk for significant complication, slow response to therapy, and prolonged viral shedding in this population.[91] Changes in the susceptibility of influenza virus strains should guide the antiviral therapy.[92] Ribavirin administration in patients with parainfluenza did not prove highly effective in decreasing viral shedding, duration of symptoms, progression of infection to lower respiratory airways, length of hospital stay, or mortality in HSCT recipients[92]; it is still used in lung transplant recipients based on in vitro susceptibility data, because of the high risk of complications and poor outcome in these patients.[91] Progression of RSV infections to lower airways and mortality seem to be effectively prevented by ribavirin treatment, especially in HSCT recipients.[91,92] Treatment of severe adenovirus infections includes a combination of supportive therapy, reduction of immunosuppression, and sometimes use of cidofovir (with probenecid and aggressive hydration).[95,96]

Noroviruses

Noroviruses have a highly variable incidence from 3% to 60% in immunocompromised patients.[97–100] Norovirus enteritis is diagnosed at a median 1.2 months after HSCT, whereas SOT recipients are diagnosed much later (mean 37–42 months).[98–102] Patients usually present with nausea, vomiting, diarrhea, and abdominal pain; fever is an uncommon feature.[103] A high proportion (55%–80%) of patients required hospitalization because of severe diarrhea that led to significant dehydration, and renal failure, with 27% of them being admitted to the intensive care unit.[100] Nausea at time of presentation and prior CMV infection seem to be independent risk factors for prolonged diarrhea.[103] Patients with norovirus compared with patients with other infectious enteritis are more likely to be admitted to intensive care, and to have renal failure and weight loss.[100] Complications have been well described: acute renal failure requiring hemodialysis, malnutrition, pneumatosis intestinalis, peritonitis, bacteremia, and death.[100,104–109] Treatment is supportive: fluid administration, dietary manipulations (changes in enteral nutrition or total parenteral nutrition), nonspecific antidiarrheal therapy, and reduction of immunosuppressive therapy. Oral intravenous immunoglobulins and nitazoxanide treatment have been used in the attempt to shorten the duration of symptoms, but there is no evidence from clinical trials supporting their use.[89,110–112]

Strongyloidiasis

Hyperinfection with *Strongyloides* in transplant recipients is uncommon, but the true incidence remains unknown.[113] In HSCT recipients, compared with SOT recipients, the onset of *Strongyloides* hyperinfection appears to occur earlier (first 2 months vs first 3–12 months).[113] *Strongyloides* larvae migrating from the bowel through the venous system usually cause bacteremia, mainly with enteric gram-negative organisms.[14] Frequent complications of larva migrations include gram-negative sepsis, meningitis, cholecystitis, pancreatitis, liver abscess, and acute respiratory failure with migratory pulmonary infiltrates.[113] Eosinophilia may be present only intermittently. Parasitologic examination of stool or sputum can allow for rapid identification of larvae. Biopsy of the duodenum looking for rhabditiform larvae can be performed.[113] Serologic testing (enzyme-linked immunosorbent assay immunoglobulin G antibody) for *Strongyloides* has good sensitivity (~90%) and is available in reference laboratories.[113] Steroids and/or other potent immunosuppressive agents often need to be administered urgently in patients admitted to the ICU; and because serologic testing can take several days to have results back, and stool samples may not always show larvae, preemptive treatment with ivermectin is suggested in those settings until results are available. Prolonged therapy with ivermectin with or without albendazole is recommended.[114–117]

SELECTED SEVERE INFECTIONS IN PATIENTS WITH HUMAN IMMUNODEFICIENCY VIRUS

In recent years, the prevalence of human immunodeficiency virus (HIV)-infected patients admitted to the ICU has significantly decreased, especially those admissions related to opportunistic infections, due to more widespread availability and uptake of potent antiretroviral therapy.[118,119] HIV disease itself predisposes the host to a variety of infections that may occur with increased frequency compared with the immunocompetent population. Uncontrolled HIV infection ultimately leads to immunodeficiency, with significant decline in CD4 counts. In a fashion like transplant patients, several cutoffs have been classically used to identify the risk of opportunistic infections to better define the need and timing of prophylactic antibiotics. It is widely accepted that opportunistic infections, such as *Pneumocystis* pneumonia, occur when the CD4 count is less than 200 cells/mm^3, whereas other infections, such as cryptococcosis, toxoplasmosis, or endemic mycosis (histoplasmosis or coccidioidomycosis), usually occur when CD4 counts are less than 100 cells/mm^3.[118] The risk for these infections is predictable and hence preventable by using antimicrobial prophylaxis[118,120] and by treating patients with antiretroviral therapy to promote immune restoration and reduce mortality.[119,120] On the other hand, although the risk can be determined, it is more difficult to predict which patients might present with severe manifestations of these opportunistic infections.

Pneumonia and Human Immunodeficiency Virus

Pneumonia remains the most frequent clinical syndrome in patients infected with HIV. The incidence of pneumococcal disease remains 35 times higher among people infected with HIV when compared with age-matched controls.[121] Pneumococci that cause invasive disease in the HIV-infected population tend to have increased antimicrobial resistance.[122]

Pneumocystis pneumonia may present with progressive shortness of breath, fever, and nonproductive cough, especially when CD4 counts are less than 200 cells/mm^3.[118,123] The presence of bilateral granular, interstitial, or ground-glass opacities should increase the suspicion for *Pneumocystis* pneumonia.[124] Moreover, the presence of acute pneumothorax in patients infected with HIV should prompt suspicion for *Pneumocystis* pneumonia.[118] Toxoplasma usually reactivates in the CNS, causing encephalitis. Clinical manifestations include fever, focal neurologic signs, confusion, and altered mental status.[125,126] Less commonly, toxoplasma may cause a pneumonitis syndrome with clinical and radiographic features indistinguishable from *Pneumocystis* pneumonia, but BAL with Giemsa staining should readily identify the parasite, or less frequently a biopsy would reveal parasites in lung tissue.[118,127]

Sepsis and Human Immunodeficiency Virus

Despite higher risk for opportunistic infections, HIV-infected patients are not usually considered at higher risk for sepsis and may not be admitted to the ICU as frequently as patients not infected with HIV.[128] In a study comparing HIV-infected and non–HIV-infected patients admitted to the ICU, HIV-infected individuals had low CD4 counts and advanced HIV disease at presentation. Moreover, a great majority were newly diagnosed with HIV, and presented with an opportunistic infection. The organ most commonly affected was the lung, and a high proportion of fungal infections and mycobacterial infections were seen.[128] Mortality also seems to be higher among HIV-infected patients who present with sepsis, with HIV itself being an independent risk factor.[128,129]

Toxoplasmosis, Cryptococcosis, Bartonellosis, and Human Immunodeficiency Virus

Disseminated toxoplasmosis is rare, but may present with a clinical picture of septic shock and pneumonitis, progressing to acute respiratory distress syndrome. Severe thrombocytopenia and high lactate dehydrogenase (LDH) are common findings. Treatment regimens should include pyrimethamine with either sulfadiazine or alternatively clindamycin, and folinic acid as rescue agent. Alternative agents include TMP-SMX at high doses, or combinations with atovaquone, or macrolides. Duration of therapy should continue for at least 6 weeks, but it may need to be extended, depending on the response, followed by suppressive therapy.[118]

Disseminated cryptococcal disease affects patients with CD4 counts usually less than 100 cells/mm^3. Cryptococcus usually causes subacute meningitis or meningoencephalitis, but in rare instances may present with respiratory disease. Pneumonia is an unusual but severe manifestation of disseminated cryptococcal disease, presenting with fever, cough, malaise, and acute respiratory failure. CXR may show diffuse pulmonary infiltrates, similar to those of *Pneumocystis* pneumonia, although nodules, masses, and empyema also may be present. Disseminated disease usually shows positive blood cultures.[118,130]

Bartonella can cause severe infections in patients with HIV disease, including bacillary angiomatosis and peliosis hepatis.[118,131] Endocarditis, meningitis, or bacteremia may also occur in this population. Prompt suspicion is key, as these infections may be life-threatening. Tissue biopsy and Warthin-Starry staining may identify intracellular bacilli. Serology is another important diagnostic method and is readily available in reference laboratories, because blood cultures are not a useful method to diagnose this fastidious organism.[118] Doxycycline or macrolides are the treatment of choice, and rifampin should be added to doxycycline for CNS infection. Doxycycline and gentamicin are used in cases of endocarditis. Duration of therapy is usually longer than 3 months.[118]

Endemic Fungal Infections and Human Immunodeficiency Virus

Patients infected with advanced HIV infection may present with disseminated forms of endemic fungal infections. Progressive disseminated histoplasmosis is usually seen with CD4 counts less than 150 cells/mm^3, and more commonly less than 50 cells/mm^3.[118] Although histoplasmosis may present with a subacute course, fungal sepsis may be seen in a minority of the patients (<10%), presenting with shock, respiratory failure, acute renal failure, and liver involvement. Pancytopenia, elevated liver enzymes, including markedly elevated alkaline phosphatase and LDH, may be seen. Antigenemia or antigenuria are highly sensitive tests, but turnaround time may take several days.[118,132,133] Peripheral blood smears can readily identify fungal forms inside neutrophils or mononuclear cells, and may be quite useful to expedite the diagnosis.[132] In cases in which bronchoscopy and BAL are performed, *Histoplasma* also may be identified in silver stains of BAL fluid.[132,133] Therapy with liposomal amphotericin B should not be delayed; however, the mortality in these cases remains elevated due to delayed presentation to care.[118]

Severe coccidioidomycosis carries high mortality. The clinical picture is consistent with diffuse pneumonia presenting with fever, progressive weakness, and shortness of breath, and is accompanied by fungemia.[134] Diffuse pneumonia may coexist with meningitis, which is of lymphocyte predominance along with hypoglycorrhachia. An early clue to diagnosis is the presence of eosinophils in the cerebrospinal fluid (CSF). Sputum and BAL samples may readily identify the fungus in the form of spherules; however, it is rare to see *Coccidioides* in CSF samples. Serology results may take several days, but *Coccidioides* should grow in cultures.[118] Prompt therapy should include amphotericin B in cases of diffuse pneumonia or fluconazole if meningitis is present.[134]

Blastomycosis is not frequently diagnosed in patients with HIV disease; however, it can cause disseminated infection, and up to 40% of the time, progress to meningitis in patients with advanced HIV.[135] CNS infection manifests with headache, confusion, or focal neurologic sings; however, these may be absent and the sole manifestation may be a mass or abscess in the brain or vertebral spine.[135–137]

Severe disease should be treated with lipid formulations of amphotericin B, followed by an oral azole agent, such as itraconazole or alternatively fluconazole or voriconazole.[135]

Cytomegalovirus and Human Immunodeficiency Virus

CMV is an opportunistic virus that causes end-organ disease in patients with advanced HIV infection and CD4 counts less than 50 cells/mm^3.[118] The most common clinical manifestation is retinitis; however, CMV may cause severe colitis and more rarely, pneumonitis. Colitis should be suspected when patients present with progressive diarrhea, weakness, malaise, and abdominal pain. It is, however, imperative to rule out other possible pathogens, such as *Cryptosporidium*, *Microsporidium*, *Cyclospora*, *Entamoeba histolytica*, *Salmonella*, and *Shigella*. CMV may cause life-threatening lower gastrointestinal hemorrhage or colonic perforations, which may manifest as an acute abdomen and peritonitis.[118,138]

Pneumonitis caused by CMV is even more rare in the setting of HIV disease. CMV may be found in BAL specimens, but its presence does not mean clinical disease, rather viral shedding.[118,139] Most of the time, CMV will be present along with other more common opportunistic lung pathogens such as *Pneumocystis*, *Histoplasma*, *Mycobacterium tuberculosis*, and *Coccidioides*.[118] Manifestations of CMV pneumonitis include fever, cough, progressive shortness of breath, hypoxemia, and bilateral reticulo-nodular infiltrates on CXR.[118,140] Diagnosis would be supported by the presence of CMV inclusions in lung biopsy specimens and after ruling out other more common pathogens.[118,138]

SUMMARY

The clinical approach to both diagnosis and treatment of infections in the critically ill immunosuppressed patient is highly dependent on the specific cause of the immunosuppression. As described, the opportunistic infections affecting patients with HIV are different from those affecting SOT recipients, which in turn are also different from those affecting HSCT recipients. Furthermore, important epidemiologic questions, such as how advanced the HIV disease is, how far the patients with SOT is from the surgical procedure, and what type of stem cell transplant was performed, are all important to guide the clinician toward the most probable infection etiology that could be causing the critically ill status. The general treatment approach is dependent on the precision of the diagnostic approach and consists of rapid initiation of antimicrobials, source control, and minimization of immunosuppression by either reducing immuno-suppressive drugs, or reconstituting the immune system with antiretroviral drugs for patients with HIV.

REFERENCES

1. Kalil AC, Dakroub H, Freifeld AG. Sepsis and solid organ transplantation. Curr Drug Targets 2007;8(4):533–41.
2. Kalil AC, Opal SM. Sepsis in the severely immunocompromised patient. Curr Infect Dis Rep 2015;17(6):487.
3. Harpaz R, Dahl RM, Dooling KL. Prevalence of immunosuppression among US adults, 2013. JAMA 2016;316(23):2547–8.
4. Hsu RB, Chang CI, Fang CT, et al. Bloodstream infection in heart transplant recipients: 12-year experience at a university hospital in Taiwan. Eur J Cardio-thorac Surg 2011;40(6):1362–7.
5. Linares L, Garcia-Goez JF, Cervera C, et al. Early bacteremia after solid organ transplantation. Transplant Proc 2009;41(6):2262–4.
6. Kumar G, Ahmad S, Taneja A, et al. Severe sepsis in hematopoietic stem cell transplant recipients*. Crit Care Med 2015;43(2):411–21.
7. Freifeld AG, Bow EJ, Sepkowitz KA, et al. Clinical practice guideline for the use of antimicrobial agents in neutropenic patients with cancer: 2010 update by the Infectious Diseases Society of America. Clin Infect Dis 2011;52(4):e56–93.
8. Avery RK, Michaels MG, AST Infectious Diseases Community of Practice. Strategies for safe living after solid organ transplantation. Am J Transplant 2013; 13(Suppl 4):304–10.
9. Clark NM, Reid GE, AST Infectious Diseases Community of Practice. Nocardia infections in solid organ transplantation. Am J Transplant 2013;13(Suppl 4): 83–92.
10. Fishman JA. Infection in solid-organ transplant recipients. N Engl J Med 2007; 357(25):2601–14.
11. Green M. Introduction: infections in solid organ transplantation. Am J Transplant 2013;13(Suppl 4):3–8.
12. Kalil AC, Syed A, Rupp ME, et al. Is bacteremic sepsis associated with higher mortality in transplant recipients than in nontransplant patients? A matched case-control propensity-adjusted study. Clin Infect Dis 2015;60(2):216–22.
13. Florescu DF, Qiu F, Langnas AN, et al. Bloodstream infections during the first year after pediatric small bowel transplantation. Pediatr Infect Dis J 2012; 31(7):700–4.
14. Silva JT, San-Juan R, Fernandez-Caamano B, et al. Infectious complications following small bowel transplantation. Am J Transplant 2015;16(3):951–9.
15. Baden LR, Swaminathan S, Angarone M, et al. Prevention and treatment of cancer-related infections, version 2.2016, NCCN clinical practice guidelines in oncology. J Natl Compr Canc Netw 2016;14(7):882–913.
16. Mermel LA, Allon M, Bouza E, et al. Clinical practice guidelines for the diagnosis and management of intravascular catheter-related infection: 2009 update by the Infectious Diseases Society of America. Clin Infect Dis 2009;49(1):1–45.

17. Razonable RR, Findlay JY, O'Riordan A, et al. Critical care issues in patients after liver transplantation. Liver Transpl 2011;17(5):511–27.
18. Boussaud V, Guillemain R, Grenet D, et al. Clinical outcome following lung transplantation in patients with cystic fibrosis colonised with Burkholderia cepacia complex: results from two French centres. Thorax 2008;63(8):732–7.
19. Dobbin C, Maley M, Harkness J, et al. The impact of pan-resistant bacterial pathogens on survival after lung transplantation in cystic fibrosis: results from a single large referral centre. J Hosp Infect 2004;56(4):277–82.
20. Dettenkofer M, Wenzler-Rottele S, Babikir R, et al. Surveillance of nosocomial sepsis and pneumonia in patients with a bone marrow or peripheral blood stem cell transplant: a multicenter project. Clin Infect Dis 2005;40(7):926–31.
21. Tomblyn M, Chiller T, Einsele H, et al. Guidelines for preventing infectious complications among hematopoietic cell transplantation recipients: a global perspective. Biol Blood Marrow Transplant 2009;15(10):1143–238.
22. Neofytos D, Horn D, Anaissie E, et al. Epidemiology and outcome of invasive fungal infection in adult hematopoietic stem cell transplant recipients: analysis of multicenter prospective antifungal therapy (path) alliance registry. Clin Infect Dis 2009;48(3):265–73.
23. Wald A, Leisenring W, van Burik JA, et al. Epidemiology of *Aspergillus* infections in a large cohort of patients undergoing bone marrow transplantation. J Infect Dis 1997;175(6):1459–66.
24. Wong A, Marrie TJ, Garg S, et al. Increased risk of invasive pneumococcal disease in haematological and solid-organ malignancies. Epidemiol Infect 2010; 138(12):1804–10.
25. Kupeli E, Eyuboglu FO, Haberal M. Pulmonary infections in transplant recipients. Curr Opin Pulm Med 2012;18(3):202–12.
26. Musher DM, Thorner AR. Community-acquired pneumonia. N Engl J Med 2014; 371(17):1619–28.
27. Anderson TP, Werno AM, Barratt K, et al. Comparison of four multiplex PCR assays for the detection of viral pathogens in respiratory specimens. J Virol Methods 2013;191(2):118–21.
28. Salez N, Vabret A, Leruez-Ville M, et al. Evaluation of four commercial multiplex molecular tests for the diagnosis of acute respiratory infections. PLoS One 2015; 10(6):e0130378.
29. Joos L, Chhajed PN, Wallner J, et al. Pulmonary infections diagnosed by BAL: a 12-year experience in 1066 immunocompromised patients. Respir Med 2007; 101(1):93–7.
30. Bulpa PA, Dive AM, Mertens L, et al. Combined bronchoalveolar lavage and transbronchial lung biopsy: safety and yield in ventilated patients. Eur Respir J 2003;21(3):489–94.
31. Bentz MR, Primack SL. Intensive care unit imaging. Clin Chest Med 2015;36(2): 219–34, viii.
32. Ketai L, Jordan K, Busby KH. Imaging infection. Clin Chest Med 2015;36(2): 197–217, viii.
33. Godet C, Elsendoorn A, Roblot F. Benefit of CT scanning for assessing pulmonary disease in the immunodepressed patient. Diagn Interv Imaging 2012; 93(6):425–30.
34. Arendrup MC, Bille J, Dannaoui E, et al. Ecil-3 classical diagnostic procedures for the diagnosis of invasive fungal diseases in patients with leukaemia. Bone Marrow Transplant 2012;47(8):1030–45.

35. Kalil AC, Metersky ML, Klompas M, et al. Management of adults with hospital-acquired and ventilator-associated pneumonia: 2016 clinical practice guidelines by the infectious Diseases Society of America and the American Thoracic Society. Clin Infect Dis 2016;63(5):e61–111.

36. Mandell LA, Wunderink RG, Anzueto A, et al. Infectious Diseases Society of America/American Thoracic Society consensus guidelines on the management of community-acquired pneumonia in adults. Clin Infect Dis 2007;44(Suppl 2): S27–72.

37. Abid Q, Nkere UU, Hasan A, et al. Mediastinitis in heart and lung transplantation: 15 years experience. Ann Thorac Surg 2003;75(5):1565–71.

38. Diez C, Koch D, Kuss O, et al. Risk factors for mediastinitis after cardiac surgery—a retrospective analysis of 1700 patients. J Cardiothorac Surg 2007;2:23.

39. Koval CE, Rakita R, AST Infectious Diseases Community of Practice. Ventricular assist device related infections and solid organ transplantation. Am J Transplant 2013;13(Suppl 4):348–54.

40. Misawa Y, Fuse K, Hasegawa T. Infectious mediastinitis after cardiac operations: computed tomographic findings. Ann Thorac Surg 1998;65(3):622–4.

41. Yamaguchi H, Yamauchi H, Yamada T, et al. Diagnostic validity of computed tomography for mediastinitis after cardiac surgery. Ann Thorac Cardiovasc Surg 2001;7(2):94–8.

42. Benlolo S, Mateo J, Raskine L, et al. Sternal puncture allows an early diagnosis of poststernotomy mediastinitis. J Thorac Cardiovasc Surg 2003;125(3):611–7.

43. Bernabeu-Wittel M, Cisneros JM, Rodriguez-Hernandez MJ, et al. Suppurative mediastinitis after heart transplantation: early diagnosis with CT-guided needle aspiration. J Heart Lung Transplant 2000;19(5):512–4.

44. Trouillet JL, Vuagnat A, Combes A, et al. Acute poststernotomy mediastinitis managed with debridement and closed-drainage aspiration: factors associated with death in the intensive care unit. J Thorac Cardiovasc Surg 2005;129(3): 518–24.

45. Paya CV, Hermans PE, Washington JA 2nd, et al. Incidence, distribution, and outcome of episodes of infection in 100 orthotopic liver transplantations. Mayo Clin Proc 1989;64(5):555–64.

46. Aksoy DY, Tanriover MD, Uzun O, et al. Diarrhea in neutropenic patients: a prospective cohort study with emphasis on neutropenic enterocolitis. Ann Oncol 2007;18(1):183–9.

47. McCarville MB, Adelman CS, Li C, et al. Typhlitis in childhood cancer. Cancer 2005;104(2):380–7.

48. Nesher L, Rolston KV. Neutropenic enterocolitis, a growing concern in the era of widespread use of aggressive chemotherapy. Clin Infect Dis 2013;56(5):711–7.

49. Wade DS, Nava HR, Douglass HO Jr. Neutropenic enterocolitis. Clinical diagnosis and treatment. Cancer 1992;69(1):17–23.

50. Kirkpatrick ID, Greenberg HM. Gastrointestinal complications in the neutropenic patient: characterization and differentiation with abdominal ct. Radiology 2003; 226(3):668–74.

51. Parasuraman R, Julian K, AST Infectious Diseases Community of Practice. Urinary tract infections in solid organ transplantation. Am J Transplant 2013; 13(Suppl 4):327–36.

52. Abbott KC, Oliver JD 3rd, Hypolite I, et al. Hospitalizations for bacterial septicemia after renal transplantation in the United States. Am J Nephrol 2001; 21(2):120–7.

53. Wagener MM, Yu VL. Bacteremia in transplant recipients: a prospective study of demographics, etiologic agents, risk factors, and outcomes. Am J Infect Control 1992;20(5):239–47.

54. Willems L, Porcher R, Lafaurie M, et al. *Clostridium difficile* infection after allogeneic hematopoietic stem cell transplantation: incidence, risk factors, and outcome. Biol Blood Marrow Transplant 2012;18(8):1295–301.

55. Bobak D, Arfons LM, Creger RJ, et al. *Clostridium difficile*-associated disease in human stem cell transplant recipients: coming epidemic or false alarm? Bone Marrow Transplant 2008;42(11):705–13.

56. Paudel S, Zacharioudakis IM, Zervou FN, et al. Prevalence of *Clostridium difficile* infection among solid organ transplant recipients: a meta-analysis of published studies. PLoS One 2015;10(4):e0124483.

57. Boutros M, Al-Shaibi M, Chan G, et al. *Clostridium difficile* colitis: increasing incidence, risk factors, and outcomes in solid organ transplant recipients. Transplantation 2012;93(10):1051–7.

58. Dallal RM, Harbrecht BG, Boujoukas AJ, et al. Fulminant *Clostridium difficile*: an underappreciated and increasing cause of death and complications. Ann Surg 2002;235(3):363–72.

59. Alonso CD, Treadway SB, Hanna DB, et al. Epidemiology and outcomes of *Clostridium difficile* infections in hematopoietic stem cell transplant recipients. Clin Infect Dis 2012;54(8):1053–63.

60. Altclas J, Requejo A, Jaimovich G, et al. *Clostridium difficile* infection in patients with neutropenia. Clin Infect Dis 2002;34(5):723.

61. Chakrabarti S, Lees A, Jones SG, et al. *Clostridium difficile* infection in allogeneic stem cell transplant recipients is associated with severe graft-versus-host disease and non-relapse mortality. Bone Marrow Transplant 2000;26(8):871–6.

62. Dubberke ER, Burdette SD, AST Infectious Diseases Community of Practice. *Clostridium difficile* infections in solid organ transplantation. Am J Transplant 2013;13(Suppl 4):42–9.

63. Dubberke ER, Reske KA, Yan Y, et al. *Clostridium difficile*–associated disease in a setting of endemicity: identification of novel risk factors. Clin Infect Dis 2007; 45(12):1543–9.

64. Lebeaux D, Morelon E, Suarez F, et al. Nocardiosis in transplant recipients. Eur J Clin Microbiol Infect Dis 2014;33(5):689–702.

65. De Castro N, Neuville S, Sarfati C, et al. Occurrence of *Pneumocystis jiroveci* pneumonia after allogeneic stem cell transplantation: a 6-year retrospective study. Bone Marrow Transplant 2005;36(10):879–83.

66. de Boer MG, Kroon FP, le Cessie S, et al. Risk factors for *Pneumocystis jirovecii* pneumonia in kidney transplant recipients and appraisal of strategies for selective use of chemoprophylaxis. Transpl Infect Dis 2011;13(6):559–69.

67. Martin SI, Fishman JA, AST Infectious Diseases Community of Practice. *Pneumocystis* pneumonia in solid organ transplantation. Am J Transplant 2013; 13(Suppl 4):272–9.

68. Cordonnier C, Cesaro S, Maschmeyer G, et al. *Pneumocystis jirovecii* pneumonia: still a concern in patients with haematological malignancies and stem cell transplant recipients. J Antimicrob Chemother 2016;71(9):2379–85.

69. Cooley L, Dendle C, Wolf J, et al. Consensus guidelines for diagnosis, prophylaxis and management of *Pneumocystis jirovecii* pneumonia in patients with haematological and solid malignancies, 2014. Intern Med J 2014;44(12b): 1350–63.

70. Patterson TF, Thompson GR 3rd, Denning DW, et al. Practice guidelines for the diagnosis and management of aspergillosis: 2016 update by the Infectious Diseases Society of America. Clin Infect Dis 2016;63(4):e1–60.

71. Singh N, Husain S, AST Infectious Diseases Community of Practice. Aspergillosis in solid organ transplantation. Am J Transplant 2013;13(Suppl 4):228–41.

72. Ison MG, Fishman JA. Cytomegalovirus pneumonia in transplant recipients. Clin Chest Med 2005;26(4):691–705, viii.

73. Kotloff RM, Ahya VN, Crawford SW. Pulmonary complications of solid organ and hematopoietic stem cell transplantation. Am J Respir Crit Care Med 2004; 170(1):22–48.

74. Taplitz RA, Jordan MC. Pneumonia caused by herpesviruses in recipients of hematopoietic cell transplants. Semin Respir Infect 2002;17(2):121–9.

75. Razonable RR, Humar A, AST Infectious Diseases Community of Practice. Cytomegalovirus in solid organ transplantation. Am J Transplant 2013;13(Suppl 4): 93–106.

76. Florescu DF, Kalil AC. Cytomegalovirus infections in non-immunocompromised and immunocompromised patients in the intensive care unit. Infect Disord Drug Targets 2011;11(4):354–64.

77. Dee SL, Butt K, Ramaswamy G. Intestinal ischemia. Arch Pathol Lab Med 2002; 126(10):1201–4.

78. Flanigan RC, Reckard CR, Lucas BA. Colonic complications of renal transplantation. J Urol 1988;139(3):503–6.

79. Lee CJ, Lian JD, Chang SW, et al. Lethal cytomegalovirus ischemic colitis presenting with fever of unknown origin. Transpl Infect Dis 2004;6(3):124–8.

80. Iwaki Y, Starzl TE, Yagihashi A, et al. Replacement of donor lymphoid tissue in small-bowel transplants. Lancet 1991;337(8745):818–9.

81. Roche JK, Cheung KS, Boldogh I, et al. Cytomegalovirus: detection in human colonic and circulating mononuclear cells in association with gastrointestinal disease. Int J Cancer 1981;27(5):659–67.

82. Zhang Y, Ruiz P. Solid organ transplant-associated acute graft-versus-host disease. Arch Pathol Lab Med 2010;134(8):1220–4.

83. Okubo H, Nagata N, Uemura N. Fulminant gastrointestinal graft-versus-host disease concomitant with cytomegalovirus infection: case report and literature review. World J Gastroenterol 2013;19(4):597–603.

84. Clelland C, Higenbottam T, Stewart S, et al. Bronchoalveolar lavage and transbronchial lung biopsy during acute rejection and infection in heart-lung transplant patients. Studies of cell counts, lymphocyte phenotypes, and expression of HLA-DR and interleukin-2 receptor. Am Rev Respir Dis 1993;147(6 Pt 1): 1386–92.

85. Gasparetto EL, Ono SE, Escuissato D, et al. Cytomegalovirus pneumonia after bone marrow transplantation: high resolution CT findings. Br J Radiol 2004; 77(921):724–7.

86. Kotton CN. CMV: prevention, diagnosis and therapy. Am J Transplant 2013; 13(Suppl 3):24–40 [quiz: 40].

87. Korkmaz M, Kunefeci G, Selcuk H, et al. The role of early colonoscopy in CMV colitis of transplant recipients. Transplant Proc 2005;37(7):3059–60.

88. Da Ines D, Petitcolin V, Lannareix V, et al. CT imaging features of colitis in neutropenic patients. J Radiol 2010;91(6):675–86 [in French].

89. Florescu DF, Hermsen ED, Kwon JY, et al. Is there a role for oral human immunoglobulin in the treatment for norovirus enteritis in immunocompromised patients? Pediatr Transplant 2011;15(7):718–21.

90. Lee I, Barton TD. Viral respiratory tract infections in transplant patients: epidemiology, recognition and management. Drugs 2007;67(10):1411–27.

91. Manuel O, Estabrook M, AST Infectious Diseases Community of Practice. RNA respiratory viruses in solid organ transplantation. Am J Transplant 2013; 13(Suppl 4):212–9.

92. Chemaly RF, Shah DP, Boeckh MJ. Management of respiratory viral infections in hematopoietic cell transplant recipients and patients with hematologic malignancies. Clin Infect Dis 2014;59(Suppl 5):S344–51.

93. Englund JA. Diagnosis and epidemiology of community-acquired respiratory virus infections in the immunocompromised host. Biol Blood Marrow Transplant 2001;7(Suppl):2S–4S.

94. Martin ST, Torabi MJ, Gabardi S. Influenza in solid organ transplant recipients. Ann Pharmacother 2012;46(2):255–64.

95. Florescu DF, Hoffman JA, AST Infectious Diseases Community of Practice. Adenovirus in solid organ transplantation. Am J Transplant 2013;13(Suppl 4): 206–11.

96. Sandkovsky U, Vargas L, Florescu DF. Adenovirus: current epidemiology and emerging approaches to prevention and treatment. Curr Infect Dis Rep 2014; 16(8):416.

97. Lemes LG, Correa TS, Fiaccadori FS, et al. Prospective study on norovirus infection among allogeneic stem cell transplant recipients: prolonged viral excretion and viral RNA in the blood. J Clin Virol 2014;61(3):329–33.

98. Robles JD, Cheuk DK, Ha SY, et al. Norovirus infection in pediatric hematopoietic stem cell transplantation recipients: incidence, risk factors, and outcome. Biol Blood Marrow Transplant 2012;18(12):1883–9.

99. Ueda R, Fuji S, Mori S, et al. Characteristics and outcomes of patients diagnosed with norovirus gastroenteritis after allogeneic hematopoietic stem cell transplantation based on immunochromatography. Int J Hematol 2015;102(1): 121–8.

100. Ye X, Van JN, Munoz FM, et al. Noroviruses as a cause of diarrhea in immunocompromised pediatric hematopoietic stem cell and solid organ transplant recipients. Am J Transplant 2015;15(7):1874–81.

101. Saif MA, Bonney DK, Bigger B, et al. Chronic norovirus infection in pediatric hematopoietic stem cell transplant recipients: a cause of prolonged intestinal failure requiring intensive nutritional support. Pediatr Transplant 2011;15(5):505–9.

102. Schorn R, Hohne M, Meerbach A, et al. Chronic norovirus infection after kidney transplantation: molecular evidence for immune-driven viral evolution. Clin Infect Dis 2010;51(3):307–14.

103. Chong PP, van Duin D, Sonderup JL, et al. Predictors of persistent diarrhea in norovirus enteritis after solid organ transplantation. Clin Transplant 2016; 30(11):1488–93.

104. Bok K, Green KY. Norovirus gastroenteritis in immunocompromised patients. N Engl J Med 2012;367(22):2126–32.

105. Ebdrup L, Bottiger B, Molgaard H, et al. Devastating diarrhoea in a heart-transplanted patient. J Clin Virol 2011;50(4):263–5.

106. Kim MJ, Kim YJ, Lee JH, et al. Norovirus: a possible cause of pneumatosis intestinalis. J Pediatr Gastroenterol Nutr 2011;52(3):314–8.

107. Roddie C, Paul JP, Benjamin R, et al. Allogeneic hematopoietic stem cell transplantation and norovirus gastroenteritis: a previously unrecognized cause of morbidity. Clin Infect Dis 2009;49(7):1061–8.

108. Schwartz S, Vergoulidou M, Schreier E, et al. Norovirus gastroenteritis causes severe and lethal complications after chemotherapy and hematopoietic stem cell transplantation. Blood 2011;117(22):5850–6.

109. Ziring D, Tran R, Edelstein S, et al. Infectious enteritis after intestinal transplantation: incidence, timing, and outcome. Transplantation 2005;79(6):702–9.

110. Morris J, Morris CL. Nitazoxanide is effective therapy for norovirus gastroenteritis after chemotherapy and hematopoietic stem cell transplantation (HSCT). Biol Blood Marrow Transplant 2015;21(2):S255–6.

111. Available at: https://clinicaltrials.gov/ct2/results?term=NCT02371538&Search=Search. Accessed February 10, 2017.

112. Rossignol JF, El-Gohary YM. Nitazoxanide in the treatment of viral gastroenteritis: a randomized double-blind placebo-controlled clinical trial. Aliment Pharmacol Ther 2006;24(10):1423–30.

113. Roxby AC, Gottlieb GS, Limaye AP. Strongyloidiasis in transplant patients. Clin Infect Dis 2009;49(9):1411–23.

114. Marty FM. Strongyloides hyperinfection syndrome and transplantation: a preventable, frequently fatal infection. Transpl Infect Dis 2009;11(2):97–9.

115. Patel G, Arvelakis A, Sauter BV, et al. Strongyloides hyperinfection syndrome after intestinal transplantation. Transpl Infect Dis 2008;10(2):137–41.

116. Safdar A, Malathum K, Rodriguez SJ, et al. Strongyloidiasis in patients at a comprehensive cancer center in the United States. Cancer 2004;100(7):1531–6.

117. Schwartz BS, Mawhorter SD, AST Infectious Diseases Community of Practice. Parasitic infections in solid organ transplantation. Am J Transplant 2013; 13(Suppl 4):280–303.

118. Panel on Opportunistic Infections in HIV-Infected Adults and Adolescents. Guidelines for the prevention and treatment of opportunistic infections in HIV-infected adults and adolescents: recommendations from the centers for disease control and prevention, the National Institutes of Health, and the HIV Medicine Association of the Infectious Diseases Society of America. Available at: http://aidsinfo.nih.gov/contentfiles/lvguidelines/adult_oi.Pdf. Accessed February 12, 2017.

119. Zolopa A, Andersen J, Powderly W, et al. Early antiretroviral therapy reduces AIDS progression/death in individuals with acute opportunistic infections: a multicenter randomized strategy trial. PLoS One 2009;4(5):e5575.

120. Available at: https://www.aids.gov/hiv-aids-basics/staying-healthy-with-hiv-aids/potential-related-health-problems/opportunistic-infections/. Accessed February 10, 2017.

121. Heffernan RT, Barrett NL, Gallagher KM, et al. Declining incidence of invasive *Streptococcus pneumoniae* infections among persons with AIDS in an era of highly active antiretroviral therapy, 1995-2000. J Infect Dis 2005;191(12): 2038–45.

122. Crewe-Brown HH, Karstaedt AS, Saunders GL, et al. *Streptococcus pneumoniae* blood culture isolates from patients with and without human immunodeficiency virus infection: alterations in penicillin susceptibilities and in serogroups or serotypes. Clin Infect Dis 1997;25(5):1165–72.

123. Selwyn PA, Pumerantz AS, Durante A, et al. Clinical predictors of *Pneumocystis carinii* pneumonia, bacterial pneumonia and tuberculosis in HIV-infected patients. AIDS 1998;12(8):885–93.

124. DeLorenzo LJ, Huang CT, Maguire GP, et al. Roentgenographic patterns of *Pneumocystis carinii* pneumonia in 104 patients with AIDS. Chest 1987;91(3): 323–7.

125. Cohen BA. Neurologic manifestations of toxoplasmosis in AIDS. Semin Neurol 1999;19(2):201–11.
126. Luft BJ, Remington JS. Toxoplasmic encephalitis in AIDS. Clin Infect Dis 1992; 15(2):211–22.
127. Rabaud C, May T, Lucet JC, et al. Pulmonary toxoplasmosis in patients infected with human immunodeficiency virus: a French national survey. Clin Infect Dis 1996;23(6):1249–54.
128. Silva JM Jr, dos Santos Sde S. Sepsis in AIDS patients: clinical, etiological and inflammatory characteristics. J Int AIDS Soc 2013;16:17344.
129. Cribbs SK, Tse C, Andrews J, et al. Characteristics and outcomes of HIV-infected patients with severe sepsis: continued risk in the post-highly active antiretroviral therapy era. Crit Care Med 2015;43(8):1638–45.
130. Perfect JR, Dismukes WE, Dromer F, et al. Clinical practice guidelines for the management of cryptococcal disease: 2010 update by the Infectious Diseases Society of America. Clin Infect Dis 2010;50(3):291–322.
131. Perkocha LA, Geaghan SM, Yen TS, et al. Clinical and pathological features of bacillary peliosis hepatis in association with human immunodeficiency virus infection. N Engl J Med 1990;323(23):1581–6.
132. Kauffman CA. Histoplasmosis: a clinical and laboratory update. Clin Microbiol Rev 2007;20(1):115–32.
133. Wheat LJ, Freifeld AG, Kleiman MB, et al. Clinical practice guidelines for the management of patients with histoplasmosis: 2007 update by the Infectious Diseases Society of America. Clin Infect Dis 2007;45(7):807–25.
134. Galgiani JN, Ampel NM, Blair JE, et al. 2016 Infectious Diseases Society of America (IDSA) clinical practice guideline for the treatment of coccidioidomycosis. Clin Infect Dis 2016;63(6):e112–46.
135. Chapman SW, Dismukes WE, Proia LA, et al. Clinical practice guidelines for the management of blastomycosis: 2008 update by the Infectious Diseases Society of America. Clin Infect Dis 2008;46(12):1801–12.
136. Pappas PG, Pottage JC, Powderly WG, et al. Blastomycosis in patients with the acquired immunodeficiency syndrome. Ann Intern Med 1992;116(10):847–53.
137. Pappas PG, Threlkeld MG, Bedsole GD, et al. Blastomycosis in immunocompromised patients. Medicine (Baltimore) 1993;72(5):311–25.
138. Dieterich DT, Rahmin M. Cytomegalovirus colitis in aids: presentation in 44 patients and a review of the literature. J Acquir Immune Defic Syndr 1991;4(Suppl 1):S29–35.
139. Jacobson MA, Mills J, Rush J, et al. Morbidity and mortality of patients with AIDS and first-episode *Pneumocystis carinii* pneumonia unaffected by concomitant pulmonary cytomegalovirus infection. Am Rev Respir Dis 1991;144(1):6–9.
140. Rodriguez-Barradas MC, Stool E, Musher DM, et al. Diagnosing and treating cytomegalovirus pneumonia in patients with AIDS. Clin Infect Dis 1996;23(1): 76–81.

Role of Procalcitonin in the Management of Infected Patients in the Intensive Care Unit

David N. Gilbert, MD

KEYWORDS

- Procalcitonin • Multiplex PCR • Respiratory panel • Antimicrobial stewardship
- Sepsis • Septic shock • Community-acquired pneumonia

KEY POINTS

- With available diagnostic "bundles," an etiologic agent or agents can be quickly identified in 70% or more of patients with severe community-acquired pneumonia (CAP).
- In patients with CAP and a serum procalcitonin (PCT) level ≤0.25 ng/mL, the likelihood of an invasive bacterial etiology is 5% or less.
- In patients with CAP, serum PCT levels can help determine if detected potential bacterial pathogens are colonizing or invading.
- Elevated serum PCT levels do not discriminate between the major categories of shock. However, a normal serum PCT eliminates a bacterial etiology of the shock in more than 95% of patients.
- For both severe CAP and bacteremic septic shock, sequential PCT levels assist in both assessing source control and determining the duration of antimicrobial therapy.

INTRODUCTION

Approximately 70% of patients admitted to critical care units are started on some type of antimicrobial therapy.[1–4] The most common indications are empiric therapy for suspected community-acquired pneumonia (CAP) or sepsis/septic shock. Of concern, the empiric therapy was continued beyond 3 days in one study and for more than 4 days in another.[3,5]

In critically ill patients, with ultimately documented severe bacterial pneumonia or septic shock, the aggressive early use of antibacterials can decrease attributable mortality.[6] When no microbial etiology is identified, clinical uncertainty drives the

Disclosure: Served as consultant to and received research grants from Biomerieux and its subsidiary company, Biofire.
Infectious Diseases, Providence Portland Medical Center, Oregon Health and Sciences University, 5050 Northeast Hoyt, Suite 540, Portland, OR 97213, USA
E-mail address: David.gilbert@providence.org

continuation of empiric antimicrobial therapy. The goal is to quickly define etiologic pathogens, or pathogens, so as to apply individualized focused therapy.

In patients with CAP, molecular diagnostics can rapidly detect potential viral and bacterial pathogens. The biomarker procalcitonin (PCT) can help clarify if a detected bacterial pathogen is colonizing or invading. As a consequence, empiric therapy can become specific therapy in an increasing number of patients.

In patients with shock, earlier detection and rapid speciation of blood culture isolates is increasingly available. Normal serum PCT levels strongly suggest the patient's hypotension is not due to invasive bacterial infection. Sequential PCT levels assist in documenting "source" control and allow individualization of the duration of antibiotic therapy.

SEVERE COMMUNITY-ACQUIRED PNEUMONIA
Standard Diagnostic Methods

Detection of the etiology, or etiologies of CAP results in a change from empiric to specific antimicrobial therapy. The higher the diagnostic yield, the better. The traditional diagnostic bundle for patients admitted to the intensive care unit (ICU) with CAP and hypoxemic respiratory failure consists of the following:

- Sputum, or if intubated, endotracheal tube aspirate, for culture and sensitivity
- Urine to test for presence of *Streptococcus pneumoniae* antigen, and *Legionella pneumophila*, serogroup 1 antigen
- Usually 2 blood cultures

If not intubated, it is not possible to collect a valid sputum in up to half or more of the patients.[7-10] Blood cultures are easily obtainable, but blood cultures are positive in fewer than 10% of the patients.[11] *S pneumoniae* antigen is found in urine in roughly 11% of the patients.[12] Using the urine antigen for detection, *L pneumophila* is found in 1% or less of the patients with CAP.[11,13] In short, the overall diagnostic yield with the standard bundle is less than 50%.[14,15]

Further, the turnaround time is slow. Urine antigen results return in 2 to 12 hours, sputum cultures in a minimum of 2 to 3 days, and blood cultures can take many days.[15]

Addition of Molecular Diagnostics

The diagnostic yield can be increased, with fast turnaround times, by adding molecular polymerase chain reaction (PCR) probes to the diagnostic bundle.

In 2 separate studies of patients admitted with CAP, the following tests were added to the previously discussed bundle:

- Anterior nasal swab for nucleic acid amplification test (NAAT) for *Staphylococcus aureus* (results within 24 hours)
- Nasopharyngeal swab for FilmArray Multiplex PCR panel for 17 viral strains and 3 bacteria (results within 2 hours)
- Nasopharyngeal swab for NAAT for *S pneumoniae* (results within 24–48 hours)

With the enlarged bundle, a potential pathogen was detected in 70% to 80% in 2 cohorts of patients enrolled over 2 respiratory winter seasons.[14,15]

Similar results with a slightly smaller diagnostic package were reported for patients with acute exacerbations of chronic bronchitis and other lower respiratory tract infections.[16]

Gadsby and colleagues[17] retrospectively performed quantitative PCR of purulent sputum for 26 pathogens: that is, 8 bacteria, 5 atypical bacteria, and 13 respiratory viruses. Potential pathogens were detected in 87% of 323 specimens. A potential bacterial pathogen was found in 71.5% and a respiratory virus in 30%.

In sum, these results demonstrate the ability to detect the presence of potential pathogens. The next question is whether the bacteria detected is colonizing or invading.[18]

Colonization or infection: procalcitonin

Reported nasal colonization with S pneumoniae in adults varies from 0.3% to 18.0%.[19] The tracheobronchial tree of 35% of smokers with chronic bronchitis is frequently colonized with Haemophilus species.[20] S aureus colonizes the nose of 30% of the general population.[21] Traditionally, clinicians have relied on signs, symptoms, and white blood cells (WBCs) to decide if detected bacteria are colonizing or invading.

PCT serum levels may help. PCT is a biomarker of activation of the innate immune system by bacteria and serum PCT levels rise within 4 to 6 hours in response to invasive bacterial infection.[22] Serum PCT levels remain low in the presence of colonization by potential pathogens.

Further, the PCT assay is user friendly. The lower limit of sensitivity is 0.06 ng/mL, and the turnaround time is less than 2 hours. In our CAP clinical trials, if a pneumococcus was detected by PCR but the PCT serum level was low, we interpreted the pneumococcus as colonizing and not invading.[14,15]

Procalcitonin levels distinguish viral and bacterial infection

Procalcitonin levels can distinguish bacterial from viral infection. In an animal model of Escherichia coli peritonitis, transcription of the PCT gene, as evidenced by elevated PCT messenger RNA, was found in virtually all body cells, tissues, and organs.[22,23] As elevation of PCT levels does not depend solely on activation of phagocytic cells, tumor necrosis factor (TNF), or other proinflammatory cytokines, it is not surprising that PCT increases occur in profoundly neutropenic patients with focal or bloodstream infections.[24]

Further, the PCT response is rapid. Human volunteers given low doses of lipopolysaccharide (LPS) developed detectable elevations of serum PCT over 4 to 6 hours.[25] With 1 LPS injection, the PCT level peaked at 24 hours. The increase in PCT serum levels occurred several hours earlier than the increase in C-reactive protein concentration.

In contrast, pure invasive viral infection rarely increases the PCT level above 0.25 ng/mL.[26] The biologic basis of the blunted PCT response is believed to result from inhibition of PCT transcription by gamma interferon. Gamma interferon levels rise in response to most respiratory viral infections. When adipose cells were cultured in vitro in the presence of interleukin (IL)-1, PCT levels increased. If interferon gamma was added to the IL-1, virtually no PCT was synthesized.[27]

In pediatric emergency department patients with documented viral infections, the PCT levels did not increase.[26] In several European PCT trials, patients with clinical viral respiratory tract infection had PCT serum levels of ≤0.25 ng/mL.[28,29] In the latter trials, there was no systematic attempt to correlate PCT levels with the microbial etiology of the infection.

In US studies of both acute exacerbations of chronic bronchitis and CAP, low PCT levels were found in patients with detection of only a respiratory virus. Of interest, in an average of 26% of the patients, there was evidence of a mixed infection due to a respiratory virus and a bacterial pathogen.[7,9,15,17] Note, PCT levels increased in patients with viral and bacterial coinfection. It appears invasion by a bacterium nullifies the inhibitory effect of viral-induced gamma interferon on PCT increases.

Last, in patients with documented meningitis, the serum PCT concentrations were low in patients with viral meningitis and elevated in patients with bacterial meningitis.[30–32]

Value of viral detection and procalcitonin levels in patients with community-acquired pneumonia

European studies document the safety of using PCT serum levels to guide antibiotic use decisions in patients with CAP.[28,29] However, there was no systematic attempt to associate the microbial etiology of the airway infection with the PCT concentrations.[27,28] In the United States, studies have used various diagnostic bundles and then correlated the results with PCT serum levels.[7,9,15,17] The inclusion of multiplex PCR platforms for respiratory viruses plus NAATs for S pneumoniae and S aureus have identified an etiology in up to 70% of the patients, with turnaround times of only a few hours.[15] The combination of enhanced etiologic diagnosis and serum PCT levels offer significant guidance in the management of severe CAP. Suggested interpretations are summarized in **Table 1**.

Some general points:

- All the interpretations in **Table 1** assume a compatible clinical illness.
- In adults or children, detection of influenza, respiratory syncytial virus, and human metapneumovirus likely indicates an etiologic role. Other respiratory

Table 1
Suggested interpretation of microbial diagnostics and procalcitonin (PCT) levels in patients with community-acquired pneumonia

Potential Bacterial Pathogen Detected[a]	Potential Viral Pathogen Detected with Multiplex Polymerase Chain Reaction	PCT, ng/mL	Hemodynamic Shock Present	Interpretation
No	No	≤0.10	No	No infection
No	Yes	≤0.10	No	Consistent with pure viral infection
No	Yes	0.25–1000	No	Likely dual infection: virus + nondetected bacteria
Yes	No	0.25–1000	No	Consistent with pure bacterial infection
Yes	Yes	0.25–1000	No	Dural viral and bacterial infection
Yes	No	≤0.10	No	No respiratory virus; bacterial colonization
Yes	Yes	≤0.10	No	Viral infection and bacterial colonization
No	No	0.25–1000	Yes	Gastrointestinal translocation (see shock discussion) or noncultured airway bacterial pathogen

[a] Detection by some combination of nucleic acid amplification test (eg, *Streptococcus pneumoniae, Staphylococcus aureus*), detection of antigen of *S pneumoniae* or *Legionella pneumophila* serotype 1 in urine, or traditional sputum culture and sensitivity.

viruses, especially in children, may be infection or asymptomatic carriage.[33,34] For this reason, Raoult[35] has emphasized the need for negative controls in future studies assessing the role of detected viral pathogens.

- Caution is suggested in a patient with clinical features of an acute bacterial pneumonia and a PCT level of ≤ 0.25 ng/mL. As the increase in PCT levels can take 4 to 6 hours from the initiation of bacterial invasion, it is advisable to repeat the PCT level in 4 to 6 hours before concluding the infection is nonbacterial.[22]
- The magnitude of the PCT rise correlates with the acuity and severity of the infection. A mild bronchitis or a chronic walled-off infection (eg, chronic empyema) may not stimulate an increase in the serum PCT concentration.[36]
- With pure viral infection, the magnitude of the gamma interferon response varies with the strain of virus (eg, influenza A vs influenza B) and from one respiratory virus to another. The result is reflected in low but variable levels of serum procalcitonin.[37–39]
- Gamma interferon plays a role in the complex host inflammatory response to bacterial, as well as viral, pneumonia. Somewhat surprisingly, neutrophils express gamma interferon in animal models of pneumonia.[40,41] Gamma interferon was expressed in mouse pneumococcal or staphylococcal pneumonia and not *E coli* or *Pseudomonas aeruginosa* pneumonia. As evidence supports lower PCT levels in the presence of interferon gamma, there is biologic plausibility of the anecdotal reports of lower PCT levels in patients with invasive gram-positive bacteria as compared with gram-negative bacteria.[42,43]
- Even with an adequate sputum specimen, a bacterial pathogen may not be detected. An example are patients with aspiration of large volumes of saliva and/or gastric content. In such patients, we, and others, have accepted an elevated PCT level, in the absence of clinical shock, as a surrogate for likely bacterial invasive infection and justification for antibiotic therapy.[9,15]

With these caveats, the suggested interpretation of serum PCT levels is summarized in **Table 1**. PCT levels remain low with a pure viral infection and increase with either a pure bacterial or a mixed viral-bacterial infection. If a respiratory virus is detected and the PCT level increases and even if no potential bacterial pathogen is detected, and the patient has a clear CAP clinical syndrome, it is reasonable to postulate the presence of undetected invading bacteria.

PCT levels are very helpful when they remain low despite culture of potential respiratory bacterial pathogens: for example, *S pneumoniae, Haemophilus influenza,* and *Moraxella catarrhalis.* This is the classic pattern for colonization without invasion by potential bacterial pathogens.

In patients with CAP plus another site of infection (eg, urinary tract infection (UTI), peritonitis, or bacteremia), it is difficult to ascertain which process is stimulating an increase in the PCT concentration. In patients with shock, possible gastrointestinal translocation is possible as discussed later in this article under the role of PCT levels in patients with clinical shock syndromes.

For emphasis, whether a patient has CAP and/or possible septic shock, a normal PCT serum concentration strongly suggests the etiology is not a bacterial infection. The negative predictive values are 92% or greater.[44]

Influence of renal function on interpretation of serum procalcitonin levels

The serum concentration of PCT increases in patients with stage 5 end-stage renal disease (ESRD) or as defined by a creatinine clearance of less than 15 mL/min. In the absence of renal replacement therapy in uninfected patients, the reported PCT levels range from 0.12 to 1.8 ng/mL (**Table 2**).[45,46] After hemodialysis is initiated,

Table 2
Procalcitonin (PCT) serum concentrations in uninfected and infected patients with end-stage renal disease[a]

Renal Function or Renal Replacement Therapy	PCT, ng/mL Uninfected Patients	PCT, ng/mL Infected Patients
Creatinine clearance:		
15 to >90 mL/min	0.05 to <0.25	≥0.25
<15 mL/min	0.12–1.8	≥0.5
Hemodialysis patients	<0.5	≥0.5
Peritoneal dialysis patients	0.32–1.2	≥0.05
After renal transplantation[a]	≤0.25	≥0.25

[a] As OKT-3 and/or antithymocyte globulin can increase PCT levels greater than 10-fold in the absence of infection, PCT levels are not interpretable in patients on such therapy.[47,48]

Data from Grace E, Turner RM. Use of procalcitonin in patients with various degrees of chronic kidney disease including renal replacement therapy. Clin Infect Dis 2014;59:1761–7; and Dahaba AA, Rehak PH, List WF. Procalcitonin and C-reactive protein plasma concentrations in nonseptic uremic patients undergoing hemodialysis. Intensive Care Med 2003;29:579–83.

and in the absence of infection, serum PCT levels decrease to less than 0.5 ng/mL in most patients. In infected patients with ESRD, the PCT levels increase to ≥0.5 ng/mL. In patients undergoing peritoneal dialysis, with sparse available data, the PCT levels range from 0.32 to 1.2 in the absence of active infection.[45] For all patients undergoing dialysis, a reasonable "cutoff" suggesting active bacterial infection is ≥0.5 ng/mL.

PCT levels are not a valid biomarker in renal transplant patients receiving therapy with OKT-3 and/or antithymocyte globulin. The latter can, via cytokine effects, increase the PCT level greater than 10-fold.[47,48]

Two benefits of sequential procalcitonin levels

"Source" control. With the right drug in the right dose and, in the absence of confounding nonpulmonary infections, the PCT level, like the WBC, quickly trends toward normal values if the source of the infection(s) has/have been identified and controlled.

Duration of antimicrobial therapy for CAP. Management reviews and guidelines provide general suggestions for the duration of CAP antibiotic therapy. The 2007 CAP Infectious Diseases Society of America Guidelines, "UpToDate," and more recent reviews suggest a minimum of 5 days of therapy with resolution of fever for 48 to 72 hours.[49] There are many caveats. Duration can vary with the etiologic bacteria (longer for S aureus, aerobic gram-negative bacilli), presence of extrapulmonary infection, host comorbidities that impede recovery (eg, congestive heart failure, continued aspiration, immunodeficiency), and other factors.

Trending PCT levels is one way to individualize duration of therapy.[50] The usual suggestion is to repeat the PCT level every 2 to 4 days and discontinue antimicrobial therapy when the PCT concentration is ≤0.25 ng/mL. An alternative, used in Europe, is to stop when the PCT levels have decreased by ≥80% from the peak value.[51] We have not endorsed this approach, as the peak value may not be known. Numerous studies have found that this trending approach shortens treatment duration, and is safe.[51]

Community-acquired pneumonia summary

In short, the combination of expanded diagnostics, to include multiplex PCR panels plus PCT levels, rapidly provides physicians with information that

- Can decrease overuse of antibacterials for viral infections; a "normal" PCT level virtually excludes an invasive bacterial infection
- Detects coinfection due to bacteria and viruses
- Discriminates colonization from invasion by potential bacterial pathogens
- A downward trend in sequential PCT levels supports "source control" of the infection that is stimulating the innate immune system
- Trending PCT levels allows individualization of the duration of antibacterial therapy

Community-acquired pneumonia: the future of diagnostics

There is no doubt that the evolution in molecular diagnostics and understanding host genomic responses to infection will continue. We can anticipate the following:

- Discrimination of viral versus bacterial invasion based on the pattern of activated host genes[52–55]
- Discovery of biomarkers other than PCT that distinguish viral from bacterial infection
- Next-generation PCR multiplex platforms designed to detect more pathogens in sputum or sputum equivalent (endotracheal aspirate, bronchoalveolar lavage)
- Evolution of methods that quickly ascertain the presence and expression of antibiotic resistance genes
- Additional prospective trials that combine enhanced diagnostics with markers of activation of pertinent genes or gene products
- Point-of-care application of affordable multiplex PCR platforms and PCT levels in a variety of settings: primary care clinics, emergency departments, and others

SEPTIC SHOCK AND PROCALCITONIN
Case Presentations

Case 1

A 19-year-old female college coed is admitted with purpura fulminans. Within hours, blood cultures confirm the diagnosis of meningococcemia. PCT and other biomarkers are not needed to facilitate the diagnosis of bacteremic shock. The higher the peak PCT concentration, the higher the risk of patient mortality.

Case 2

A 55-year-old man with advanced alcoholic cirrhosis is admitted to the ICU with hypotension, fever, hematemesis, oliguria, and confusion. Ascites and other stigmata of cirrhosis are present. There is endoscopy evidence of bleeding varices. Echocardiogram documents an ejection fraction of 25%. His serum creatinine is 2.5 mg/dL. The serum lactate concentration is elevated. Blood pressure is 70/40 mm Hg. The ascitic fluid absolute neutrophil count is 600 cells/μL. The serum PCT is 2.0 ng/mL. The serum soluble CD14 (sCD14) level (generic name is presepsin) is 1000 pg/mL (N 48–171). What is/are the etiology/etiologies of the patient's shocklike state?

Procalcitonin and Etiology of Shock

As the example patient with cirrhosis illustrates, patients often have more than 1 process contributing to the pathogenesis of their clinical shock. The example patient with cirrhosis has findings compatible with hemorrhagic shock from bleeding esophageal varices, cardiogenic shock from alcohol-induced cardiomyopathy, and septic shock due to likely spontaneous bacterial peritonitis with or without bacteremia.

Well documented increases of serum PCT occur in all categories of shock: that is, hypovolemic, anaphylactic, cardiogenic, obstructive (tamponade, pulmonary embolus), toxic shock syndrome, and bacteremic shock.[56–62] In some patients, the elevated PCT may result from a bacterial infection complicating a noninfectious shock etiology.

Translocation of gut bacteria is an oft-suggested explanation for the PCT increase in all types of nonbacteremic shock and the associated impaired perfusion of the bowel wall.

Translocation of Gut Bacteria

The literature on translocation of gut bacteria is voluminous and increasingly sophisticated. In early studies in humans and animals, translocation was detected by finding bacteria in mesenteric lymph nodes or in portal venous blood.[63] Serum was tested for the presence of bacterial lipopolysaccharide using the Limulus amebocyte lysate assay, which is fraught with risk of contamination by environmental LPS.

More recently, blood specimens were tested with primers and a probe that targeted the conserved region of the 16s ribosomal DNA.[64] Testing takes days and there is risk of bacterial DNA contamination of the specimen or the PCR reagents.

Current literature criteria for translocation of gut bacteria is some combination of the following:[65]

- An increase in serum concentration of LPS-LPS–binding protein complex[66]
- In the absence of overt pneumonia, UTI, or other bacterial infection, an increase in the serum concentration of sCD14 (generic name, presepsin)[67]
- In the absence of invasive bacterial infection, elevated concentration of serum PCT[68]

Serum Soluble CD14 (Presepsin)

The CD14 gene encodes a cluster-of-differentiation glycoprotein found on the surface of monocytes, macrophages, and dendritic cells.[67,68] CD14-encoded protein is a high-affinity receptor for the complex of LPS with LPS-binding protein. Binding of the complex to the CD14 receptor activates Toll-like receptor (pattern recognition receptor) 4. The result is twofold: signal transduction to initiate nuclear transcription of proinflammatory cytokines and concomitantly, the release of a soluble form of CD14 (sCD14) into the circulation.

In volunteers given endotoxin, sCD14 levels rose within 2 hours.[69] It is possible to quantitate the sCD14 level with a chemiluminescence enzyme immunoassay (PATH-FAST [Mitsubishi Chemical Corporation, Tokyo, Japan]). Results are available in 17 minutes using an automated instrument.[70]

In addition, the proinflammatory cytokines (TNF, IL-1, IL-2, IL-6), stimulated by membrane activation in turn stimulate transcription of the PCT gene.

Example: the following are clinical syndromes with documented translocation of gut bacteria in animals and patients:

- All categories of clinical shock[65]
- Neutropenia[71]
- Low-level translocation documented in
  - Hepatic cirrhosis[72,73]
  - Incompletely controlled human immunodeficiency virus infection[74,75]

Translocation of gut bacteria may not be the sole explanation for an increase in PCT serum levels in the absence of overt invasive bacterial infection. The host response to mitochondrial DNA may help explain PCT increases in patients with massive organ necrosis: for example, trauma-associated rhabdomyolysis, severe burns, large myocardial infarction, and liver necrosis due to mushroom poisoning. Shock may or may not be present.

Mitochondria were originally saprophytic bacteria that eukaryotic cells captured with eventual evolution to a critical intracellular eukaryotic organelle.[76] The circular DNA of mitochondria retains some characteristics of bacterial DNA. In a series of experiments, Zhang and colleagues[77] demonstrated the rapid appearance of mitochondrial DNA in the plasma of 15 patients who suffered major trauma. The data are consistent with the release of DNA that initiated an innate immune-type inflammatory response as would occur in bacterial invasive infection. It is postulated that tissues either directly respond to the bacterialike DNA with a rise in PCT levels or the proinflammatory cytokines indirectly increase PCT levels.[78,79]

Negative Predictive Value in Patients with Shock

One of the benefits of serum PCT levels in patients with shock is the power of the negative predictive value. With a few caveats, a normal PCT concentration in a hypotensive patient virtually excludes bacteremia as an etiology (**Table 3**).[24,80–84]

Two cautions are in order. It takes 4 to 5 hours for the serum level of PCT to increase after an initial microbial stimulus.[22] With an acute illness, we suggest a second PCT serum level after 4 to 6 hours. Acute appendicitis is a good example. With early, less than transmural inflammation, the PCT concentration may not increase, as clearly happens with transmural inflammation or perforation of the appendix.[85]

Procalcitonin, Source Control, and Mortality

Source control is a major objective in the management of clinical sepsis. Sequential PCT serum levels, in concert with clinical assessment and normalization of the WBCs, are an objective measurement of the degree of source control.

In a study from France, the magnitude of the decrease in serum PCT between days 2 and 3 of therapy correlated with survival.[86] Similar results were reported from Australia[87] and the Netherlands.[88]

There is no known toxic effect of elevated PCT levels. To the contrary, there is in vitro evidence of an anti-inflammatory function.[89] Our current view is that PCT serum levels are best considered as a marker of activation of the host innate immune response.

Table 3
Representative negative predictive values (NPV) of serum procalcitonin levels in patients with possible severe sepsis

Ref No.	Clinical Setting	Clinical Endpoint	Procalcitonin "Cutoff" Concentration, ng/mL	NPV, %
Reitman et al,[24] 2012	Febrile neutropenia in children	Bacteremia	<0.5	93
Riedel et al,[80] 2011	Sepsis in emergency department	Bacteremia	<0.1	98
Garcia-Granero et al,[81] 2013	Gastrointestinal surgery	Anastomotic leak	<0.35	100
Markogiannakis et al,[82] 2011	Bowel obstruction	Ischemic bowel	<0.25	95
Menacci et al,[83] 2012	Hospitalized with sepsis syndrome	Bacteremia	<0.25	99
Menendez et al,[84] 2012	Community-acquired pneumonia	Bacteremia	<0.36	98

A recent Cochrane Review concluded that PCT-guided antimicrobial therapy did not lower the risk of death.[90] Mortality risk and source control is multifactorial. In the septic patient, source control often requires some combination of surgery, prompt and appropriate antibacterial therapy, reversal of organ failure, successful treatment of a concomitant malignancy, and a long list of other potential confounders. In short, PCT levels alone do not influence mortality; rising or persistently high PCT levels indicate a failure to control the process triggering the PCT genes, which in turn reflects poor source control and is associated with an increased risk of mortality.[89,90]

Procalcitonin Levels and Individualization of Treatment

Guidelines on how long to treat bacteremia vary with the following:

- The source of the bacteremia: for example, uncomplicated versus complicated UTI
- The etiologic organism
- The immune status of the host and other factors[91]

In theory, sequential serum PCT levels create the potential to individualize the duration of therapy. The goal is to treat until the innate immune system is no longer activated.

In prospective clinical trials, duration of therapy was guided by sequential PCT serum levels or by physician choice without knowledge of the PCT values. In the PCT-guided patients, treatment was continued until the PCT level fell by 80% from its peak or reached a concentration in the range of ≤ 5.0 or ≤ 2.5 ng/mL.

The results consistently showed that patients in the PCT guidance group discontinued antibacterial therapy roughly 2 days sooner than patients with no PCT levels available to guide duration.[88,91–94] Of import, the PCT guidance was safe with no infection relapses reported. The results have been consistent, as reflected in systematic reviews and meta-analyses.[94,95]

Subsummary: What Does, and What Does Not, Increase the Serum Concentration of Procalcitonin?

Knowledge as to what increases, or does not increase, the PCT serum concentration is constantly changing. The current status is summarized in **Table 4** with the caveat that some of the conclusions need validation. The summary is organized by microorganisms, clinical syndromes, neoplasms, and drugs. In **Table 4**, we selected a PCT concentration of ≥ 0.25 ng/mL as the usual or mean "cutoff" for a meaningful PCT elevation. Some literature may use cutoff levels as high as 0.50, or rarely 1.0, as definition of a low PCT category. Such levels are hard to interpret, as often important details like patients' renal function and possible concomitant viral and bacterial infection are not provided.

Perhaps most useful is the list of microorganisms, inflammatory clinical syndromes, neoplasms and drugs that DO NOT substantively activate the PCT gene: for example, pure viral infection,[25–32] Chlamydia species,[26] and Mycoplasma species[26] do not stimulate PCT increases. Yet, other intracellular bacterial pathogens, like Scrub typhus, do increase PCT serum levels.[96] Mycobacteria may or may not stimulate PCT.[97,98]

Note the list of inflammatory conditions that do not substantively increase PCT:

- Chronic walled-off infections: for example, chronic empyema[36]
- Edematous/necrotizing pancreatitis unless secondary bacterial infection is present[99,100]
- Uncomplicated regional enteritis or ulcerative colitis[101–103]

Table 4 Summary of microorganisms, clinical syndromes, neoplasms, and drugs that DO or DO NOT increase serum levels of procalcitonin (PCT)	
DO Increase Serum PCT to ≥0.25 ng/mL	**DO NOT Increase Serum PCT to ≥0.25 ng/mL**
Microorganisms	
Bacteria: • Alone or with viral coinfection[9,15,16] • Gram-positive and gram-negative pathogens • *Legionella* species[118,119] • *Mycobacteria* species[a,97,98] • Scrub typhus[96] Bacterial toxin-mediated inflammation: • *Clostridium difficile* toxin[120] • Toxic shock syndrome toxins[62] Fungi: *Candida* species[122] Parasites: *Plasmodium* species (malaria)[121] Viruses: None, so far	Bacteria: • *Chlamydia* species[26] • *Mycoplasma pneumoniae*[26] • *Mycobacteria* species[a,97,98] • Lyme borreliosis[131] Fungi[122–124]: • Aspergillosis • Coccidioidomycosis[123] • Mucormycosis[124] Viruses: Virtually all, so far
Clinical Syndromes	
Bacterial: • Aspiration pneumonia[125–127] • Bacterial meningitis[30–32] • Bacterial pancreatitis[99,100] • Bacterial peritonitis[132] • Bacterial pneumonia[7,9,15,17] • Bacterial septic shock[135] • Febrile neutropenia[24,128] • Mushroom poisoning[130] • Pyelonephritis[129] • Renal insufficiency[45,46] • Septic arthritis[108,109] • Shock[54–62,117,133]: anaphylactic, bacteremic, cardiogenic, toxic shock syndrome, adrenal insufficiency, hemorrhagic, obstructive • Thermal injury, burns[133] • Trauma: crush injury (case reports)[134]	Viral: respiratory tract infections[9,15,17] • Meningitis[30–32] Abscess, chronic: for example, empyema[36] Gout, pseudogout[108] Inflammatory bowel disease[101–103] Rheumatic diseases[104–108]: • Behcet syndrome • Polyarteritis nodosa • Rheumatoid arthritis • Systemic lupus erythematosus • Still disease • Temporal arteritis • Wegener granulomatosis
Neoplasms	
Medullary thyroid cancer[23,110,111]	[110,111] Lymphomas Pancreas Renal cell Sarcomas
Drugs[47,48,114–116]	
Alemtuzumab (CD52 antibody) Granulocyte transfusions Interleukin-2 Rituximab (anti-CD20 antibody) T-cell antibodies	Most have no effect unless influence innate immune inflammatory response NOTE: glucocorticoids do not impede a PCT response[111]

[a] Reports of Mycobacterial infections either increasing or decreasing serum levels of PCT.

- Viral meningitis or pericarditis[30–32]
- Rheumatologic syndromes: for example, gout/pseudogout, temporal arteritis, systemic lupus erythematosus, polyarteritis nodosa, rheumatoid arthritis, reactive arthritis, Behcet syndrome, adult Still disease[104–109]
- Neoplasms associated with a fever of unknown origin syndrome (lymphoma, renal cell carcinoma, sarcomas, pancreatic carcinoma) do not cause a substantive increase in the PCT serum level[110,111]
- Of interest, glucocorticoids do not block an increase in PCT concentrations.[112,113] In one report, nonsteroidal anti-inflammatory drugs increased the peak PCT level in human volunteers given endotoxin.[114] In contrast, a variety of immune-modulating drugs are reported to increase PCT levels.[47,48,115,116]

Much of the data in **Table 4** derive from uncontrolled observational studies of small numbers of patients. Hence, conclusions are guarded and confirmatory studies needed.

SUMMARY

More than half of the patients admitted to a critical care unit are administered empiric antimicrobial therapy. The most common empiric indications are CAP or "sepsis." The combination of multiplex PCR platforms and biomarkers like PCT are powerful tools that allow quick and precise identification of etiologic pathogens. The result is transition to specific or directed therapy. The anticipated result is fewer days of antimicrobial therapy, fewer drug-related adverse effects, and, hopefully, greater therapeutic efficacy with slower emergence of resistance pathogens. Better panels, better understanding of host genomic responses to infection, and controlled prospective studies are needed to better understand the strengths and weaknesses of our new tool box. As to PCT, there is need for further basic study to clarify its role in the host inflammatory response.

REFERENCES

1. Polk RE, Hohmann SF, Medvedev S, et al. Benchmarking risk-adjusted adult antibacterial drug use in 70 US academic medical center hospitals. Clin Infect Dis 2011;53(11):1100–10.
2. Gilbert DN. Influence of an infectious diseases specialist on ICU multidisciplinary rounds. Crit Care Res Pract 2014;2014:307817.
3. Thomas Z, Bandali F, Sankaranarayanan J, et al. A multicenter evaluation of prolonged empiric antibiotic therapy in adult ICUs in the United States. Crit Care Med 2015;43:2527–34.
4. Vincent JL, Rello J, Marshall J, et al. International study of the prevalence and outcomes of infection in intensive care units. JAMA 2009;302:2323–9.
5. Aarts MA, Brun-Buisson C, Cook DJ, et al. Antibiotic management of suspected nosocomial ICU-acquired infection: does prolonged empiric therapy improve outcome? Intensive Care Med 2007;33:1369–78.
6. Kumar A, Roberts D, Wood KE, et al. Duration of hypotension before initiation of effective antimicrobial therapy is the critical determinant of survival in human septic shock. Crit Care Med 2006;34:1589–96.
7. Musher DM, Roig IL, Cazares G, et al. Can an etiologic agent be identified in adults who are hospitalized for community-acquired pneumonia: results of a one year study. J Infect 2013;67:11–8.

8. Musher DM. Quantitative molecular approach to diagnosing pneumonia. Clin Infect Dis 2016;62:824–5.

9. Falsey AR, Becker KL, Swinburne AJ, et al. Bacterial complications of respiratory tract viral illness. A comprehensive evaluation. J Infect Dis 2013;208: 432–41.

10. Jain S, Williams DJ, Arnold SR, et al. Community-acquired pneumonia requiring hospitalization among U.S. children. N Engl J Med 2015;372:835–45.

11. Jain WH, Wunderink RG, Kakhran S, et al. Community-acquired pneumonia requiring hospitalization among U.S. adults. N Engl J Med 2015;373:415–27.

12. Albrich WC, Madhi SA, Adrian PV, et al. Use of a rapid test of pneumococcal colonization density to diagnose pneumococcal pneumonia. Clin Infect Dis 2012;54:601–9.

13. Johansson N, Kalin M, Tiveljung-Lindell A, et al. Etiology of community-acquired pneumonia: increased microbiological yield with new diagnostic methods. Clin Infect Dis 2010;50:202–9.

14. Gelfer G, Leggett J, Myers J, et al. The clinical impact of the detection of potential etiologic pathogens of community-acquired pneumonia. Diagn Microbiol Infect Dis 2015;83:400–6.

15. Gilbert D, Gelfer G, Wang L, et al. The potential of molecular diagnostics and serum procalcitonin levels to change the antibiotic management of community-acquired pneumonia. Diagn Microbiol Infect Dis 2016;86:102–7.

16. Branche AR, Walsh EE, Vargas R, et al. Serum procalcitonin measurement and viral testing to guide antibiotic use for respiratory infections in hospitalized adults: a randomized controlled trial. J Infect Dis 2015;212:1692–700.

17. Gadsby NJ, Russell CD, McHugh MP, et al. Comprehensive molecular testing for respiratory pathogens in community-acquired pneumonia. Clin Infect Dis 2016;62:817–23.

18. Jain S, Pavia AT. The modern quest for the "Holy Grail" of pneumonia etiology. Clin Infect Dis 2016;62:826–8.

19. Collins AM, Johnstone CMK, Gritzfeld JF, et al. Pneumococcal colonization rates in patients admitted to a United Kingdom hospital with lower respiratory tract infection: a prospective case-control study. J Clin Microbiol 2016;54:944–9.

20. Sethi S, Maloney J, Grove L, et al. Airway inflammation and bronchial colonization in chronic obstructive pulmonary disease. Am J Respir Crit Care Med 2016; 173:991–8.

21. Gorwitz RJ, Kruszon-Moran D, McAllister SK, et al. Changes in the prevalence of nasal colonization with *Staphylococcus aureus* in the United States, 2001-2004. J Infect Dis 2008;19:1226–34.

22. Becker KL, Nylen ES, White JC, et al. Procalcitonin and the calcitonin gene family of peptides in inflammation, infection, and sepsis: a journey from calcitonin back to its precursors. J Clin Endocrinol Metab 2004;89:1512–25.

23. Muller B, White JC, Nylen ES, et al. Ubiquitous expression of the calcitonin-I gene in multiple tissues in response to sepsis. J Clin Endocrinol Metab 2001; 86:396–403.

24. Reitman AJ, Pisk RM, Gates JV 3rd, et al. Serial procalcitonin levels to detect bacteremia in febrile neutropenia. Clin Pediatr (Phila) 2012;51:1175–83.

25. Becker KL, Snider R, Nylen ES. Procalcitonin assay in systemic inflammation, infection, and sepsis: clinical utility and limitations. Crit Care Med 2008;36: 941–52.

26. Schutzle H, Forster J, Superti-Furga A, et al. Is serum procalcitonin a reliable diagnostic marker in children with acute respiratory tract infections? A retrospective analysis. Eur J Pediatr 2009;168:1117–24.

27. Linscheid P, Seboek D, Nylen ES, et al. In vitro and in vivo calcitonin I gene expression in parenchymal cells: a novel product of human adipose tissue. Endocrinology 2003;144:5578–84.

28. Schuetz P, Matthias B, Christ-Grain M, et al. Procalcitonin to guide initiation and duration of antibiotic treatment in acute respiratory infections: an individual patient data meta-analysis. Clin Infect Dis 2012;55:651–62.

29. Schuetz P, Briel M, Mueller B. Clinical outcomes associated with procalcitonin algorithms to guide antibiotic therapy in respiratory tract infections. JAMA 2013;309:717–8.

30. Schwarz S, Bertram M, Schwab S, et al. Serum procalcitonin levels in bacterial and abacterial meningitis. Crit Care Med 2000;28:1828–32.

31. Vikse J, Henry M, Roy J, et al. The role of serum procalcitonin in the diagnosis of bacterial meningitis in adults: a systemic review and meta-analysis. Int J Infect Dis 2015;38:68–76.

32. Wei TT, Hu ZD, Qin BD, et al. Diagnostic accuracy of procalcitonin in bacterial meningitis versus nonbacterial meningitis. Medicine 2016;95(11):e3079.

33. Self WH, Williams DJ, Zhu Y, et al. Respiratory viral detection in children and adults: comparing asymptomatic controls and patients with community-acquired pneumonia. J Infect Dis 2016;213:584–91.

34. Bxington CL, Ampofo K, Stockman F, et al. Community surveillance of respiratory viruses among families in the Utah Better Identification of Germs– Longitudinal Viral Epidemiology (BIG-LOVE) Study. Clin Infect Dis 2015;61:1217–24.

35. Raoult D. The new diagnostic techniques highlight the need for negative controls. Clin Infect Dis 2016;62:809.

36. Lin MC, Chen YC, Wu JT, et al. Diagnostic and prognostic values of pleural fluid procalcitonin in parapneumonic pleural effusions. Chest 2009;136:205–11.

37. Sato M, Hasoxa M, Wright PF. Differences in serum cytokine levels between influenza virus A and B infections in children. Cytokine 2009;47:65–8.

38. Melendi G, Laham A, Monsalvo FR, et al. Cytokine profiles in the respiratory tract during primary infection with human metapneumovirus, respiratory syncytial virus, or influenza virus in infants. Pediatrics 2007;120:e410–5.

39. Henriquez K, Hayney MS, Rakel DP, et al. Procalcitonin levels in acute respiratory infection. Viral Immunol 2016;29:128–31.

40. Yamada M, Gomez JC, Chugh PE, et al. Interferon-γ production by neutrophils during bacterial pneumonia in mice. Am J Respir Crit Care Med 2011;183:1391–401.

41. Gomez JC, Yamada M, Martin JR, et al. Mechanisms of interferon-γ production by neutrophils and its function during *Streptococcus pneumoniae* pneumonia. Am J Respir Cell Mol Biol 2015;52:349–64.

42. Brodska H, Malickova K, Adamkova V, et al. Significantly higher procalcitonin levels could differentiate gram-negative sepsis from gram-positive and fungal sepsis. Clin Exp Med 2013;13:165–70.

43. Charles PE, Ladaire S, Aho S, et al. Serum procalcitonin elevation in critically ill patients at the onset of bacteremia caused by either gram-negative or gram-positive bacteria. BMC Infect Dis 2008;8:38.

44. Rodriguez AH, Aviles-Jurado ED, Schuetz P, et al. Procalcitonin (PCT) levels for ruling out bacterial co-infection in ICU patients with influenza: a CHAID decision tree analysis. J Infect 2016;72:143–51.

45. Grace E, Turner RM. Use of procalcitonin in patients with various degrees of chronic kidney disease including renal replacement therapy. Clin Infect Dis 2014;59:1761–7.

46. Dahaba AA, Rehak PH, List WF. Procalcitonin and C-reactive protein plasma concentrations in nonseptic uremic patients undergoing hemodialysis. Intensive Care Med 2003;29:579–83.

47. Sabat R, Hoflich C, Docke WD, et al. Massive elevation of procalcitonin plasma levels in the absence of infection in kidney transplant patients treated with pan-T-cell antibodies. Intensive Care Med 2001;27:987–91.

48. Brodska H, Drabek T, Malickova K, et al. Marked increase of procalcitonin after the administration of anti-thymocyte globulin in patients before hematopoietic stem cell transplantation does not indicate sepsis: a prospective study. Crit Care 2009;13:RF37.

49. Musher DM, Thorner AR. Community-acquired pneumonia. N Engl J Med 2014; 37:1619–28.

50. Mitsuma SF, Mansour MK, Dekker JP, et al. Promising new assays and technologies for the diagnosis and management of infectious disease. Clin Infect Dis 2013;56:996.

51. Schuetz P, Muller B, Christ-Crain M, et al. Procalcitonin to initiate or discontinue antibiotics in acute respiratory tract infections. Cochrane Database Syst Rev 2012;(9):CD007498.

52. Suarez NM, Bunsaw E, Falsey AR, et al. Superiority of transcriptional profiling over procalcitonin for distinguishing bacterial from viral lower respiratory tract infections in adults. J Infect Dis 2015;212(2):213–22.

53. Tsalik EL, McClain M, Zaas A. Moving toward prime time: host signatures for diagnosis of respiratory infection. Clin Infect Dis 2015;212:173–5.

54. Tsalik EL, Henao R, Nichols M, et al. Host gene expression classifiers diagnose acute respiratory illness etiology. Sci Transl Med 2016;8(322):322ra11.

55. Sweeney TE, Shidham A, Wong HR, et al. A comprehensive time-course-based multicohort analysis of sepsis and sterile inflammation reveals a robust diagnostic gene set. Sci Transl Med 2015;7(287):287ra71.

56. Kafkas N, Venetsanon K, Patsilinakos S, et al. Procalcitonin in acute myocardial infarction. Aucte Card Care 2008;10:30–6.

57. Mann J, Cavallazzi R. Marked serum procalcitonin in response to isolated anaphylactic shock. Am J Emerg Med 2015;33:1256.e5-6.

58. Picariello C, Lazzeri C, Valente S, et al. Procalcitonin in cardiac patients. Intern Emerg Med 2011;6:245–52.

59. Ates H, Ates I, Bozkurt B, et al. What is the most reliable marker in the differential diagnosis of pulmonary embolism and community-acquired pneumonia? Blood Coagul Fibrinolysis 2016;27:252–8.

60. Clech C, Ferriere F, Karoubi P, et al. Diagnostic and prognostic value of procalcitonin in patients with septic shock. Crit Care Med 2004;32:1166–9.

61. Meisner M, Adim H, Schmidt J. Correlation of procalcitonin and C-reactive protein to inflammation, complications, and outcome during the intensive care unit course of multiple-trauma patients. Crit Care 2006;10(1):R1.

62. Kato M, Kaneko S, Takagaki K, et al. Procalcitonin as a biomarker for toxic shock syndrome. Acta Derm Venereol 2010;90:441–3.

63. Schoeffel U, Pelz K, Haring RU, et al. Inflammatory consequences of the translocation of bacteria and endotoxin to mesenteric lymph nodes. Am J Surg 2000; 180:66–71.

64. Nikkari S, McLoughlin IJ, Bi W, et al. Does blood of healthy subjects contain bacterial ribosomal DNA? J Clin Microbiol 2001;39:1956–9.
65. Vaishnavi C. Translocation of gut flora and its role in sepsis. Indian J Med Microbiol 2013;31:334–42.
66. Elsing C, Ernst S, Kayali N, et al. Lipopolysaccharide binding protein, interleukin-6 and C-reaction protein in acute gastrointestinal infections: value as biomarker to reduce unnecessary antibiotic therapy. Infection 2011;39: 327–31.
67. Kitchens R. Role of CD14 in cellular recognition of bacterial lipopolysaccharides. Chem Immunol 2000;74:71–82.
68. Kautsoumas I, Kaltsa G, Siakavellar SI, et al. Markers of bacterial translocation in end-stange liver disease. World J Hepatol 2015;7:2264–73.
69. Pajkrt D, Doran JE, Koster F. Antiinflammatory effects of reconstituted high-density lipoprotein during human endotoxemia. J Exp Med 1996;184:1601–8.
70. Ulla M, Pizzolato E, Lucchiari M, et al. Diagnostic and prognostic value of pre-sepsin in the management of sepsis in the emergency department: a multi-center prospective study. Crit Care 2013;17:R168.
71. Wong M, Barqasho B, Ohrmalm L, et al. Microbial translocation contribute to febrile episodes in adults with chemotherapy-induced neutropenia. PLoS One 2013;8(7):e68056.
72. Sandler NG, Koh C, Roque A, et al. Host response to translated microbial products predicts outcomes of patients with HBV or HCV infection. Gastroenterology 2011;141:1220–30.
73. de Oca Arjona MM, Marquez M, Soto MJ, et al. Bacterial translocation in HIV-infected patients with HCV cirrhosis. Implications in hemodynamic alterations and mortality. J Acquir Immune Defic Syndr 2011;56:420–7.
74. Jiang W, Lederman MM, Hunt P, et al. Plasma levels of bacterial DNA correlate with immune activation and magnitude of immune restoration in persons with antiretroviral-treated HIV infection. J Infect Dis 2009;199:1177–85.
75. Nowroozalizadeh S, Mansson F, de Silva Z, et al. Microbial translocation correlates with the severity of both HIV-1 and HIV-2 infections. J Infect Dis 2010;201: 1150–4.
76. Manfredi A, Rovere-Querini P. The mitochrondion–a Trojan horse that kicks off inflammation? N Engl J Med 2010;362:2132–4.
77. Zhang Q, Raoof M, Chen Y, et al. Circulating mitochondrial DAMPs cause inflammatory responses to injury. Nature 2010;464:104–8.
78. Morganthaler NG, Struck J, Chancerelle Y, et al. Production of procalcitonin (PCT) in non-thyroidal tissue after LPS injection. Horm Metab Res 2003;35: 290–5.
79. Matwiyoff GN, Prahl JD, Miller RJ, et al. Immune regulation of procalcitonin: a biomarker and mediator of inflammation. Inflamm Res 2012;61:401–9.
80. Riedel S, Melendez JH, An AT, et al. Procalcitonin as a marker for the detection of bacteremia and sepsis in the emergency department. Am J Clin Pathol 2011; 135:182–9.
81. Garcia-Granero A, Frasson M, Flor-Lorente B, et al. Procalcitonin and C-reactive protein as early predictors of anastomotic tear in colorectal surgery: a prospective observational study. Dis Colon Rectum 2013;56:475–83.
82. Markogiannakis H, Memos N, Messaris E, et al. Predictive value of procalcitonin for bowel ischemia and necrosis in bowel obstruction. Surgery 2011;149: 394–403.

83. Menacci A, Leli C, Cardaccia A, et al. Procalcitonin predicts real-time PCR results in blood samples from patients with suspected sepsis. PLoS One 2012; 7(12):e53279.
84. Menendez R, Sahuquillo-Arce M, Reyes S, et al. Cytokine activation patterns and biomarkers are influenced by microorganisms in community-acquired pneumonia. Chest 2012;141:1537–45.
85. Sand M, Trullen XV, Bechara FG, et al. A prospective bicenter study investigating the diagnostic value of procalcitonin in patients with acute appendicitis. Eur Surg Res 2009;43:291–7.
86. Charles PE, Tinel C, Barbar S, et al. Procalcitonin kinetics within the first days of sepsis: relationship with the appropriateness of antibiotic therapy and outcome. Crit Care 2009;13:R38.
87. Shehabi Y, Sterba M, Garrett PM, et al. Procalcitonin algorithm in critically ill adults with undifferentiated infection or suspected sepsis. Am J Respir Crit Care Med 2014;190:1102–10.
88. DeJong E, vanOers JA, Beishinzen A, et al. Efficacy and safety of procalcitonin guidance in reducing the duration of antibiotic treatment in critically ill patients: a randomized, controlled, open-label trial. Lancet Infect Dis 2016;16:819–27.
89. Matera G, Quirino A, Giancotti A, et al. Proacalcitonin neutralizes bacterial LPS and reduces LPS-induced cytokine release in human peripheral mononuclear cells. BMC Microbiol 2012;12:68.
90. Andriolo BNG, Andriolo RB, Salomao R, et al. Effectiveness and safety of procalcitonin evaluation for reducing mortality in adults with sepsis, severe sepsis or septic shock [review]. Cochrane Database Syst Rev 2017;(1):CD010959.
91. Harvey TC, Fowler RA, Daneman N. Duration of antibiotic therapy for bacteremia: a systematic review and meta-analysis. Crit Care 2011;15:R267.
92. Nobre V, Harbarth S, Graf JD, et al. Use of procalcitonin to shorten antibiotic treatment duration in septic patients. Am J Respir Crit Care Med 2008;177: 498–505.
93. Bouadma L, Luxt CE, Tubach F, et al. Use of procalcitonin to reduce patients' exposure to antibiotics in intensive care units (PRORATA trial): a multicentre randomized controlled trial. Lancet 2010;375:463–74.
94. Agarwal R, Schwartz DN. Procalcitonin to guide duration of antimicrobial therapy in intensive care units: a systematic review. Clin Infect Dis 2011;53:379–87.
95. Kopterides P, Siempos II, Tsangaris I, et al. Procalcitonin-guided algorithms of antibiotic therapy in the intensive care unit: a systematic review and meta-analysis of randomized controlled trials. Crit Care Med 2010;38:2229–41.
96. Peter JV, Karthik G, Ramakrishna K, et al. Elevated procalcitonin is associated with increased mortality in patients with scrub typhus infection needing intensive care admission. Indian J Crit Care Med 2013;17:174–7.
97. Schleicher GK, Herbert V, Brink A, et al. Procalcitonin and c-reactive protein levels in HIV positive subjects with tuberculosis and pneumonia. Eur Respir J 2005;25:688–92.
98. Nyamande K, Lalloo UG. Serum procalcitonin distinguishes CAP due to bacteria, *Mycobacterium tuberculosis* and PJP. Int J Tuberc Lung Dis 2006;10:510–5.
99. Li HC, Fan XJ, Chen YF, et al. Early prediction of intestinal mucosal barrier function impairment by elevated serum procalcitonin in rats with severe acute pancreatitis. Pancreatology 2016;16:211–7.
100. Yang CJ, Chen J, Phillips ARJ, et al. Predictors of severe and critical acute pancreatitis. Dig Liver Dis 2014;46:446–51.

101. Koido S, Ohkusa T, Takakura K, et al. Clinical significance of procalcitonin (PCT) with ulcerative colitis (UC) activity. World J Gastroenterol 2013;19:8335–41.

102. Kim SE. Serum procalcitonin is a candidate biomarker to differentiate bacteremia from disease flares in patients with inflammatory bowel disease. Gut Liver 2016;10:491–2.

103. Chung SH, Lee HW, Kim SW, et al. Usefulness of measuring serum procalcitonin levels in patients with inflammatory bowel disease. Gut Liver 2016;10:574–80.

104. Bador KM, Intan S, Hussin S, et al. Serum procalcitonin has negative predictive value for bacterial infection in active systemic lupus erythematosus. Lupus 2012;21:1172–7.

105. Quintana G, Medina Y, Rojas C, et al. The use of procalcitonin determinations in evaluation of systemic lupus erythematosus. J Clin Rheumatol 2008;14:138–42.

106. Limper M, deKruif MD, Duits AJ, et al. The diagnostic role of procalcitonin and other biomarkers in discriminating infectious from non-infectious fever. J Infect 2010;60:409–16.

107. Chen DY, Chen YM, Ho WL, et al. Diagnostic value of procalcitonin for differentiation between bacterial infection and non-infectious inflammation in febrile patients with active adult-onset Still's disease. Ann Rheum Dis 2009;68:1074–5.

108. Hugle T, Schuetz P, Mueller B, et al. Serum procalcitonin for discrimination between septic and non-septic arthritis. Clin Exp Rheumatol 2008;26:305–8.

109. Maharajan K, Patro DK, Merron J, et al. Serum procalcitonin is a sensitive and specific marker in the diagnosis of septic arthritis and acute osteomyelitis. J Orthop Surg Res 2013;8:19.

110. Schuthrumpf S, Binder L, Hagemann T, et al. Utility of procalcitonin concentration in the evaluation of patients with malignant diseases and elevated C-reactive protein plasma concentrations. Clin Infect Dis 2006;43:468–73.

111. Hangai S, Nannya Y, Kurokawa M. Role of procalcitonin and C-reactive protein for discrimination between tumor fever and infection in patients with hematological diseases. Leuk Lymphoma 2015;56:910–4.

112. Tamaki K, Kogata Y, Sugiyama D, et al. Diagnostic accuracy of serum procalcitonin concentrations for detecting systemic bacterial infection in patients with systemic autoimmune diseases. J Rheumatol 2008;35:114–9.

113. Pihusch M, Pihusch R, Faunberger P, et al. Evaluation of C-reactive protein, interleukin-6 and procaclitonin levels in allogenic hematopoietic stem cell recipients. Eur J Hematol 2006;76:96–101.

114. Preas HL, Nylen ES, Snider RH, et al. Effects of anti-inflammatory agents on serum levels of calcitonin precursors during human experimental endotoxemia. J Infect Dis 2001;184:373–6.

115. Dornbusch HJ, Strenger V, Sovinz P, et al. Non-infectious causes of elevated procalcitonin and C-reactive protein serum levels in pediatric patients with hematologic and oncologic disorders. Support Care Cancer 2008;16:1035–40.

116. Robier C, Neubauer M, Reicht G. Marked elevation of procalcitonin in a patient with a drug-related infusion reaction to rituximab. Clin Chem Lab Med 2016;54:e101–3.

117. Schumm J, Pfeifer R, Ferrari M, et al. An unusual case of progressive shock and highly elevated procalcitonin level. Am J Crit Care 2010;19:96–103.

118. Haeuptle J, Zaborsky R, Fiumefreddo R, et al. Prognostic value of procalcitonin in Legionella pneumonia. Eur J Clin Microbiol Infect Dis 2009;28:55–60.

119. Bellman-Weiler R, Ausserwinkler M, Kurz K, et al. Clinical potential of C-reactive protein and procalcitonin serum concentrations to guide differential diagnosis

and clinical management of pneumococcal and *Legionella* pneumonia. J Clin Microbiol 2010;48:1915–7.

120. Rao K, Walk ST, Micic D, et al. Procalcitonin levels associate with severity of *Clostridium difficile* infection. PLoS One 2013;8(3):e58265.

121. Righi E, Merelli M, Arzese A, et al. Determination of PCT on admission is a useful tool for the assessment of disease severity in travelers with imported *Plasmodium falciparum* malaria. Acta Parasitol 2016;61:412–8.

122. Dou YH, Du JK, Liu HL, et al. The role of procalcitonin in the identification of invasive fungal infection–a systemic review and meta-analysis. Diagn Microbiol Infect Dis 2013;76:464–9.

123. Sakata KK, Grys TE, Chang YHH, et al. Serum procalcitonin levels in patients with primary pulmonary coccidioidomycosis. Ann Am Thorac Soc 2014;11: 1239–43.

124. Roques M, Chretien ML, Favennec C, et al. Evolution of procalcitonin, C-reactive protein and fibrinogen levels in neutropenic leukemic patients with invasive pulmonary aspergillosis or mucormycosis. Mycoses 2016;59:383–90.

125. El-Solh AA, Vora H, Knight RR III, et al. Diagnostic use of serum procalcitonin levels in pulmonary aspiration syndromes. Crit Care Med 2011;39:1251–6.

126. Niederman MS. Distinguishing chemical pneumonitis from bacterial aspiration: still a clinical determination. Crit Care Med 2011;39:1543–4.

127. Gilbert DN. Procalcitonin and pulmonary aspiration. Another possible interpretation. Crit Care Med 2011;39:2019–21.

128. Aimoto M, Koh H, Katayama T, et al. Diagnostic performance of serum high-sensitivity procalcitonin and serum C-reactive protein tests for detecting bacterial infection in febrile neutropenia. Infection 2014;42:971–9.

129. Park JH, Wee JH, Choi SP, et al. Serum procalcitonin level for the prediction of severity in women with acute pyelonephritis in the ED: value of procalcitonin in acute pyelonephritis. Am J Emerg Med 2013;31:1092–7.

130. Merlet A, Dauchy FA, Dupon M. Hyperprocalcitonemia due to mushroom poisoning. Clin Infect Dis 2012;54:307–8.

131. Lotric-Furlan S, Maraspin-Carman V, Cimperman J, et al. Procalcitonin levels in patients with Lyme borreliosis. Wien Klin Wochenschr 2002;114:530–2.

132. Watkins RR, Lemonovich TL. Serum procalcitonin in the diagnosis and management of intra-abdominal infections. Expert Rev Anti Infect Ther 2012;10: 197–203.

133. Paratz JD, Lipman J, Boots RJ, et al. A new marker of sepsis post burn injury. Crit Care Med 2014;42:2029–36.

134. Redi H, Schlag G, Togel E, et al. Procalcitonin release patterns in a baboon model of trauma and sepsis: relationship to cytokines and neopterin. Crit Care Med 2000;28:3659–63.

135. Wacker C, Prkno A, Brunkhorst FM, et al. Procalcitonin as a diagnostic marker for sepsis: a systematic review and meta-analysis. Lancet Infect Dis 2013;13: 426–35.

Severe Respiratory Viral Infections

New Evidence and Changing Paradigms

James M. Walter, MD[1], Richard G. Wunderink, MD, FCCP*

KEYWORDS

- Viral pneumonia • Community-acquired pneumonia • Rhinovirus
- Human adenovirus • Respiratory syncytial virus • Human metapneumovirus

KEY POINTS

- The epidemiology of severe lower respiratory tract infection is changing due in part to the aging of the US population and the success of childhood vaccination programs.
- Diagnostic advances including nucleic acid amplification platforms have greatly improved the detection of respiratory viral pathogens.
- Respiratory viral pathogens are now recognized as an important cause of severe respiratory infection in both immunocompetent and immunocompromised adults.
- Despite advances in diagnostic testing, a large number of patients with severe community-acquired respiratory infections do not have a causative pathogen identified.
- Better characterizing this group of patients remains an ongoing challenge.

Lower respiratory tract infection (LRTI) is a leading cause of death in the United States and the most common infection identified in patients admitted to the intensive care unit (ICU).[1,2] This burden will only increase as the population ages.[3]

The diagnosis and treatment of LRTIs including community-acquired pneumonia (CAP) has focused traditionally on bacterial pathogens.[4] Enthusiasm for the study of respiratory viral pathogens in severe respiratory illness has been tempered in the past by cumbersome diagnostic techniques and limited pharmacologic therapies. However, as pneumonia epidemiology and diagnostic platforms evolve, this focus has begun to change. The success of childhood vaccination programs and the aging of the US population have altered the landscape of severe respiratory infection.

Disclosure Statement: Dr J.M. Walter has nothing to disclose. Dr R.G. Wunderink has consulted for Genmark and Accelerate Diagnostics.
Division of Pulmonary and Critical Care, Department of Medicine, Northwestern University Feinberg School of Medicine, 676 North St Clair Street, Arkes 14-000, Chicago, IL 60611, USA
[1] Present address: 240 E. Huron, McGaw M-300, Chicago, IL 60611.
* Corresponding author. 676 North St. Clair Street, Arkes Pavilion 14-015, Chicago, IL 60611.
E-mail address: r-wunderink@northwestern.edu

Infect Dis Clin N Am 31 (2017) 455–474
http://dx.doi.org/10.1016/j.idc.2017.05.004
0891-5520/17/© 2017 Elsevier Inc. All rights reserved.

id.theclinics.com

Invasive pneumococcal disease has declined dramatically and viral pathogens that particularly impact the elderly are now recognized as common causal pathogens in severe disease.[5,6] Concurrently, the widespread use of nucleic acid amplification testing has markedly improved the detection of viral pathogens.[7]

This review focuses on the importance of respiratory viral pathogens in the pathogenesis of severe respiratory infections with a particular emphasis on community-acquired infections. Given widespread knowledge of influenza's important role in severe respiratory infections, we will focus on the noninfluenza viruses rhinovirus, human adenovirus (HAdV), respiratory syncytial virus (RSV), and human metapneumovirus (hMPV; **Table 1**).[8]

THE EVOLVING EPIDEMIOLOGY OF SEVERE RESPIRATORY INFECTIONS

As the US population ages, the number of homebound elderly, patients discharged to long-term care facilities, and adults with chronic medical conditions has increased.[3,9,10] It is, therefore, not surprising that the number of elderly patients admitted to the hospital with pneumonia is increasing. In 1 study, hospitalizations for pneumonia in patients 65 years of age or older increased by 20% over a 15-year period with an 11% increase in the number of patients with chronic cardiac or pulmonary disease.[3] Elderly and functionally limited adults are particularly prone to severe viral infection.[11] The incidence of rhinovirus infection in patients 65 years of age or older is 10 times higher than in younger adults; likewise, the majority of deaths attributable to RSV infection occur in patients older than 65 years of age.[12,13] Outbreaks of severe viral infections at long-term care facilities are common for numerous respiratory viral pathogens.[14–16]

As the number of adults susceptible to severe viral infections has increased, the incidence of invasive bacterial pneumonia has decreased owing to widespread pneumococcal vaccination, increased awareness of the importance of early antimicrobial therapy, and decreased rates of cigarette smoking. In 1 study, the incidence of invasive pneumococcal disease decreased by almost 30% over a 5-year period in adults greater than 50 years of age.[17] This shift in CAP pathogenesis may in part explain why the percentage of pneumonia hospitalizations with no reported pathogen increased by almost 20% from 1993 to 2011 despite improvements in diagnostic testing.[18]

Concurrently, our ability to diagnose viral infections rapidly and accurately has improved. Conventional diagnostic tests for respiratory viral pathogens include viral culture, acute and convalescent phase viral serologies, and direct fluorescence antibody staining. These methods are limited by slow turnaround time and limited sensitivity.[19] Nucleic acid amplification testing with the use of polymerase chain reaction (PCR) platforms has greatly improved the diagnosis of respiratory viral infections. The sensitivity of PCR testing is up to 5 times higher than conventional diagnostic methods, which may be particularly important in elderly patients who shed lower titers of virus.[20–23] PCR can also aid with viral subtyping and quantification of viral burden. Multiplex assays are now available, which allow for the testing of up to 19 viruses simultaneously.[19] Numerous clinical samples can be used for PCR testing including nasopharyngeal swabs, tracheal aspirates, bronchoalveolar lavage fluid, and pleural fluid.

The widespread use of PCR-based testing has allowed for a more accurate assessment of the role respiratory viral pathogens play in severe disease. In studies of hospitalized patients with CAP, between 15% and 35% have evidence of a viral infection.[21,24–27] This was best illustrated in the recent Centers for Disease Control and Prevention (CDC) EPIC study (Etiology of Pneumonia in the Community), a multicenter

Table 1
Characteristics of common noninfluenza respiratory viral pathogens

Virus	Structure	Peak Infectivity	Notable Groups at Risk	Notable Features	Preferred Diagnostic Test	Investigational Therapies
Rhinovirus	Single-stranded negative-sense RNA virus	Late spring and early fall	• Immunocompromised patients • Patients with COPD	• Common cause of asthma exacerbations in children • Most common pathogen isolated in CDC EPIC study	RT-PCR	Pegylated interferon-α2A + ribavirin
Human adenovirus	Nonenveloped double-stranded DNA virus	No seasonal peak	• Immunocompromised patients • Adults in crowded living environments including military barracks and long-term care facilities	• HAdV-14 linked to outbreaks of severe respiratory infection in the US • HAdV-55 an important cause of CAP in China	PCR	Cidofivir
Respiratory syncytial virus	Enveloped negative-sense single-stranded RNA virus	December to February	• Immunocompromised patients • Elderly patients • Patients with COPD	• Most common cause of LRTIs in children • Commonly presents with wheezing	RT-PCR	• Ribavirin ± IVIG • Viral replication inhibitor ALS-008176
Human metapneumovirus	Single-stranded negative-sense RNA virus	Winter to spring	• Immunocompromised patients • Residents of long-term care facilities • Patients with COPD	• Commonly presents with wheezing	RT-PCR	Ribavirin + IVIG

Abbreviations: CAP, community-acquired pneumonia; COPD, chronic obstructive pulmonary disease; EPIC, Etiology of Pneumonia in the Community; IVIG, intravenous immunoglobulin; LRTI, lower respiratory tract infection; PCR, polymerase chain reaction; RT-PCR, reverse-transcriptase polymerase chain reaction.

population-based surveillance study conducted in the United States, which used rigorous microbiologic testing in 2259 hospitalized adults with CAP.[12] Viruses were the most common type of pathogen isolated, found in 23% of patients compared with just 11% of patients with bacterial pathogens (**Fig. 1**).

Viral pathogens are also frequently isolated in patients with severe CAP requiring ICU admission. In a single-site study from Korea, viral pathogens were isolated by reverse transcription PCR (RT-PCR) from nasopharyngeal swabs or lavage fluid in 72 of 198 (36%) patients with severe CAP or health care-associated pneumonia.[28] Viral detection rates in similar studies of ICU patients have ranged from 16% to 41%.[29–31]

Studies have also found respiratory viral pathogens present in over 20% of patients with hospital-acquired pneumonia (HAP)[32,33] and between 14% and 29% of patients undergoing bronchoalveolar lavage for suspected infection.[22,34]

As our understanding of the importance of respiratory viral pathogens in the pathogenesis of severe respiratory infection continues to evolve, it is important for clinicians to be familiar with the unique characteristics of the most commonly identified pathogens.

RHINOVIRUS

Rhinoviruses are singe-stranded negative-sense RNA viruses that are divided into 3 species (rhinovirus-A, -B, -C) and more than 160 distinct serotypes.[35] Rhinovirus infections occur throughout the year with increased prevalence noted in the late spring and early fall.[36] Transmission occurs most commonly through autoinoculation after contact with contaminated objects, although aerosolization also contributes to viral spread.[37] Nosocomial outbreaks of rhinovirus have been reported and highlight the importance of infection control protocols when caring for infected patients.[38]

The clinical importance of rhinovirus is well described in children where it may be responsible for more than 70% of asthma exacerbations in children greater than

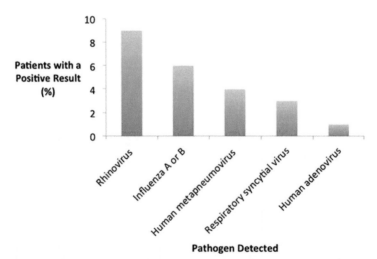

Fig. 1. Percentage of all adults in the Centers for Disease Control and Prevention EPIC (Etiology of Pneumonia in the Community) study in whom specific respiratory viral pathogens were detected. (*Data from* Jain S, Self WH, Wunderink RG, et al. Community-acquired pneumonia requiring hospitalization among U.S. adults. N Engl J Med 2015;373(5):415–27.)

2 years of age.[39] Infection with rhinovirus early in childhood has been linked to asthma pathogenesis, particularly in children with a genetic predisposition to the disease.[40,41] Rhinovirus is also recognized as an important cause of pediatric CAP.[42]

Rhinovirus Infection in Adults

In immunocompetent adults, rhinovirus most commonly causes a self-limited upper respiratory tract infection (URI) and may be responsible for more than 80% of common colds during the fall and spring.[43] The frequent association with benign URIs has led many clinicians to question its relevance to pneumonia. However, rather than simply a precursor to more serious infections, rhinovirus can itself be an important pathogen. In the clearest example, immunocompromised patients are particularly prone to severe rhinovirus infection. Infection after lung transplantation is common and may contribute to graft dysfunction.[44] Rhinovirus is also a common cause of severe LRTIs in adults with hematologic malignancies, commonly in association with bacterial coinfection.[45–47]

In patients with chronic obstructive pulmonary disease (COPD), rhinovirus is an important cause of exacerbations. In a study of 77 patients with COPD and frequent exacerbations, rhinovirus prevalence and viral load, measured in sputum by quantitative RT-PCR, were significantly higher in patients during acute exacerbations. Of patients with rhinoviral infection, 73% were found to have bacteria in their sputum by day 14.[48] This association between rhinovirus and bacterial coinfection may be due in part to changes in the host microbiome. A recent study of rhinovirus infection in patients with COPD and healthy controls found that rhinovirus altered the microbiome of COPD patients, allowing for an increase in pathogenic bacterial species such as *Haemophilus influenzae*.[49] Rhinovirus may also degrade antimicrobial peptides in the lung, predisposing susceptible patients to bacterial coinfection.[50]

Rhinovirus is isolated frequently in adult patients with CAP. In the CDC EPIC study, rhinovirus was the most common pathogen identified and was found in 9% of all patients.[12] Importantly, rhinovirus was rarely isolated in the study's healthy controls. In a single-center prospective study of 304 hospitalized patients with CAP in New Zealand, rhinovirus was also the most frequently identified pathogen and was isolated in 10% of patients.[26] The incidence of rhinovirus in other studies of CAP both in the United States and around the world have ranged from 1% to 4%.[24,25,27]

Several studies have focused specifically on patients with severe CAP requiring admission to the ICU. In a prospective multicenter study from Kentucky, rhinovirus was identified from nasopharyngeal swab in 33 of 393 patients (36%) with severe CAP.[31] In a study of 49 patients with CAP requiring mechanical ventilation in Finland, 15 (31%) were found to be infected with rhinovirus.[51] Similarly, rhinovirus was identified in 4 of 64 patients (6%) with severe CAP in Korea.[28]

Rhinovirus also plays an important role in HAP. Rhinovirus was identified in 15 of 262 patients (6%) with HAP requiring admission to an ICU in Korea.[28] Similarly, a retrospective single-center study found rhinovirus in 19 (11%) of 174 patients with nonventilated HAP.[33]

Clinical Presentation and Diagnosis

Sore throat and rhinorrhea are typical early symptoms of rhinovirus infection.[52] Common presenting symptoms in patients with CAP secondary to rhinovirus are not well-described. In 1 study of 304 hospitalized patients with CAP, the most common symptoms in 31 patients with documented rhinovirus infection were cough (94%), lethargy (87%), anorexia (77%), sputum production (74%), and pleuritic pain (58%).[26]

RT-PCR is the preferred diagnostic test for severely ill patients with rhinovirus owing to improved sensitivity and more rapid turnaround time than conventional culture-based diagnostic methods.[53] In the future, identifying specific host transcriptional changes may help to differentiate between true infection and asymptomatic carriage.[54]

Treatment

Treatment of even severe rhinoviral infection is supportive. Case reports have described the use of pegylated interferon-α2A and ribavirin in immunosuppressed patients with evidence of persistent infection, but this strategy has not been tested in randomized trials.[55]

HUMAN ADENOVIRUSES

HAdVs are nonenveloped double-stranded DNA viruses that have long been recognized as an important cause of respiratory tract infections in children.[56] HAdVs are divided into seven species (HAdV-A through HAdV-G) with species B, C, and E most commonly associated with respiratory infections.[57] Based on serotypes and genomic analysis, 67 subtypes of adenovirus have been identified.[58]

Unlike other respiratory viruses, HAdV infections do not demonstrate clear seasonal variation.[58] Transmission can occur via inhalation of aerosolized droplets, direct conjunctival inoculation, fecal–oral spread, and contact with infected environmental surfaces.[59] HAdVs are resistant to many common disinfectants, so rigorous infection control policies, including the use of 95% ethanol for decontamination, are essential to prevent nosocomial spread of infection.[59,60]

Human Adenovirus Infection in Adults

Severe HAdV infection is most commonly encountered in immunocompromised hosts, where disease can range from asymptomatic viremia to invasive multiorgan disease. Patients with human immunodeficiency virus and those who have undergone solid organ transplantation or allogeneic stem cell transplantation are particularly at risk.[61] Common disease manifestations in the immunocompromised patient include pneumonia, colitis, hemorrhagic cystitis, hepatitis, and graft dysfunction.[58]

By adulthood, almost all immunocompetent individuals have evidence of prior HAdV exposure and exhibit HAdV-specific T cells.[57] As a result, HAdV infection is usually mild and self-limited. However, outbreaks of severe respiratory infection are well-described and it is important for clinicians to be aware of recent trends in HAdV epidemiology.

Crowded living environments are a risk factor for outbreaks of severe HAdV in otherwise healthy individuals. The best documented example is US military recruits who for decades have been found to be at high risk for severe HAdV infection.[61] Recognition of this association led to routine vaccination of military trainees against HAdV-4 and HAdV-7, which produced a dramatic decrease in HAdV disease.[62] However, a recent epidemic of HAdV pneumonia at a US Air Force base in Texas was found to be caused by HAdV-14, an uncommon subtype not usually associated with severe disease.[63] Of 66 hospitalized trainees, 23 (35%) were found to have HAdV-14 infection, including 4 (17%) who required ICU admission. HAdV infection has been responsible for outbreaks of febrile respiratory infections at military training facilities outside of the United States.[64–67] and infections requiring hospitalization at mental health facilities,[68] job training sites,[69] and boarding schools.[70]

Recent community outbreaks of HAdV-14 in the United States emphasize the increasing importance of this particular subtype even outside of communal living environments. In Oregon, 28 cases of HAdV-14 pneumonia were identified including 18 (47%) who required admission to the ICU and 7 (18%) who died.[71] Similarly, 46 cases of HAdV-14 respiratory illness were recently documented in an Alaskan community, including 11 patients who required hospitalization.[72] In both of these outbreaks, elderly patients with underlying lung disease and other chronic health problems were at particular risk.

Outside of the United States, HAdV has emerged as an increasingly important cause of CAP. A recent multicenter surveillance study in China documented HAdV as a causative pathogen in 5% of all cases of CAP and found that infection with serotype HAdV-55 was associated with a particularly high pneumonia severity index score.[73] A retrospective analysis of all cases of CAP caused by HAdV-55 at 2 hospitals in northern China noted a 27% mortality rate.[74] Interestingly, 2 cases of severe CAP secondary to HAdV-55 were also recently described in France, perhaps signaling the importance of this serotype outside of Asia.[75]

Clinical Presentation and Diagnosis

Patients with pneumonia owing to HAdV present with symptoms indistinguishable from other types of pneumonia, including fever, cough, and shortness of breath.[71,72] No clinical factors reliably discriminate between pneumonia caused by HAdV and pneumonia caused by other pathogens. In a study of infected military personnel, those with HAdV infection were more likely to have cytopenias than those without HAdV infection.[76] This association between HAdV infection and cytopenias has been documented in other studies, but not with enough consistency to impact clinical practice.[68,77] Although chest imaging is usually abnormal, findings are nonspecific and can include focal areas of consolidation or interstitial abnormalities.[71,78]

Numerous methods are available to diagnose HAdV infection, although PCR is the most practical choice for acutely ill patients. Viral culture was previously considered the "gold standard" although the time needed to observe the characteristic cytopathic effect in human epithelial cells makes it impractical for use in critically ill patients.[61] Shell vial cultures have improved turnaround time although may have lower sensitivity.[58] HAdV-specific antigens can be identified by enzyme-specific immunoassays, although this method is not recommended in immunocompromised patients owing to poor sensitivity.[79] Although tissue sampling is rarely pursued in immunocompetent patients, HAdV can be diagnosed readily on histopathology by visualizing characteristic intranuclear viral inclusions. In recent years, PCR has become the test of choice owing to rapid turnaround time and high sensitivity and specificity.[80] Molecular typing, although helpful for epidemiologic studies, is not recommended for individual patients.

Treatment

The mainstay of therapy for immunocompetent patients with HAdV infection is supportive care. No high-quality randomized trials inform the decision to use pharmacologic therapy in any patient population. Of available antiviral agents, cidofovir, the nucleoside analogue of cytidine monophosphate, has the most supporting data and several case reports have described the safe and successful use of cidofovir in the treatment of severe HAdV infection in immunocompromised patients.[81,82] However, routine use is limited by significant side effects, including nephrotoxicity and neutropenia.[83,84]

RESPIRATORY SYNCYTIAL VIRUS

RSV is an enveloped, negative-sense, single-stranded RNA virus first identified more than 50 years ago.[85] The 2 serotypes, RSV-A and RSV-B, are discriminated by reactivity to monoclonal antibodies. RSV has a worldwide circulation and peak infectivity in temperate climates between December and February.[86] Exposure to the virus by 2 years of age is nearly universal.[85] RSV is highly infectious and can spread via aerosolized droplets or contact with infected secretions.[87] Outbreaks of RSV infections in hospitalized patients are well-described and strict infection control protocols are essential when caring for infected patients.[88]

The clinical and economic burden of RSV infection in children is substantial. Globally, RSV is the most common cause of LRTIs in children, with more than 3 million hospitalizations and up to 200,000 deaths in children less than 5 years of age per year.[89] Annual direct medical costs in the United States are estimated at more than $650 million.[90] Respiratory bronchiolitis, characterized by inflammation and obstruction of the small airways, is one of the most common manifestations of RSV infection and is a significant cause of pediatric morbidity and mortality in the United States.[91] Children with Down syndrome seem to be at particular risk of severe infection.[92] RSV infection early in life has also been associated with the development of asthma.[93] RSV can cause numerous extrapulmonary diseases in children, including myocarditis, hepatitis, and seizures.[94]

Respiratory Syncytial Virus Infection in Adults

As with other respiratory viruses, immunocompromised patients are at particular risk of severe RSV infection. Severe LRTIs have been described in multiple patient populations, including after hematopoietic stem cell transplantation, patients with hematologic malignancies, and after solid organ transplantation, where infection may predispose to graft dysfunction.[95–98] Outbreaks of severe RSV infections in bone marrow transplantation wards highlight the susceptibility of this patient population to infection.[99]

In otherwise healthy adults, RSV infection typically produces a URI characterized by a productive cough, nasal congestion, and sinus involvement.[100] In elderly patients and those with underlying cardiac and pulmonary disease, RSV is an important cause of LRTIs and pneumonia (**Fig. 2**). Studies using national mortality and viral surveillance data have found that more than 75% of deaths attributable to RSV infection occur in patients older than 65 years of age.[101] In this age group, RSV is responsible for an estimated 62,000 hospitalizations per year and 9% of all hospitalizations for pneumonia.[102] The numerous reports of RSV outbreaks at long-term care facilities highlight the susceptibility of elderly patients to severe RSV infection.[15,103]

In one of the most rigorous studies to date, Falsey and colleagues[13] prospectively evaluated the impact of RSV infection over 4 consecutive winters in 3 patient cohorts: healthy adults 65 years of age or older, elderly adults with chronic cardiac or pulmonary disease, and adult patients hospitalized with acute respiratory symptoms. Importantly, in addition to viral culture and serologies, RT-PCR was used to aid the diagnosis of RSV infection. The annual rate of RSV infection was 3% to 7% in healthy elderly patients and 4% to 10% in high-risk adults. Of 56 high-risk patients with RSV infection, 25 (45%) were unable to perform activities of daily living owing to their acute illness, 9 (16%) required hospitalization, and 2 (4%) died. In the cohort of hospitalized patients with confirmed RSV infection, 20 (15%) required ICU admission, 17 (13%) required mechanical ventilation, and 10 (8%) died. During the study period, RSV accounted for 11% of hospitalizations for pneumonia, 11% for COPD, 5% for congestive heart failure, and 7% for asthma.

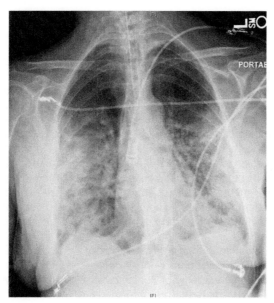

Fig. 2. Posteroanterior chest radiograph in an elderly woman with acute hypoxemic respiratory failure secondary to respiratory syncytial virus pneumonia demonstrating dense bilateral airspace disease.

In studies of CAP, RSV has been found to be an important pathogen. In the CDC EPIC study, RSV was detected in 3% of adults hospitalized with CAP with detection rates varying significantly by season.[12] A similar detection rate has been found in other studies.[25,104] In patients with severe CAP requiring admission to the ICU, RSV may be responsible for up to 10% of cases.[28,29,31]

Patients with COPD seem to be at particular risk of RSV infection. Although persistent RSV infection in stable COPD seems to be uncommon,[105,106] RSV is a common trigger for COPD exacerbations.[107] COPD is frequently identified as a risk factor for severe RSV infection[108] and mortality rates in infected COPD patients may eclipse those of infected patients after stem cell transplantation.[109]

Clinical Presentation and Diagnosis

Among adults presenting to the hospital with confirmed RSV infection, wheezing is encountered more frequently than with other viral infections, including influenza.[104,110,111] Cough, shortness of breath, and fever are other common presenting symptoms.[13,104] Chest radiography is frequently normal, although radiographic evidence of pneumonia may be found more frequently than in patients with influenza.[13,104] On chest computed tomography scans, tree-in-bud opacities and abnormalities in a bronchocentric distribution are more common in RSV infection than with other respiratory viruses.[112,113]

As with other respiratory viruses, nucleic acid amplification, specifically with RT-PCR, has become the test of choice for suspected RSV infection in adults.[114] Culture techniques including shell vial culture are challenging given the unstable nature of the RSV virus and lack sensitivity.[85] Rapid antigen detection tests, which are used commonly in children, perform less well in adults likely owing to lower viral titers present in the secretions of elderly patients.[115] Detection of acute and convalescent phase serologies is useful for epidemiologic study and may increase the yield of RT-PCR, but is not widely used in clinical practice.[85]

Treatment

The mainstay of therapy for immunocompetent adults with severe RSV infection is supportive care. In immunocompromised patients and other select high-risk adult groups, additional therapy may be considered. The guanosine analogue ribavirin has been used with some success in patients with RSV infection after hematopoietic stem cell transplantation. In a recent single-center study of 280 patients after alloge-neic stem cell transplantation, early use of aerosolized ribavirin was associated with a reduction in progression to LRTI and improved mortality.[116] Similar results were found in a recent review of published case series.[117] Concerns regarding cost, teratoge-nicity, and adverse effects including hemolytic anemia have limited routine use in adults.[118] Immunotherapy with intravenous immunoglobulin in combination with riba-virin has been described in case reports, but has not been studied in randomized trials.[119]

In children, passive immunoprophylaxis with palivizumab, a monoclonal antibody directed against the RSV F glycoprotein, has been used with success and is recom-mended by the American Academy of Pediatrics for use in infants with hemodynam-ically significant heart disease or chronic lung disease of prematurity.[120] Unfortunately, results with the use of palivizumab in at-risk adult patients have been disappointing.[117,121] A novel oral viral replication inhibitor ALS-008176 was recently used with encouraging results in a small RSV challenge study in healthy adults, but further trials are required before it can be recommended for routine use.[122]

The substantial morbidity and mortality associated with RSV infection in the elderly has heightened calls for the development of an RSV vaccine.[13] Although progress has been made, no vaccines are currently available.[123]

HUMAN METAPNEUMOVIRUS

hMPV is a single-stranded, negative-sense RNA virus first isolated in 2001 from chil-dren with respiratory tract infections in the Netherlands.[124] The virus is present world-wide and exhibits clear seasonality with peak circulation in temperate climates between winter and spring.[125] Exposure to the virus by 5 years of age is nearly univer-sal.[126] Modes of transmission are not well-described, but outbreaks of hMPV at long-term care facilities and hospital wards highlight the importance of infection control protocols when caring for infected patients.[14,16,127]

The clinical importance of hMPV is well-documented in children. In a recent prospective study in the United States, hMPV was identified in 6% of all children hospitalized with an acute respiratory illness and associated with increased ICU duration of stay.[128] hMPV may be responsible for more than 10% of all LRTIs in chil-dren in the United States and 5% to 7% of all pediatric respiratory tract infections worldwide.[129,130] Disease manifestations in children range from croup and bronchio-litis to exacerbations of asthma and severe pneumonia requiring mechanical ventilation.[129]

Human Metapneumovirus Infection in Adults

hMPV is recognized as an important respiratory pathogen in immunocompromised adults. Studies using RT-PCR have identified hMPV as the cause of severe pneumonia in hematopoietic stem cell transplant recipients,[131] patients with hematologic malig-nancies,[132] and solid organ transplant recipients where infection may increase the risk of graft dysfunction.[133–135] A recent systematic review found a 26% mortality in immunocompromised patients with hMPV LRTI.[135]

In immunocompetent adults with suspected viral infection, the incidence of hMPV ranges from 2% to 9%.[136–138] In the recent CDC EPIC study, hMPV was identified in 4% of hospitalized adults with CAP.[12] Although severe hMPV infection in immuno-competent adults is uncommon, several at-risk patient populations deserve mention. Outbreaks of hMPV are common at long-term acute care facilities. In California, 26 residents and staff were infected with hMPV including 8 (31%) who developed radio-graphically confirmed pneumonia and 2 (5%) who required hospitalization.[14] Similarly, during an outbreak of severe respiratory infection at a long-term care facility in Quebec, hMPV was identified in 6 of 96 infected patients, with a 50% mortality.[16] Out-breaks have also been described at long-term care facilities in Oregon,[139] the Netherlands,[140] and Japan.[141]

Limited data suggest that hMPV may be an important cause of hospitalizations in patients with COPD. In a single-center, observational study of 50 adults hospitalized for a COPD exacerbation, RT-PCR of nasopharyngeal specimens identified 6 patients (12%) with hMPV infection.[142] Documented hMPV infection rates in other studies of patients with COPD exacerbations have ranged from 2.3% to 5.5%.[143,144]

Clinical Presentation and Diagnosis

Patients hospitalized with hMPV present with nonspecific symptoms. In 1 study of 91 hospitalized adults with hMPV, the most common symptoms were dyspnea (98%), cough (94%), wheezing (79%), and sputum production (74%).[145] High rates of wheezing have been noted in other studies and are similar to the incidence of bron-chospasm found with RSV infection.[138,146] Chest imaging is similarly nonspecific and may be normal in more than one-third of hospitalized patients.[145] Reports of chest computed tomography findings in hPMV infection are limited. In 1 study of high-resolution computed tomography findings in 4 patients with hMPV, ground-glass opacities, consolidation, and parenchymal bands were present in all patients.[147]

Although uncommon, hMPV infection can lead to severe disease. In a single study from Korea of 198 patients with severe pneumonia requiring admission to the ICU, hMPV infection was identified by RT-PCR in 13 patients including 5 (8%) with CAP.[28] Similarly, in a recent review of all admissions to a single ICU over 4 years, 40 cases of hMPV infection were identified, of which 55% required mechanical venti-lation, 23% developed shock, and 48% met criteria for acute respiratory distress syn-drome.[148] Importantly, 6 of these 40 patients (15%) had only minor comorbidities. Finally, in a study of 91 patients hospitalized with hMPV, 12 (13%) required admission to the ICU, 11 (12%) required mechanical ventilation, and 6 (7%) died.[145]

hMPV replicates slowly and is difficult to isolate with typical cell culture techniques, making viral culture impractical for routine use in the ICU.[149] RT-PCR is the preferred diagnostic test for hMPV and is now available as part of a multiplex PCR panel for simultaneous testing with other viruses.[138]

Treatment

Treatment of severe hMPV infection is supportive and no pharmacologic therapies are currently approved for use. Ribavirin has shown promising activity in murine models of infection[150] and several case reports describe the drug's potential efficacy in humans when used in conjunction with intravenous immunoglobulins.[151,152] However, con-cerns regarding the cost of ribaviran, teratogenicity and reports showing underwhelm-ing clinical results have tempered enthusiasm for more routine use.[153]

CHALLENGES AND FUTURE DIRECTIONS

With the improved sensitivity of PCR-based testing, a major challenge in the diagnosis and treatment of viral pneumonia is distinguishing true infection from asymptomatic carriage or isolated URI.[6] This is especially true for samples obtained from the upper respiratory tract in patients with suspected LRTI. The specificity of PCR testing likely depends on both the age of the patient and the pathogen identified and further studies are needed to refine test interpretation.[154] The results of the CDC EPIC study, where only 2% of 238 asymptomatic control subjects had a pathogen identified, suggest that the majority of identified respiratory viral pathogens play a causal role in disease pathogenesis.[12]

Measuring convalescent phase serum antibodies may help to improve the diagnostic yield and specificity of PCR-based testing although further studies are needed to validate this approach.[155] Transcriptional profiling of the host response to infection may also aid the diagnosis of viral pneumonia. Recently, an 11-gene influenza virus-specific host response signature was identified in human blood that accurately diagnosed influenza infection, identified bacterial coinfection, and predicted outcomes in patients with influenza pneumonia.[156] Similarly, a host transcriptional signature defined largely by the overexpression of interferon-related genes was found to discriminate between viral and bacterial pneumonia.[157]

Perhaps the greatest challenge facing both clinicians and researchers is the large number of patients with a clinical diagnosis of pneumonia in whom a causative pathogen is never identified. Of the more than 2000 patients in the CDC EPIC study, 62% had no identifiable pathogen despite a degree of microbiologic testing that exceeded usual clinical practice.[12] Over the past 2 decades, the percentage of patients hospitalized with pneumonia who had no reported pathogen increased by almost 20% in the United States.[18] Research that better characterizes this large group of patients has the potential to profoundly impact health care costs and antimicrobial stewardship.[158] Our evolving understanding of the link between the respiratory microbiome and pneumonia pathogenesis may prove an important engine of innovation in the coming years.[159]

REFERENCES

1. Vincent JL, Rello J, Marshall J, et al. International study of the prevalence and outcomes of infection in intensive care units. JAMA 2009;302(21):2323–9.
2. Xu J, Murphy SL, Kochanek KD, et al. Deaths: final data for 2013. Natl Vital Stat Rep 2016;64(2):1–119.
3. Fry AM, Shay DK, Holman RC, et al. Trends in hospitalizations for pneumonia among persons aged 65 years or older in the United States, 1988-2002. JAMA 2005;294(21):2712–9.
4. Bartlett JG, Mundy LM. Community-acquired pneumonia. N Engl J Med 1995; 333(24):1618–24.
5. Griffin MR, Zhu Y, Moore MR, et al. U.S. hospitalizations for pneumonia after a decade of pneumococcal vaccination. N Engl J Med 2013;369(2):155–63.
6. Ruuskanen O, Lahti E, Jennings LC, et al. Viral pneumonia. Lancet 2011; 377(9773):1264–75.
7. Somerville LK, Ratnamohan VM, Dwyer DE, et al. Molecular diagnosis of respiratory viruses. Pathology 2015;47(3):243–9.
8. Chowell G, Bertozzi SM, Colchero MA, et al. Severe respiratory disease concurrent with the circulation of H1N1 influenza. N Engl J Med 2009;361(7):674–9.

9. Ornstein KA, Leff B, Covinsky KE, et al. Epidemiology of the homebound population in the United States. JAMA Intern Med 2015;175(7):1180–6.
10. Kahn JM, Benson NM, Appleby D, et al. Long-term acute care hospital utilization after critical illness. JAMA 2010;303(22):2253–9.
11. Falsey AR, Walsh EE. Viral pneumonia in older adults. Clin Infect Dis 2006;42(4): 518–24.
12. Jain S, Self WH, Wunderink RG, et al. Community-acquired pneumonia Requiring hospitalization among U.S. adults. N Engl J Med 2015;373(5):415–27.
13. Falsey AR, Hennessey PA, Formica MA, et al. Respiratory syncytial virus infection in elderly and high-risk adults. N Engl J Med 2005;352(17):1749–59.
14. Louie JK, Schnurr DP, Pan CY, et al. A summer outbreak of human metapneumovirus infection in a long-term-care facility. J Infect Dis 2007;196(5):705–8.
15. Sorvillo FJ, Huie SF, Strassburg MA, et al. An outbreak of respiratory syncytial virus pneumonia in a nursing home for the elderly. J Infect 1984;9(3):252–6.
16. Boivin G, De Serres G, Hamelin ME, et al. An outbreak of severe respiratory tract infection due to human metapneumovirus in a long-term care facility. Clin Infect Dis 2007;44(9):1152–8.
17. Lexau CA, Lynfield R, Danila R, et al. Changing epidemiology of invasive pneumococcal disease among older adults in the era of pediatric pneumococcal conjugate vaccine. JAMA 2005;294(16):2043–51.
18. Smith SB, Ruhnke GW, Weiss CH, et al. Trends in pathogens among patients hospitalized for pneumonia from 1993 to 2011. JAMA Intern Med 2014; 174(11):1837–9.
19. Mahony JB, Petrich A, Smieja M. Molecular diagnosis of respiratory virus infections. Crit Rev Clin Lab Sci 2011;48(5–6):217–49.
20. Diederen BM, Van Der Eerden MM, Vlaspolder F, et al. Detection of respiratory viruses and Legionella spp. by real-time polymerase chain reaction in patients with community acquired pneumonia. Scand J Infect Dis 2009;41(1):45–50.
21. Templeton KE, Scheltinga SA, van den Eeden WC, et al. Improved diagnosis of the etiology of community-acquired pneumonia with real-time polymerase chain reaction. Clin Infect Dis 2005;41(3):345–51.
22. Garbino J, Gerbase MW, Wunderli W, et al. Lower respiratory viral illnesses: improved diagnosis by molecular methods and clinical impact. Am J Respir Crit Care Med 2004;170(11):1197–203.
23. She RC, Polage CR, Caram LB, et al. Performance of diagnostic tests to detect respiratory viruses in older adults. Diagn Microbiol Infect Dis 2010;67(3): 246–50.
24. Qu JX, Gu L, Pu ZH, et al. Viral etiology of community-acquired pneumonia among adolescents and adults with mild or moderate severity and its relation to age and severity. BMC Infect Dis 2015;15:89.
25. Johnstone J, Majumdar SR, Fox JD, et al. Viral infection in adults hospitalized with community-acquired pneumonia: prevalence, pathogens, and presentation. Chest 2008;134(6):1141–8.
26. Jennings LC, Anderson TP, Beynon KA, et al. Incidence and characteristics of viral community-acquired pneumonia in adults. Thorax 2008;63(1):42–8.
27. Zhan Y, Yang Z, Chen R, et al. Respiratory virus is a real pathogen in immunocompetent community-acquired pneumonia: comparing to influenza like illness and volunteer controls. BMC Pulm Med 2014;14:144.
28. Choi SH, Hong SB, Ko GB, et al. Viral infection in patients with severe pneumonia requiring intensive care unit admission. Am J Respir Crit Care Med 2012;186(4):325–32.

29. Ostby AC, Gubbels S, Baake G, et al. Respiratory virology and microbiology in intensive care units: a prospective cohort study. APMIS 2013;121(11):1097–108.

30. Cilloniz C, Ewig S, Ferrer M, et al. Community-acquired polymicrobial pneumonia in the intensive care unit: aetiology and prognosis. Crit Care 2011; 15(5):R209.

31. Wiemken T, Peyrani P, Bryant K, et al. Incidence of respiratory viruses in patients with community-acquired pneumonia admitted to the intensive care unit: results from the severe influenza pneumonia surveillance (SIPS) project. Eur J Clin Microbiol Infect Dis 2013;32(5):705–10.

32. Hong HL, Hong SB, Ko GB, et al. Viral infection is not uncommon in adult patients with severe hospital-acquired pneumonia. PLoS One 2014;9(4):e95865.

33. Shorr AF, Zilberberg MD, Micek ST, et al. Viruses are prevalent in non-ventilated hospital-acquired pneumonia. Respir Med 2017;122:76–80.

34. Garbino J, Soccal PM, Aubert JD, et al. Respiratory viruses in bronchoalveolar lavage: a hospital-based cohort study in adults. Thorax 2009;64(5):399–404.

35. Greenberg SB. Update on Human Rhinovirus and Coronavirus Infections. Semin Respir Crit Care Med 2016;37(4):555–71.

36. Turner RB. Rhinovirus: more than just a common cold virus. J Infect Dis 2007; 195(6):765–6.

37. Musher DM. How contagious are common respiratory tract infections? N Engl J Med 2003;348(13):1256–66.

38. Reese SM, Thompson M, Price CS, et al. Evidence of nosocomial transmission of human rhinovirus in a neonatal intensive care unit. Am J Infect Control 2016; 44(3):355–7.

39. Rakes GP, Arruda E, Ingram JM, et al. Rhinovirus and respiratory syncytial virus in wheezing children requiring emergency care. IgE and eosinophil analyses. Am J Respir Crit Care Med 1999;159(3):785–90.

40. Caliskan M, Bochkov YA, Kreiner-Moller E, et al. Rhinovirus wheezing illness and genetic risk of childhood-onset asthma. N Engl J Med 2013;368(15):1398–407.

41. Camargo CA Jr. Human rhinovirus, wheezing illness, and the primary prevention of childhood asthma. Am J Respir Crit Care Med 2013;188(11):1281–2.

42. Jain S, Williams DJ, Arnold SR, et al. Community-acquired pneumonia requiring hospitalization among U.S. children. N Engl J Med 2015;372(9):835–45.

43. Arruda E, Pitkaranta A, Witek TJ Jr, et al. Frequency and natural history of rhinovirus infections in adults during autumn. J Clin Microbiol 1997;35(11):2864–8.

44. Kaiser L, Aubert JD, Pache JC, et al. Chronic rhinoviral infection in lung transplant recipients. Am J Respir Crit Care Med 2006;174(12):1392–9.

45. Jacobs SE, Lamson DM, Soave R, et al. Clinical and molecular epidemiology of human rhinovirus infections in patients with hematologic malignancy. J Clin Virol 2015;71:51–8.

46. Jacobs SE, Soave R, Shore TB, et al. Human rhinovirus infections of the lower respiratory tract in hematopoietic stem cell transplant recipients. Transpl Infect Dis 2013;15(5):474–86.

47. Malcolm E, Arruda E, Hayden FG, et al. Clinical features of patients with acute respiratory illness and rhinovirus in their bronchoalveolar lavages. J Clin Virol 2001;21(1):9–16.

48. George SN, Garcha DS, Mackay AJ, et al. Human rhinovirus infection during naturally occurring COPD exacerbations. Eur Respir J 2014;44(1):87–96.

49. Molyneaux PL, Mallia P, Cox MJ, et al. Outgrowth of the bacterial airway microbiome after rhinovirus exacerbation of chronic obstructive pulmonary disease. Am J Respir Crit Care Med 2013;188(10):1224–31.

50. Mallia P, Footitt J, Sotero R, et al. Rhinovirus infection induces degradation of antimicrobial peptides and secondary bacterial infection in chronic obstructive pulmonary disease. Am J Respir Crit Care Med 2012;186(11):1117–24.
51. Karhu J, Ala-Kokko TI, Vuorinen T, et al. Lower respiratory tract virus findings in mechanically ventilated patients with severe community-acquired pneumonia. Clin Infect Dis 2014;59(1):62–70.
52. Harris JM 2nd, Gwaltney JM Jr. Incubation periods of experimental rhinovirus infection and illness. Clin Infect Dis 1996;23(6):1287–90.
53. Hammond SP, Gagne LS, Stock SR, et al. Respiratory virus detection in immunocompromised patients with FilmArray respiratory panel compared to conventional methods. J Clin Microbiol 2012;50(10):3216–21.
54. Heinonen S, Jartti T, Garcia C, et al. Rhinovirus detection in symptomatic and asymptomatic children: value of host transcriptome analysis. Am J Respir Crit Care Med 2016;193(7):772–82.
55. Ruuskanen O, Waris M, Kainulainen L. Treatment of persistent rhinovirus infection with pegylated interferon alpha2a and ribavirin in patients with hypogammaglobulinemia. Clin Infect Dis 2014;58(12):1784–6.
56. Gardner PS. Virus infections and respiratory disease of childhood. Arch Dis Child 1968;43(232):629–45.
57. Lion T. Adenovirus infections in immunocompetent and immunocompromised patients. Clin Microbiol Rev 2014;27(3):441–62.
58. Ison MG, Hayden RT. Adenovirus. Microbiol Spectr 2016;4(4).
59. Sandrock C, Stollenwerk N. Acute febrile respiratory illness in the ICU: reducing disease transmission. Chest 2008;133(5):1221–31.
60. Cassir N, Hraiech S, Nougairede A, et al. Outbreak of adenovirus type 1 severe pneumonia in a French intensive care unit, September-October 2012. Euro Surveill 2014;19(39) [pii:20914].
61. Lynch JP 3rd, Kajon AE. Adenovirus: epidemiology, global spread of novel serotypes, and advances in treatment and prevention. Semin Respir Crit Care Med 2016;37(4):586–602.
62. Potter RN, Cantrell JA, Mallak CT, et al. Adenovirus-associated deaths in US military during postvaccination period, 1999-2010. Emerg Infect Dis 2012;18(3):507–9.
63. Tate JE, Bunning ML, Lott L, et al. Outbreak of severe respiratory disease associated with emergent human adenovirus serotype 14 at a US air force training facility in 2007. J Infect Dis 2009;199(10):1419–26.
64. Kurian PV, Lal R, Pandit V. Adenovirus infections in Indian army personnel. Indian J Med Res 1966;54(9):812–8.
65. Pavilanis V, Davignon L, Podoski MO. Incidence of Adenovirus Infections in a Camp of Canadian Recruits. Rev Can Biol 1964;23:291–8 [in French].
66. Hierholzer JC, Pumarola A, Rodriguez-Torres A, et al. Occurrence of respiratory illness due to an atypical strain of adenovirus type 11 during a large outbreak in Spanish military recruits. Am J Epidemiol 1974;99(6):434–42.
67. Kajon AE, Dickson LM, Metzgar D, et al. Outbreak of febrile respiratory illness associated with adenovirus 11a infection in a Singapore military training cAMP. J Clin Microbiol 2010;48(4):1438–41.
68. Klinger JR, Sanchez MP, Curtin LA, et al. Multiple cases of life-threatening adenovirus pneumonia in a mental health care center. Am J Respir Crit Care Med 1998;157(2):645–9.

69. Centers for Disease Control and Prevention (CDC). Civilian outbreak of adenovirus acute respiratory disease–South Dakota, 1997. MMWR Morb Mortal Wkly Rep 1998;47(27):567–70.
70. Zhu Z, Zhang Y, Xu S, et al. Outbreak of acute respiratory disease in China caused by B2 species of adenovirus type 11. J Clin Microbiol 2009;47(3): 697–703.
71. Lewis PF, Schmidt MA, Lu X, et al. A community-based outbreak of severe respiratory illness caused by human adenovirus serotype 14. J Infect Dis 2009; 199(10):1427–34.
72. Centers for Disease Control and Prevention (CDC). Outbreak of adenovirus 14 respiratory illness–Prince of Wales Island, Alaska, 2008. MMWR Morb Mortal Wkly Rep 2010;59(1):6–10.
73. Cao B, Huang GH, Pu ZH, et al. Emergence of community-acquired adenovirus type 55 as a cause of community-onset pneumonia. Chest 2014;145(1):79–86.
74. Tan D, Zhu H, Fu Y, et al. Severe community-acquired pneumonia caused by human adenovirus in immunocompetent adults: a multicenter case series. PLoS One 2016;11(3):e0151199.
75. Lafolie J, Mirand A, Salmona M, et al. Severe pneumonia associated with adenovirus type 55 infection, France, 2014. Emerg Infect Dis 2016;22(11):2012–4.
76. Vento TJ, Prakash V, Murray CK, et al. Pneumonia in military trainees: a comparison study based on adenovirus serotype 14 infection. J Infect Dis 2011; 203(10):1388–95.
77. Yoon H, Jhun BW, Kim SJ, et al. Clinical characteristics and factors predicting respiratory failure in adenovirus pneumonia. Respirology 2016;21(7):1243–50.
78. Tan D, Fu Y, Xu J, et al. Severe adenovirus community-acquired pneumonia in immunocompetent adults: chest radiographic and CT findings. J Thorac Dis 2016;8(5):848–54.
79. Ison MG. Adenovirus infections in transplant recipients. Clin Infect Dis 2006; 43(3):331–9.
80. Damen M, Minnaar R, Glasius P, et al. Real-time PCR with an internal control for detection of all known human adenovirus serotypes. J Clin Microbiol 2008; 46(12):3997–4003.
81. Kim SJ, Kim K, Park SB, et al. Outcomes of early administration of cidofovir in non-immunocompromised patients with severe adenovirus pneumonia. PLoS One 2015;10(4):e0122642.
82. Lee M, Kim S, Kwon OJ, et al. Treatment of adenoviral acute respiratory distress syndrome using cidofovir with extracorporeal membrane oxygenation: case series and literature review. J Intensive Care Med 2016;32:231–8.
83. Ison MG, Green M. Practice ASTIDCo. Adenovirus in solid organ transplant recipients. Am J Transplant 2009;9(Suppl 4):S161–5.
84. Ljungman P, Ribaud P, Eyrich M, et al. Cidofovir for adenovirus infections after allogeneic hematopoietic stem cell transplantation: a survey by the infectious diseases working party of the European Group for Blood and Marrow Transplantation. Bone Marrow Transplant 2003;31(6):481–6.
85. Griffiths C, Drews SJ, Marchant DJ. Respiratory syncytial virus: infection, detection, and new options for prevention and treatment. Clin Microbiol Rev 2017; 30(1):277–319.
86. Bont L, Checchia PA, Fauroux B, et al. Defining the epidemiology and burden of severe respiratory syncytial virus infection among infants and children in western countries. Infect Dis Ther 2016;5(3):271–98.

87. Drysdale SB, Green CA, Sande CJ. Best practice in the prevention and management of paediatric respiratory syncytial virus infection. Ther Adv Infect Dis 2016;3(2):63–71.
88. Bont L. Nosocomial RSV infection control and outbreak management. Paediatr Respir Rev 2009;10(Suppl 1):16–7.
89. Nair H, Nokes DJ, Gessner BD, et al. Global burden of acute lower respiratory infections due to respiratory syncytial virus in young children: a systematic review and meta-analysis. Lancet 2010;375(9725):1545–55.
90. Paramore LC, Ciuryla V, Ciesla G, et al. Economic impact of respiratory syncytial virus-related illness in the US: an analysis of national databases. Pharmacoeconomics 2004;22(5):275–84.
91. Hall CB, Weinberg GA, Iwane MK, et al. The burden of respiratory syncytial virus infection in young children. N Engl J Med 2009;360(6):588–98.
92. Stagliano DR, Nylund CM, Eide MB, et al. Children with down syndrome are high-risk for severe respiratory syncytial virus disease. J Pediatr 2015;166(3): 703–9.e2.
93. Sigurs N, Aljassim F, Kjellman B, et al. Asthma and allergy patterns over 18 years after severe RSV bronchiolitis in the first year of life. Thorax 2010; 65(12):1045–52.
94. Bohmwald K, Espinoza JA, Rey-Jurado E, et al. Human respiratory syncytial virus: infection and pathology. Semin Respir Crit Care Med 2016;37(4):522–37.
95. Englund JA, Sullivan CJ, Jordan MC, et al. Respiratory syncytial virus infection in immunocompromised adults. Ann Intern Med 1988;109(3):203–8.
96. Hertz MI, Englund JA, Snover D, et al. Respiratory syncytial virus-induced acute lung injury in adult patients with bone marrow transplants: a clinical approach and review of the literature. Medicine (Baltimore) 1989;68(5):269–81.
97. Khanna N, Widmer AF, Decker M, et al. Respiratory syncytial virus infection in patients with hematological diseases: single-center study and review of the literature. Clin Infect Dis 2008;46(3):402–12.
98. Gottlieb J, Zamora MR, Hodges T, et al. ALN-RSV01 for prevention of bronchiolitis obliterans syndrome after respiratory syncytial virus infection in lung transplant recipients. J Heart Lung Transplant 2016;35(2):213–21.
99. Kelly SG, Metzger K, Bolon MK, et al. Respiratory syncytial virus outbreak on an adult stem cell transplant unit. Am J Infect Control 2016;44(9):1022–6.
100. Hall CB, Long CE, Schnabel KC. Respiratory syncytial virus infections in previously healthy working adults. Clin Infect Dis 2001;33(6):792–6.
101. Thompson WW, Shay DK, Weintraub E, et al. Mortality associated with influenza and respiratory syncytial virus in the United States. JAMA 2003;289(2):179–86.
102. Han LL, Alexander JP, Anderson LJ. Respiratory syncytial virus pneumonia among the elderly: an assessment of disease burden. J Infect Dis 1999; 179(1):25–30.
103. Hart RJ. An outbreak of respiratory syncytial virus infection in an old people's home. J Infect 1984;8(3):259–61.
104. Dowell SF, Anderson LJ, Gary HE Jr, et al. Respiratory syncytial virus is an important cause of community-acquired lower respiratory infection among hospitalized adults. J Infect Dis 1996;174(3):456–62.
105. Falsey AR, Formica MA, Hennessey PA, et al. Detection of respiratory syncytial virus in adults with chronic obstructive pulmonary disease. Am J Respir Crit Care Med 2006;173(6):639–43.
106. Giannakaki S, Politi L, Antonogiannaki EM, et al. Absence of human rhinovirus and respiratory syncytial virus from bronchoalveolar lavage and bronchial

biopsies of selected patients with stable chronic obstructive pulmonary disease. Respir Res 2016;17:11.

107. Ramaswamy M, Groskreutz DJ, Look DC. Recognizing the importance of respiratory syncytial virus in chronic obstructive pulmonary disease. COPD 2009; 6(1):64–75.

108. Walsh EE, Peterson DR, Falsey AR. Risk factors for severe respiratory syncytial virus infection in elderly persons. J Infect Dis 2004;189(2):233–8.

109. Anderson NW, Binnicker MJ, Harris DM, et al. Morbidity and mortality among patients with respiratory syncytial virus infection: a 2-year retrospective review. Diagn Microbiol Infect Dis 2016;85(3):367–71.

110. O'Shea MK, Ryan MA, Hawksworth AW, et al. Symptomatic respiratory syncytial virus infection in previously healthy young adults living in a crowded military environment. Clin Infect Dis 2005;41(3):311–7.

111. Wald TG, Miller BA, Shult P, et al. Can respiratory syncytial virus and influenza a be distinguished clinically in institutionalized older persons? J Am Geriatr Soc 1995;43(2):170–4.

112. Mayer JL, Lehners N, Egerer G, et al. CT-morphological characterization of respiratory syncytial virus (RSV) pneumonia in immune-compromised adults. Rofo 2014;186(7):686–92.

113. Miller WT Jr, Mickus TJ, Barbosa E Jr, et al. CT of viral lower respiratory tract infections in adults: comparison among viral organisms and between viral and bacterial infections. AJR Am J Roentgenol 2011;197(5):1088–95.

114. Falsey AR, Formica MA, Walsh EE. Diagnosis of respiratory syncytial virus infection: comparison of reverse transcription-PCR to viral culture and serology in adults with respiratory illness. J Clin Microbiol 2002;40(3):817–20.

115. Chartrand C, Tremblay N, Renaud C, et al. Diagnostic accuracy of rapid antigen detection tests for respiratory syncytial virus infection: systematic review and meta-analysis. J Clin Microbiol 2015;53(12):3738–49.

116. Shah DP, Ghantoji SS, Shah JN, et al. Impact of aerosolized ribavirin on mortality in 280 allogeneic haematopoietic stem cell transplant recipients with respiratory syncytial virus infections. J Antimicrob Chemother 2013;68(8):1872–80.

117. Shah JN, Chemaly RF. Management of RSV infections in adult recipients of hematopoietic stem cell transplantation. Blood 2011;117(10):2755–63.

118. Chemaly RF, Aitken SL, Wolfe CR, et al. Aerosolized ribavirin: the most expensive drug for pneumonia. Transpl Infect Dis 2016;18(4):634–6.

119. Ghosh S, Champlin RE, Englund J, et al. Respiratory syncytial virus upper respiratory tract illnesses in adult blood and marrow transplant recipients: combination therapy with aerosolized ribavirin and intravenous immunoglobulin. Bone Marrow Transplant 2000;25(7):751–5.

120. Ralston SL, Lieberthal AS, Meissner HC, et al. Clinical practice guideline: the diagnosis, management, and prevention of bronchiolitis. Pediatrics 2014; 134(5):e1474–502.

121. de Fontbrune FS, Robin M, Porcher R, et al. Palivizumab treatment of respiratory syncytial virus infection after allogeneic hematopoietic stem cell transplantation. Clin Infect Dis 2007;45(8):1019–24.

122. DeVincenzo JP, McClure MW, Symons JA, et al. Activity of oral ALS-008176 in a respiratory syncytial virus challenge study. N Engl J Med 2015;373(21): 2048–58.

123. Chiu C. Novel immunological insights in accelerating RSV vaccine development. Vaccine 2017;35(3):459–60.

124. van den Hoogen BG, de Jong JC, Groen J, et al. A newly discovered human pneumovirus isolated from young children with respiratory tract disease. Nat Med 2001;7(6):719–24.

125. Haynes AK, Fowlkes AL, Schneider E, et al. Human Metapneumovirus Circulation in the United States, 2008 to 2014. Pediatrics 2016;137(5) [pii:e20152927].

126. Falsey AR. Human metapneumovirus infection in adults. Pediatr Infect Dis J 2008;27(10 Suppl):S80–3.

127. Kim S, Sung H, Im HJ, et al. Molecular epidemiological investigation of a nosocomial outbreak of human metapneumovirus infection in a pediatric hemato-oncology patient population. J Clin Microbiol 2009;47(4):1221–4.

128. Edwards KM, Zhu Y, Griffin MR, et al. Burden of human metapneumovirus infection in young children. N Engl J Med 2013;368(7):633–43.

129. Williams JV, Harris PA, Tollefson SJ, et al. Human metapneumovirus and lower respiratory tract disease in otherwise healthy infants and children. N Engl J Med 2004;350(5):443–50.

130. van den Hoogen BG, Osterhaus DM, Fouchier RA. Clinical impact and diagnosis of human metapneumovirus infection. Pediatr Infect Dis J 2004;23(1 Suppl):S25–32.

131. Englund JA, Boeckh M, Kuypers J, et al. Brief communication: fatal human metapneumovirus infection in stem-cell transplant recipients. Ann Intern Med 2006;144(5):344–9.

132. Godet C, Le Goff J, Beby-Defaux A, et al. Human metapneumovirus pneumonia in patients with hematological malignancies. J Clin Virol 2014;61(4):593–6.

133. Hopkins P, McNeil K, Kermeen F, et al. Human metapneumovirus in lung transplant recipients and comparison to respiratory syncytial virus. Am J Respir Crit Care Med 2008;178(8):876–81.

134. Larcher C, Geltner C, Fischer H, et al. Human metapneumovirus infection in lung transplant recipients: clinical presentation and epidemiology. J Heart Lung Transplant 2005;24(11):1891–901.

135. Shah DP, Shah PK, Azzi JM, et al. Human metapneumovirus infections in hematopoietic cell transplant recipients and hematologic malignancy patients: a systematic review. Cancer Lett 2016;379(1):100–6.

136. Gray GC, Capuano AW, Setterquist SF, et al. Multi-year study of human metapneumovirus infection at a large US midwestern medical referral center. J Clin Virol 2006;37(4):269–76.

137. Stockton J, Stephenson I, Fleming D, et al. Human metapneumovirus as a cause of community-acquired respiratory illness. Emerg Infect Dis 2002;8(9):897–901.

138. Falsey AR, Erdman D, Anderson LJ, et al. Human metapneumovirus infections in young and elderly adults. J Infect Dis 2003;187(5):785–90.

139. Liao RS, Appelgate DM, Pelz RK. An outbreak of severe respiratory tract infection due to human metapneumovirus in a long-term care facility for the elderly in Oregon. J Clin Virol 2012;53(2):171–3.

140. Te Wierik MJ, Nguyen DT, Beersma MF, et al. An outbreak of severe respiratory tract infection caused by human metapneumovirus in a residential care facility for elderly in Utrecht, the Netherlands, January to March 2010. Euro Surveill 2012;17(13) [pii:20132].

141. Honda H, Iwahashi J, Kashiwagi T, et al. Outbreak of human metapneumovirus infection in elderly inpatients in Japan. J Am Geriatr Soc 2006;54(1):177–80.

142. Martinello RA, Esper F, Weibel C, et al. Human metapneumovirus and exacerbations of chronic obstructive pulmonary disease. J Infect 2006;53(4):248–54.

143. Rohde G, Borg I, Arinir U, et al. Relevance of human metapneumovirus in exacerbations of COPD. Respir Res 2005;6:150.
144. Vicente D, Montes M, Cilla G, et al. Human metapneumovirus and chronic obstructive pulmonary disease. Emerg Infect Dis 2004;10(7):1338–9.
145. Walsh EE, Peterson DR, Falsey AR. Human metapneumovirus infections in adults: another piece of the puzzle. Arch Intern Med 2008;168(22):2489–96.
146. Boivin G, Abed Y, Pelletier G, et al. Virological features and clinical manifestations associated with human metapneumovirus: a new paramyxovirus responsible for acute respiratory-tract infections in all age groups. J Infect Dis 2002; 186(9):1330–4.
147. Wong CK, Lai V, Wong YC. Comparison of initial high resolution computed tomography features in viral pneumonia between metapneumovirus infection and severe acute respiratory syndrome. Eur J Radiol 2012;81(5):1083–7.
148. Hasvold J, Sjoding M, Pohl K, et al. The role of human metapneumovirus in the critically ill adult patient. J Crit Care 2016;31(1):233–7.
149. Wen SC, Williams JV. New approaches for immunization and therapy against human metapneumovirus. Clin Vaccine Immunol 2015;22(8):858–66.
150. Hamelin ME, Prince GA, Boivin G. Effect of ribavirin and glucocorticoid treatment in a mouse model of human metapneumovirus infection. Antimicrob Agents Chemother 2006;50(2):774–7.
151. Bonney D, Razali H, Turner A, et al. Successful treatment of human metapneumovirus pneumonia using combination therapy with intravenous ribavirin and immune globulin. Br J Haematol 2009;145(5):667–9.
152. Kitanovski L, Kopriva S, Pokorn M, et al. Treatment of severe human metapneumovirus (hMPV) pneumonia in an immunocompromised child with oral ribavirin and IVIG. J Pediatr Hematol Oncol 2013;35(7):e311–3.
153. Renaud C, Xie H, Seo S, et al. Mortality rates of human metapneumovirus and respiratory syncytial virus lower respiratory tract infections in hematopoietic cell transplantation recipients. Biol Blood Marrow Transplant 2013;19(8):1220–6.
154. Self WH, Williams DJ, Zhu Y, et al. Respiratory viral detection in children and adults: comparing asymptomatic controls and patients with community-acquired pneumonia. J Infect Dis 2016;213(4):584–91.
155. Zhang Y, Sakthivel SK, Bramley A, et al. Serology enhances molecular diagnosis of respiratory virus infections other than influenza in children and adults hospitalized with community-acquired pneumonia. J Clin Microbiol 2017;55(1):79–89.
156. Andres-Terre M, McGuire HM, Pouliot Y, et al. Integrated, multi-cohort analysis identifies conserved transcriptional signatures across multiple respiratory viruses. Immunity 2015;43(6):1199–211.
157. Suarez NM, Bunsow E, Falsey AR, et al. Superiority of transcriptional profiling over procalcitonin for distinguishing bacterial from viral lower respiratory tract infections in hospitalized adults. J Infect Dis 2015;212(2):213–22.
158. Nathan C, Cars O. Antibiotic resistance–problems, progress, and prospects. N Engl J Med 2014;371(19):1761–3.
159. Yan Q, Cui S, Chen C, et al. Metagenomic analysis of sputum microbiome as a tool toward culture-independent pathogen detection of patients with ventilator-associated pneumonia. Am J Respir Crit Care Med 2016;194(5):636–9.

Invasive Fungal Infections in the Intensive Care Unit

Luis Ostrosky-Zeichner, MD, Mohanad Al-Obaidi, MD*

KEYWORDS

- ICU • Fungal infection • Antifungal • Candidiasis • Aspergillosis

KEY POINTS

- The 2 major fungal pathogens in immunocompetent intensive care unit (ICU) patients are *Candida* spp and *Aspergillus* spp.
- Invasive candidiasis develops in patients with specific risk factors, and most of those risk factors occur in critically ill patients.
- Invasive aspergillosis is encountered in ICU settings in patients with certain risk factors, such as chronic obstructive pulmonary disease, liver cirrhosis, and diabetes.
- Microbiological cultures have been the main diagnostic method for invasive fungal infections for many years; however, new rapid tests can help achieve a faster diagnosis.
- Antifungals have different spectra of activity. Knowledge of the mechanism of action, efficacy, and adverse effects is crucial in managing ICU patients.

INVASIVE CANDIDIASIS

Candida are ubiquitous yeasts and part of the human microbiome; they are also linked to multiple nosocomial infections. Invasive candidiasis (IC) is a spectrum of syndromes, including blood stream infection (BSI) or candidemia, deep-seated candida infections in the presence of BSI, and deep-seated infections without BSI, each contributing of almost a third of intensive care unit (ICU) IC.[1] The incidence of infections by non-*albicans Candida* species has increased in recent years. *Candida* is currently one of the most frequent causes of BSI in US hospitals.[2] Attributable mortality can be up to 40%.[2,3] The main species of *Candida* that are found to cause IC are *Candida albicans*, *Candida glabrata*, *Candida parapsilosis*, *Candida krusei*, and *Candida tropicalis*. *Candida parapsilosis* has the tendency to cause device and central catheters infections.

Disclosure: M. Al-Obaidi has no conflicts of interest. L. Ostrosky-Zeichner has received research funding and/or honoraria from Astellas, Merck, Pfizer, Gilead, Scynexis, and Cidara.
Division of Infectious Diseases, Department of Internal Medicine, University of Texas Health Science Center at Houston, 6431 Fannin MSB 2.112, Houston, TX 77030, USA
* Corresponding author.
E-mail address: mohanad.m.alobaidi@uth.tmc.edu

Infect Dis Clin N Am 31 (2017) 475–487
http://dx.doi.org/10.1016/j.idc.2017.05.005
0891-5520/17/© 2017 Elsevier Inc. All rights reserved.

id.theclinics.com

RISK FACTORS

IC pathophysiology is thought to be related to the translocation of *Candida* spp from their colonization sites (gastrointestinal tract or skin) to achieve hematogenous or contiguous spread. Up to 80% of ICU patients can be colonized with *Candida* spp; however, it has been shown that only 10% of them develop IC.[4] Bronchial *Candida* isolates are generally considered nonpathogenic and reflect colonization. Pulmonary IC is very rare and, even in the rare reported cases, the source of infection can be traced back to hematogenous spread.[4,5]

Efforts have been made to recognize ICU patients at risk of developing IC. In one study, Candida score, which uses risk factors of surgery on ICU admission, multifocal *Candida* colonization, severe sepsis or septic shock, and total parenteral nutrition, was used to predict invasive candida infection.[6] Although it had been a topic of research, *Candida* colonization as a risk factor needs surveillance cultures from different bodily sites, which are not readily available in most centers, and adds to the cost of health care.[4]

In a multicenter study, risk factors that could predict IC infection included antibiotics use combined with central venous catheter placement within the last 3 days, in addition to 2 of the following risk factors: surgery, immunosuppression, immunosuppression, steroid use, and pancreatitis, within the last 7 days, in addition to total parenteral nutrition and/or dialysis within last 3 days. By implementing this rule, clinicians can safely rule out patients who are not at high risk of IC (negative predictive value of 97%).[7]

The authors believe that patients are at greatest risk of IC when they have been in the ICU on mechanical ventilation, with a recent history of major abdominal surgery, on broad-spectrum antibiotics, with a central venous line, total parenteral nutrition, pancreatitis, dialysis, severity of illness, immunosuppression, and steroid use. However, the ability of these risk factors to predict IC depends in part on each unit's IC incident rates.[6–11]

DIAGNOSIS

The management of IC is time sensitive, because delaying diagnosis and starting the right antifungal therapy carries a high mortality risk.[3,12–14] Among all diagnostic methods, microbiological culture still plays a major role and is considered the cornerstone for diagnosis. However, blood culture sensitivity varies depending on the type of IC. It can achieve up to 80% sensitivity in cases of candidemia, but it can be as low as 21% in deep-seated IC. The overall combined sensitivity of blood cultures in BSI and deep-seated IC is thought to be ~50%.[5,15,16] Furthermore, cultures have long turn-around times (2–5 days) and therefore carry the risk of delayed diagnosis and treatment.[5]

Several non–culture-based diagnostic methods have been proposed to tackle this problem (**Table 1**).

β-D-Glucan is an important component of the fungal cell wall that has been targeted for detection of invasive fungal infections (IFIs). It has a rapid turn-around time and has a high sensitivity (up to 75% when used in serial testing[17,18]). However, it can yield low specificity, especially in critically ill patients.[19] False-positives can occur in the presence of other fungal infections (eg, molds, *Pneumocystis jiroveci* and *Trichosporon* species), mucositis, bacterial infections, use of some antibacterial agents (piperacillin-tazobactam and amoxicillin-clavulanate), glucan-containing surgical objects (gauzes), blood products, or hemodialysis using cellulose membranes.[17]

If properly used, β-D-glucan can be used to rule out IC, and can be used as a tool to recognize high-risk patients who would benefit from empiric antifungal therapy.[20,21] In addition, β-D-glucan has been shown to be helpful in assessing the patient's response to therapy.[22]

Table 1
Contemporary diagnostic methods in medical mycology

Diagnostic Method	Sensitivity and Specificity (%)	Turn-Around Time	Comments
Candida			
Blood culture	50 and 100[15]	2–3 d	Sensitivity depends on the source of infection
β-ᴅ-Glucan	75 and 80[18]	2–4 h	Risk of false-positives in ICU patients is high. Specificity is improved with consecutive repeated tests, and is affected by presence of other fungal infections
Mannan/ antimannan	83 and 75–86[80,81]	2–4 h	Not available in United States
Polymerase chain reaction	80–95 and 70–90[23,82]	4–5 h	Lack of consensus regarding standardization. Sensitivity and specificity vary among the available commercial tests
T2Candida Panel	91 and 99[83]	4 h	New technology. Limited availability because of cost
Aspergillus			
Serum galactomannan	20–80 and 80–90[57,64]	4 h	Sensitivity increases in the presence of angioinvasion and is mainly used in hematological malignancies population. Specificity increases with consecutive tests
BAL galactomannan	80 and 95[82]	4 h	May be more sensitive than serum
BAL PCR	85 and 95[82]	12 h	Lacks standardization
BAL culture	50 and 100[64]	5–10 d	*Aspergillus* often colonize upper respiratory tract and EORTC/MSG criteria should be implemented
Histopathology	—	Many days	Requires experienced pathologist. EORTC/MSG criteria should be considered. Tissue biopsy is sometimes needed to identify acute angle branching septate hyphae

For invasive fungal infections diagnostic tests, see Refs.[5,15–18,20,21,23,59,60,62,64,66,82,83]
Abbreviations: BAL, bronchoalveolar lavage; EORTC/MSG, European Organization for Research and Treatment of Cancer/Mycoses Study Group; PCR, polymerase chain reaction.

The mannan antigen and antimannan antibodies tests measure the *Candida* cell wall constituent (mannan) and immunoglobulin G antibodies to mannan antigen. They have a fast turn-around time and have approximately 60% and 90% sensitivity and specificity, respectively, or up to 80% sensitivity and specificity if combined. This combined test is approved for use in Europe but not in the United States.[15]

Polymerase chain reaction (PCR) is another diagnostic method to consider when available. PCR has a high sensitivity of up to 90% and specificity (70–99%)[23,83] in the diagnosis of IC. However, there is no consensus regarding method standardization. It also has the advantage of detecting nonviable *Candida* compared with culture-based methods and it has a faster turn-around time. There are currently 2 commercially available methods: the T2Candida Panel is approved by the US Food and Drug Administration and it can detect 5 *Candida* species (*C albicans*, *C glabrata*, *C krusei*, *C parapsilosis*, and *C tropicalis*), and SeptiFast is approved in Europe to detect certain bacterial and fungal species (*C albicans*, *C glabrata*, *C krusei*, *C parapsilosis*, *C tropicalis*, and *Aspergillus fumigatus*).[15,23] Further studies on large cohorts of patients are necessary before this becomes standard practice.

PROPHYLAXIS AND TREATMENT

Candidemia carries high mortality risk,[3] and any delay in the administration of the proper antifungal therapy could lead to a 2-fold increase in death. There was an increase in survival rates when the proper antifungal therapy was given within 12 to 24 hours of the episode of candidemia.[14,24–27] Hence, efforts have been directed toward an early intervention with antifungal therapy in high-risk populations (prophylactically or empirically), including nonneutropenic ICU patients. Early studies involving surgical ICU patients who underwent abdominal surgical procedures and/or recurrent gastrointestinal perforations or anastomotic leakage found that daily fluconazole prophylaxis, compared with placebo, reduced the overall risk of IC.[28] Furthermore, follow-up studies concluded similar observations in surgical ICU patients, although there was no evidence of any difference between the use of empiric fluconazole versus placebo therapy on mortality.[29,30]

Subsequent prospective studies that implemented antifungal therapy (triazole or caspofungin) in high-risk ICU patients have shown a decrease in the overall incidence of IC.[31,32]

In a recent Cochrane Review that included 22 randomized clinical trials, prophylactic, preemptive, and empiric therapy in ICU patients showed a trend toward lower incidence of IC compared with no intervention, although there was no difference in survival.[33] Recent data from a large French multicenter study that investigated the impact of empiric antifungal therapy by using micafungin versus placebo in a high-risk ICU population did not find a difference in the main outcome of a 28-day IFI-free survival period, but it did show a statistically significant decrease in the rate of IFI.[34] In contrast, another recent meta-analysis for trauma and surgical ICUs showed a survival benefit.[35]

Although the lack of survival benefits in most studies might be explained by factors related to the study population, such as age, underlying renal failure, and severity of illness,[25] this area of uncertainty is not well understood because multiple studies adjusted for such risk factors with no significant change in the outcome.

Given the significant evidence of IC rate reductions from using prophylactic/empiric antifungal therapy in high-risk critically ill patients who fail to respond to proper antibacterial therapy, the authors believe that empiric antifungal therapy is recommended and should be continued until the risk and/or other sources of infections are identified.[5]

TREATMENT

Knowledge of local epidemiology, antibiogram, and the patient's antifungal exposure history are imperative for proper management of IC. The increase in the incidence of non-*albicans Candida* IC has made therapy more complicated. Broad-spectrum empiric antifungal therapy should be considered initially, followed by narrowing therapy once the *Candida* species is identified and antifungal susceptibility is known.[36] Hence, the recommended drug of choice in almost all IC cases is an echinocandin.[5] Echinocandin efficacy has been validated in multiple clinical trials. Caspofungin showed a success rate of 73.4% versus 61.7% with fewer adverse events compared with amphotericin B.[37] A comparison of caspofungin at a high dose of 150 mg daily dose versus a regular dose of 50 mg daily (after a loading dose of 70 mg) did not show significant difference in outcome or adverse event incidence.[38] Although micafungin was noninferior compared with liposomal amphotericin B, with a success rate of 89.6% versus 89.5%, respectively, liposomal amphotericin B had more adverse events.[39] Anidulafungin efficacy was investigated in a noninferiority study against fluconazole and it was superior to fluconazole in a preplanned post-hoc analysis in IC, with an 81.1% versus 62.3% success rate compared with fluconazole.[40–42] A patient-level meta-analysis of major trials in IC showed that echinocandins have a mortality benefit compared with other drug classes,[43] therefore they have become the treatment of choice as recommended by US and European treatment guidelines.[5,44]

It is recommended to change antifungal therapy once antifungal susceptibilities are available. However, other antifungal drug classes carry the risk of more adverse events and drug-drug interactions.[5] For other therapeutic options, please refer to **Table 2**.

In addition, it is recommended to control the source of infection by removing infected devices or drainage of collections. It is recommended in cases of candidemia to continue therapy for at least 2 weeks from the first negative blood cultures.[5] Therapy is usually extended to 4 to 6 weeks when dissemination and end-organ infection has occurred.

Patients with candidemia risk the development of ophthalmic candida infection; the rate ranges between 1% and 5%.[45,46] Given that ICU patients may not be able to communicate visual symptoms, all patients with candidemia need a dilated ophthalmic examination within 1 week of the diagnosis of candida BSI, to rule out ocular involvement.[5] In cases of ophthalmic involvement, therapy should be coordinated with an ophthalmologist to assess the need for vitrectomy or intravitreal therapy, and a triazole or liposomal amphotericin B with or without flucytosine should be considered. As discussed earlier, treatment duration should be extended to 4 to 6 weeks.[5]

ASPERGILLOSIS

Invasive aspergillosis (IA) is recognized as one of the IFIs that can affect nonneutropenic critically ill patients. *Aspergillus fumigatus* is the main pathogen to consider, followed by *Aspergillus niger* and *Aspergillus flavus*.[47]

Not only do patients with proven IA have higher mortalities but ICU patients colonized with *Aspergillus* also tend to do poorly, because almost half of these patients develop or may already have IA.[48–50] It is estimated that 4% of nonhematological ICU patients develop IA. Other risk factors for ICU patients include chronic obstructive pulmonary disease, malnutrition, diabetes mellitus, and liver cirrhosis. More recently, influenza infection has also been associated with IA.[47,49–53] In addition, IA has been described in patients who underwent abdominal surgical interventions and in those on peritoneal dialysis.[54–56]

DIAGNOSIS

Radiological findings can be seen on a plain radiograph or computed tomography study, such as pulmonary nodules or halo sign.[57] However, these are not very specific. At present, the diagnosis of IA infection is based on the European Organisation for Research and Treatment of Cancer (EORTC)/Invasive Fungal Infections Cooperative Group and

Table 2
Antifungal drugs used in invasive fungal infections in the intensive care unit

Antifungal Class	Dose	Spectrum	Comments
Triazoles			
Fluconazole	400–800 mg/d	C albicans, C glabrata, C parapsilosis, C tropicalis, not C krusei	Cytochrome P450 inducers can cause increased liver function enzyme levels
Voriconazole	200 (3–4 mg) mg/ twice a day (loading dose of 400 mg (6 mg/kg) twice a day for 2 doses)	C albicans, C glabrata, C parapsilosis, C tropicalis, C krusei Aspergillus spp	
Posaconazole	Delayed release 300 mg/d (loading dose 300 mg twice a day for 2 doses)		
Isavuconazonium sulfate	372 mg/d (loading dose 3 times a day for 6 doses)		
Echinocandins			
Micafungin	100 mg/d	C albicans, C glabrata, C parapsilosis, C tropicalis, C krusei Aspergillus spp	Caspofungin may need dose adjustment in severe hepatic dysfunction
Caspofungin	50 mg/d (70-mg loading dose)		
Anidulafungin	100 mg/d (200-mg loading dose)		
Amphotericin			
Deoxycholate formulation	0.1–1.5 mg/kg/d	C albicans, C glabrata, C parapsilosis, C tropicalis, C krusei Aspergillus spp (except Aspergillus terreus)	Nephrotoxic
Liposomal formulation (AmBisome)	3–5 mg/kg/d		Less nephrotoxic
Flucytosine	25 mg/kg in 4 divided doses daily	C albicans, C glabrata, C parapsilosis, C tropicalis, C krusei	High concentration can lead to hepatitis and bone marrow suppression Should be used in combination with another antifungal therapy

Dosing assumes normal renal and hepatic functions.
Data from Refs.[5,57,75]

the National Institute of Allergy and Infectious Diseases Mycoses Study Group (MSG) definition for IFIs. IA can be defined as proven, probable, and possible,[58] as follows:

- Proven IA: risk factors and specimens are acquired from sterile sites (excluding bronchoalveolar lavage [BAL], sinus cavity, and urine) that show abnormal clinical or radiological findings that are positive on microbiological and/or histopathologic testing.
- Probable IA: risk factors and clinical and radiological findings backed by positive cultures of nonsterile sites or indirect test (β-D-glucan or galactomannan [GM]).

- Possible IA: cases that have risk factors, clinical findings, and radiological findings but lack microbiological, histopathologic, or indirect mycological tests.

Although, EORTC/MSG definitions were not intended for immunocompetent ICU hosts, they have been validated for ICU patients.[52]

Microbiological cultures lack sensitivity and can take up to 10 days for the diagnosis of *Aspergillus* spp.[59] The same can be said about histopathologic examination because it also lacks the sensitivity and specificity, is pathologist dependent,[60] and is contingent on accurate sampling of the affected area.

Aspergillus GM has been investigated in multiple studies in patients with proven or probable pulmonary IA. BAL GM has high sensitivity and specificity, whereas serum GM had lower sensitivity,[61] which can be increased to about 70% on serial tests.[62] Serum GM variability can be explained by the difference in the burden of the infection and host neutrophils clearing up the GM antigen. Studies of GM have also shown that exposure to antifungal therapy can affect the results as well.[63] GM is not specific to *Aspergillus* spp because other molds may lead to false-positive results, such as *Histoplasma*, *Alternaria*, *Fusarium*, and *Penicillium*. Moreover, like the β-D-glucan test, certain antibiotics, most notably β-lactams, can cause a false-positive GM tests.[64]

Combining BAL PCR and *Aspergillus* GM has been shown to have a sensitivity and specificity of about 97% each, both of which are higher than the GM test alone[65,66] (see **Table 1** for all IA diagnostics).

TREATMENT

There are no current recommendations for IA prophylaxis in nonneutropenic ICU patients.[57] Itraconazole has activity against *Aspergillus* spp; however, its limited oral bioavailability in ICU patients limits its usefulness in that population. Voriconazole, currently the gold standard, has been shown to be more efficacious than amphotericin B deoxycholate, with a response rate of 52.8% versus 31.6%, respectively, at the end of 12 weeks, and it had higher survival rate of 70.8% versus 57.9%.[67] Therefore, voriconazole is considered the first-line therapy for IA.[57] Therapeutic drug monitoring is recommended because voriconazole pharmacokinetics (PK) is nonlinear and drug levels can fluctuate throughout the treatment. Several side effects should be considered when using voriconazole, such as hallucinations, photosensitivity, QT interval prolongation, and nausea and vomiting, with rare effects like periostitis, skin cancer, and liver failure after prolonged use of voriconazole. Intravenous voriconazole is not recommended if renal function is less than 50 mL/min because it leads to the accumulation of the excipient sulfobutylether-beta-cyclodextrin (SBECD).[57,67,68]

Isavuconazonium sulfate (isavuconazole) is a new triazole with a long half-life and does not need therapeutic drug level monitoring. It has better side effects profile than voriconazole, and it showed noninferiority in the treatment of IA compared with voriconazole.[69] It was recently approved for IA; however, it is recommended as an alternative therapy because of lack of clinical experience.[57] Isavuconazonium shares some of the side effects from the triazole group, such as gastrointestinal symptoms, and it may cause corrected QT interval shortening.[70]

Posaconazole is another triazole that was first studied as an oral solution for IA prophylaxis in hematological malignancies patients.[71,72] However, posaconazole is being investigated as a second-line therapy in patients who failed or could not tolerate first-line IA therapy. In a study comparing posaconazole with a control group that received amphotericin-based therapy, there was a better response rate (39% vs 22%) in the nonneutropenic populations, with better 30-day survival rate (74% vs 49%) in all groups (neutropenic and nonneutropenic). However, because of the lack of major randomized trials, posaconazole is currently recommended as a second-line therapy for IAs.[57,73] Such trials are currently underway.

Among the polyene antifungal class, liposomal amphotericin B has shown good outcomes when used for IA in hematological malignancy. A lower dose of 3 mg/mL not only carried lesser nephrotoxicity but had better overall outcome, with 50% response and 72% survival rate at 12 weeks compared with the higher dose with 46% and 59%, respectively.[74] Amphotericin B is active against all *Aspergillus* species except *Aspergillus terreus*.[75]

All 3 echinocandins (micafungin, caspofungin, and anidulafungin) are active in vitro against *Aspergillus* spp and are thought to have a fungistatic effect.[76] However, caspofungin is the most studied echinocandin in the setting of IA. Although studies of caspofungin as first-line monotherapy for IA have shown efficacy, they lack consistency because response rates vary between 27% and 83%.[77] Caspofungin has been shown to have some efficacy as a salvage therapy when there are contraindications to other antifungal therapies, with a 30% to 40% response rate by end of therapy and a 50% survival rate.[78,79] It is currently not recommended to use caspofungin monotherapy for treatment of IAs unless there are contraindications to the use of other agents.[57] **Table 2** contrasts current antifungal agents.

SUMMARY

ICU patients are at risk of developing infections, and this article focuses on the most encountered IFIs in the ICU. Knowledge of risk factors helps in identifying patients at risk of IFI and determining who might benefit from prophylaxis or empiric antifungal therapy. Proper implementation of rapid diagnostic methods helps in the decision of when to start and stop antifungal therapy. There are different antifungal medications that can be used and hence knowing their activity spectrum, efficacy, and adverse effects is key to achieving better outcomes in ICU patients with IFIs.

REFERENCES

1. Leroy O, Gangneux JP, Montravers P, et al. Epidemiology, management, and risk factors for death of invasive *Candida* infections in critical care: a multicenter, prospective, observational study in France (2005-2006). Crit Care Med 2009;37(5):1612–8.
2. Magill SS, Edwards JR, Bamberg W, et al. Multistate point-prevalence survey of health care–associated infections. N Engl J Med 2014;370:1198–208.
3. Wisplinghoff H, Bischoff T, Tallent SM, et al. Nosocomial bloodstream infections in US hospitals: analysis of 24,179 cases from a prospective nationwide surveillance study. Clin Infect Dis 2004;39(3):309–17.
4. Eggimann P, Pittet D. Candida colonization index and subsequent infection in critically ill surgical patients: 20 years later. Intensive Care Med 2014;40(10): 1429–48.
5. Pappas PG, Kauffman CA, Andes DR, et al. Clinical practice guideline for the management of candidiasis: 2016 update by the Infectious Diseases Society of America. Clin Infect Dis 2016;62(4):e1–50.
6. León C, Ruiz-Santana S, Saavedra P, et al. A bedside scoring system ("Candida score") for early antifungal treatment in nonneutropenic critically ill patients with Candida colonization. Crit Care Med 2006;34(3):730–7.
7. Ostrosky-Zeichner L, Sable C, Sobel J, et al. Multicenter retrospective development and validation of a clinical prediction rule for nosocomial invasive candidiasis in the intensive care setting. Eur J Clin Microbiol Infect Dis 2007;26(4):271–6.

8. Shorr AF, Tabak YP, Johannes RS, et al. Candidemia on presentation to the hospital: development and validation of a risk score. Crit Care 2009;13(5):R156.

9. Hermsen ED, Zapapas MK, Maiefski M, et al. Validation and comparison of clinical prediction rules for invasive candidiasis in intensive care unit patients: a matched case-control study. Crit Care 2011;15(4):R198.

10. Leroy G, Lambiotte F, Thévenin D, et al. Evaluation of "Candida score" in critically ill patients: a prospective, multicenter, observational, cohort study. Ann Intensive Care 2011;1(1):50.

11. Dupont H, Paugam-Burtz C, Muller-Serieys C, et al. Predictive factors of mortality due to polymicrobial peritonitis with *Candida* isolation in peritoneal fluid in critically ill patients. Arch Surg 2002;137(12):1341–6 [discussion: 1347].

12. Guzman JA, Tchokonte R, Sobel JD. Septic shock due to candidemia: outcomes and predictors of shock development. J Clin Med Res 2011;3(2):65–71.

13. Kumar A, Roberts D, Wood KE, et al. Duration of hypotension before initiation of effective antimicrobial therapy is the critical determinant of survival in human septic shock. Crit Care Med 2006;34(6):1589–96.

14. Taur Y, Cohen N, Dubnow S, et al. Effect of antifungal therapy timing on mortality in cancer patients with candidemia. Antimicrob Agents Chemother 2010;54(1): 184–90.

15. Clancy CJ, Nguyen MH. Finding the missing 50% of invasive candidiasis: how nonculture diagnostics will improve understanding of disease spectrum and transform patient care. Clin Infect Dis 2013;56(9):1284–92.

16. Cavling Arendrup M, Sulim S, Holm A, et al. Diagnostic issues, clinical characteristics and outcome for patients with fungaemia. Clin Microbiol Infect 2011; 17:S786–7.

17. Karageorgopoulos DE, Vouloumanou EK, Ntziora F, et al. β-D-glucan assay for the diagnosis of invasive fungal infections: a meta-analysis. Clin Infect Dis 2011;52(6):750–70.

18. Ellis M, Al-Ramadi B, Finkelman M, et al. Assessment of the clinical utility of serial beta-D-glucan concentrations in patients with persistent neutropenic fever. J Med Microbiol 2008;57(Pt 3):287–95.

19. Wheat LJ. Approach to the diagnosis of invasive aspergillosis and candidiasis. Clin Chest Med 2009;30(2):367–77.

20. Pickering JW, Sant HW, Bowles CAP, et al. Evaluation of a (1->3)-beta-D-glucan assay for diagnosis of invasive fungal infections. J Clin Microbiol 2005;43(12): 5957–62.

21. León C, Ruiz-Santana S, Saavedra P, et al. Usefulness of the "Candida score" for discriminating between *Candida* colonization and invasive candidiasis in non-neutropenic critically ill patients: a prospective multicenter study. Crit Care Med 2009;37(5):1624–33.

22. Jaijakul S, Vazquez JA, Swanson RN, et al. (1,3)-β-D-glucan as a prognostic marker of treatment response in invasive candidiasis. Clin Infect Dis 2012; 55(4):521–6.

23. Nguyen MH, Wissel MC, Shields RK, et al. Performance of candida real-time polymerase chain reaction, β-D-glucan assay, and blood cultures in the diagnosis of invasive candidiasis. Clin Infect Dis 2012;54(9):1240–8.

24. Morrell M, Fraser VJ, Kollef MH. Delaying the empiric treatment of *Candida* bloodstream infection until positive blood culture results are obtained: a potential risk factor for hospital mortality. Antimicrob Agents Chemother 2005;49(9):3640–5.

25. Blot SI, Vandewoude KH, Hoste EA, et al. Effects of nosocomial candidemia on outcomes of critically Ill patients. Am J Med 2002;113(6):480–5.

26. Parkins MD, Sabuda DM, Elsayed S, et al. Adequacy of empirical antifungal therapy and effect on outcome among patients with invasive *Candida* species infections. J Antimicrob Chemother 2007;60(3):613–8.

27. Garey KW, Rege M, Pai MP, et al. Time to initiation of fluconazole therapy impacts mortality in patients with candidemia: a multi-institutional study. Clin Infect Dis 2006;43(1):25–31.

28. Eggimann P, Francioli P, Bille J, et al. Fluconazole prophylaxis prevents intra-abdominal candidiasis in high-risk surgical patients. Crit Care Med 1999;27(6): 1066–72.

29. Pelz RK, Hendrix CW, Swoboda SM, et al. Double-blind placebo-controlled trial of fluconazole to prevent candidal infections in critically ill surgical patients. Ann Surg 2001;233(4):542–8.

30. Garbino J, Lew DP, Romand JA, et al. Prevention of severe *Candida* infections in nonneutropenic, high-risk, critically ill patients: a randomized, double-blind, placebo-controlled trial in patients treated by selective digestive decontamination. Intensive Care Med 2002;28(12):1708–17.

31. Schuster MG, Edwards JE, Sobel JD, et al. Empirical fluconazole versus placebo for intensive care unit patients: a randomized trial. Ann Intern Med 2008;149(2): 83–90.

32. Ostrosky-Zeichner L, Shoham S, Vazquez J, et al. MSG-01: a randomized, double-blind, placebo-controlled trial of caspofungin prophylaxis followed by preemptive therapy for invasive candidiasis in high-risk adults in the critical care setting. Clin Infect Dis 2014;58(9):1219–26.

33. Cortegiani A, Russotto V, Maggiore A, et al. Antifungal agents for preventing fungal infections in non-neutropenic critically ill patients. Cochrane Database Syst Rev 2016;(1):CD004920.

34. Timsit J-F, Azoulay E, Schwebel C, et al. Empirical micafungin treatment and survival without invasive fungal infection in adults with ICU-acquired sepsis, candida colonization, and multiple organ failure. JAMA 2016;316(15):1555.

35. Cruciani M, De Lalla F, Mengoli C. Prophylaxis of *Candida* infections in adult trauma and surgical intensive care patients: a systematic review and meta-analysis. Intensive Care Med 2005;31(11):1479–87.

36. Pfaller M, Neofytos D, Diekema D, et al. Epidemiology and outcomes of candidemia in 3648 patients: data from the prospective antifungal therapy (PATH Alliance®) registry, 2004-2008. Diagn Microbiol Infect Dis 2012;74(4):323–31.

37. Mora-Duarte J, Betts R, Rotstein C, et al. Comparison of caspofungin and amphotericin B for invasive candidiasis. N Engl J Med 2002;347(1533–4406):2020–9.

38. Betts RF, Nucci M, Talwar D, et al. A multicenter, double-blind trial of a high-dose caspofungin treatment regimen versus a standard caspofungin treatment regimen for adult patients with invasive candidiasis. Clin Infect Dis 2009;48: 1676–84.

39. Kuse ER, Chetchotisakd P, da Cunha CA, et al. Micafungin versus liposomal amphotericin B for candidaemia and invasive candidosis: a phase III randomised double-blind trial. Lancet 2007;369(9572):1519–27.

40. Reboli AC, Rotstein C, Pappas PG, et al. Anidulafungin versus fluconazole for invasive candidiasis. N Engl J Med 2007;356(24):2472–82.

41. Reboli AC, Shorr AF, Rotstein C, et al. Anidulafungin compared with fluconazole for treatment of candidemia and other forms of invasive candidiasis caused by *Candida albicans*: a multivariate analysis of factors associated with improved outcome. BMC Infect Dis 2011;11:261.

42. Krause DS, Simjee AE, van Rensburg C, et al. A randomized, double-blind trial of anidulafungin versus fluconazole for the treatment of esophageal candidiasis. Clin Infect Dis 2004;39(6):770–5.

43. Andes DR, Safdar N, Baddley JW, et al. Impact of treatment strategy on outcomes in patients with candidemia and other forms of invasive candidiasis: a patient-level quantitative review of randomized trials. Clin Infect Dis 2012;54(8): 1110–22.

44. Cornely OA, Bassetti M, Calandra T, et al. ESCMID* guideline for the diagnosis and management of candida diseases 2012: non-neutropenic adult patients. Clin Microbiol Infect 2012;18:19–37 *This guideline was presented in part at ECCMID 2011. European Society for Clinical Microbiology and Infectious Diseases.

45. Dozier CC, Tarantola RM, Jiramongkolchai K, et al. Fungal eye disease at a tertiary care center: the utility of routine inpatient consultation. Ophthalmology 2011;118(8):1671–6.

46. Adam MK, Vahedi S, Nichols MM, et al. Inpatient ophthalmology consultation for fungemia: prevalence of ocular involvement and necessity of funduscopic screening. Am J Ophthalmol 2015;160(5):1078–83.e2.

47. Taccone FS, Van den Abeele AM, Bulpa P, et al. Epidemiology of invasive aspergillosis in critically ill patients: clinical presentation, underlying conditions, and outcomes. Crit Care 2015;19(1):7.

48. Khasawneh F, Mohamad T, Moughrabieh MK, et al. Isolation of *Aspergillus* in critically ill patients: a potential marker of poor outcome. J Crit Care 2006;21(4): 322–7.

49. Vandewoude KH, Blot SI, Depuydt P, et al. Clinical relevance of *Aspergillus* isolation from respiratory tract samples in critically ill patients. Crit Care 2006;10(1):R31.

50. Meersseman W, Vandecasteele SJ, Wilmer A, et al. Invasive aspergillosis in critically ill patients without malignancy. Am J Respir Crit Care Med 2004;170(6): 621–5.

51. Crum-Cianflone NF. Invasive aspergillosis associated with severe influenza infections. Open Forum Infect Dis 2016;3(3):ofw171.

52. Blot SI, Taccone FS, Van Den Abeele AM, et al. A clinical algorithm to diagnose invasive pulmonary aspergillosis in critically ill patients. Am J Respir Crit Care Med 2012;186(1):56–64.

53. Garnacho-Montero J, Amaya-Villar R, Ortiz-Leyba C, et al. Isolation of *Aspergillus* spp. from the respiratory tract in critically ill patients: risk factors, clinical presentation and outcome. Crit Care 2005;9(3):R191–9.

54. Dichtl K, Wagener J, Tschöp J, et al. Analysis of peritoneal galactomannan for the diagnosis of *Aspergillus* peritonitis. Infection 2016;44(5):683–6.

55. Dimopoulos G, Piagnerelli M, Berré J, et al. Disseminated aspergillosis in intensive care unit patients: an autopsy study. J Chemother 2003;15(1):71–5.

56. Garbino J, Fluckiger U, Elzi L, et al. Survey of aspergillosis in non-neutropenic patients in Swiss teaching hospitals. Clin Microbiol Infect 2011;17(9):1366–71.

57. Patterson TF, Thompson GR, Denning DW, et al. Practice guidelines for the diagnosis and management of aspergillosis: 2016 update by the infectious diseases society of America. Clin Infect Dis 2016;63(4):e1–60.

58. De Pauw B, Walsha TJ, Donnellya JP, et al. Revised definitions of invasive fungal disease from the European Organization for research and treatment of cancer/invasive fungal infections cooperative group and the National Institute of Allergy and Infectious Diseases Mycoses Study Group (EORTC/MSG) Consensus Group. Clin Infect Dis 2008;46(12):1813–21.

59. Mortensen KL, Johansen HK, Fuursted K, et al. A prospective survey of *Aspergillus* spp. in respiratory tract samples: prevalence, clinical impact and antifungal susceptibility. Eur J Clin Microbiol Infect Dis 2011;30(11):1355–63.

60. Shah AA, Hazen KC. Diagnostic accuracy of histopathologic and cytopathologic examination of *Aspergillus* species. Am J Clin Pathol 2013;139(1):55–61.

61. Meersseman W, Lagrou K, Maertens J, et al. Galactomannan in bronchoalveolar lavage fluid. Am J Respir Crit Care Med 2008;177(1):27–34.

62. He H, Ding L, Chang S, et al. Value of consecutive galactomannan determinations for the diagnosis and prognosis of invasive pulmonary aspergillosis in critically ill chronic obstructive pulmonary disease. Med Mycol 2011;49(4):345–51.

63. Mennink-Kersten MA, Donnelly JP, Verweij PE. Detection of circulating galactomannan for the diagnosis and management of invasive aspergillosis. Lancet Infect Dis 2004;4(6):349–57.

64. Barton RC. Laboratory diagnosis of invasive aspergillosis: from diagnosis to prediction of outcome. Scientifica (Cairo) 2013;2013:459405.

65. Avni T, Leibovici L, Paul M. PCR diagnosis of invasive candidiasis: systematic review and meta-analysis. J Clin Microbiol 2011;49(2):665–70.

66. Heng SC, Morrissey O, Chen SCA, et al. Utility of bronchoalveolar lavage fluid galactomannan alone or in combination with PCR for the diagnosis of invasive aspergillosis in adult hematology patients: a systematic review and meta-analysis. Crit Rev Microbiol 2015;41(1):124–34.

67. Herbrecht R, Denning DW, Patterson TF, et al. Voriconazole versus amphotericin B for primary therapy of invasive aspergillosis. N Engl J Med 2002;347(6):408–15.

68. Mikulska M, Novelli A, Aversa F, et al. Voriconazole in clinical practice. J Chemother 2012;24(6):311–27.

69. Maertens JA, Raad II, Marr KA, et al. Isavuconazole versus voriconazole for primary treatment of invasive mould disease caused by *Aspergillus* and other filamentous fungi (SECURE): a phase 3, randomised-controlled, non-inferiority trial. Lancet 2016;387(10020):760–9.

70. Shirley M, Scott LJ. Isavuconazole: a review in invasive aspergillosis and mucormycosis. Drugs 2016;76(17):1647–57.

71. Ullmann AJ, Lipton JH, Vesole DH, et al. Posaconazole or fluconazole for prophylaxis in severe graft-versus-host disease. N Engl J Med 2007;356(4):335–47.

72. Cornely OA, Maertens J, Winston DJ, et al. Posaconazole vs. fluconazole or itraconazole prophylaxis in patients with neutropenia. N Engl J Med 2007;356(4):348–59.

73. Walsh TJ, Raad I, Patterson TF, et al. Treatment of invasive aspergillosis with posaconazole in patients who are refractory to or intolerant of conventional therapy: an externally controlled trial. Clin Infect Dis 2007;44(1):2–12.

74. Cornely OA, Maertens J, Bresnik M, et al. Liposomal amphotericin B as initial therapy for invasive mold infection: a randomized trial comparing a high-loading dose regimen with standard dosing (AmBiLoad trial). Clin Infect Dis 2007;44(10):1289–97.

75. Pfaller M, Messer S. Antifungal activities of posaconazole, ravuconazole, and voriconazole compared to those of itraconazole and amphotericin B against 239 clinical isolates of *Aspergillus* spp. and other filamentous fungi: report from SENTRY antimicrobial surveillance program. Antimicrob Agents Chemother 2002;46(4):1032–7.

76. Pfaller MA, Boyken L, Hollis RJ, et al. In vitro susceptibility of clinical isolates of *Aspergillus* spp. to anidulafungin, caspofungin, and micafungin: a head-to-

head comparison using the CLSI M38-A2 broth microdilution method. J Clin Microbiol 2009;47(10):3323–5.

77. Heinz WJ, Buchheidt D, Ullmann AJ. Clinical evidence for caspofungin monotherapy in the first-line and salvage therapy of invasive *Aspergillus* infections. Mycoses 2016;59(8):480–93.

78. Herbrecht R, Maertens J, Baila L, et al. Caspofungin first-line therapy for invasive aspergillosis in allogeneic hematopoietic stem cell transplant patients: an European Organisation for research and treatment of cancer study. Bone Marrow Transplant 2010;45(7):1227–33.

79. Maertens J, Raad I, Petrikkos G, et al. Efficacy and safety of caspofungin for treatment of invasive aspergillosis in patients refractory to or intolerant of conventional antifungal therapy. Clin Infect Dis 2004;39(11):1563–71.

80. Mikulska M, Calandra T, Sanguinetti M, et al, Third European Conference on Infections in Leukemia Group. The use of mannan antigen and anti-mannan antibodies in the diagnosis of invasive candidiasis: recommendations from the Third European Conference on Infections in Leukemia. Crit Care 2010;14(6): R222.

81. Duettmann W, Koidl C, Krause R, et al. Specificity of mannan antigen and anti-mannan antibody screening in patients with haematological malignancies at risk for fungal infection. Mycoses 2016;59(6):374–8.

82. Avni T, Levy I, Sprecher H, et al. Diagnostic accuracy of PCR alone compared to galactomannan in bronchoalveolar lavage fluid for diagnosis of invasive pulmonary aspergillosis: a systematic review. J Clin Microbiol 2012;50(11):3652–8.

83. Mylonakis E, Clancy CJ, Ostrosky-Zeichner L, et al. T2 magnetic resonance assay for the rapid diagnosis of candidemia in whole blood: a clinical trial. Clin Infect Dis 2015;60(6):892–9.

Clostridium difficile Infection

John G. Bartlett, MD*

KEYWORDS

- *Clostridium difficile* • Intensive care units • White blood cell
- Centers for Disease Control and Prevention

KEY POINTS

- *Clostridium difficile* infection is now recognized as a major health care challenge in terms of patient and economic consequences.
- For the patient, it is a morbid and sometimes a life-threatening iatrogenic complication of antibiotic treatment.
- In the United States, the provider's institution may face financial penalties, because the Centers for Disease Control and Prevention now views this as an iatrogenic health care-associated complication that may not be reimbursable by the Centers for Medicare and Medicaid Services.
- This has resulted in substantial incentives for new approaches to prevention and treatment.

HISTORICAL BACKGROUND

Clostridium difficile was originally reported by Hall and O'Toole in 1935 as a component of stool fora of healthy newborn infants.[1] It was shown at that time to produce a toxin that was highly lethal to experimental animals, but its role in clinical care was unknown until 1978, when it was implicated as the cause of what was called at the time "clindamycin colitis".[2] This early work also demonstrated the production of "A" and "B" toxins. The cytopathic activity became the standard diagnostic test at that time; oral vancomycin became standard treatment, and the problem of relapsing *C difficile* infection (CDI) was recognized.[3] The subsequent history of this pathogen in the disease it causes following antibiotic use is now recognized as a major concern with antibiotic management throughout the world. A Centers for Disease Control and Prevention analysis for the United States based on review of 15,461 cases in 10 geographic areas showed 66% were health care associated; there were an

Division of Infectious Diseases, Johns Hopkins University School of Medicine, 1830 Orleans Street, Baltimore MD, 2128, USA
* Corresponding author. Johns Hopkins University School of Medicine, Post Office Box 10, Belden, MS 38826.
E-mail address: jb@jhmi.edu

Infect Dis Clin N Am 31 (2017) 489–495
http://dx.doi.org/10.1016/j.idc.2017.05.012
0891-5520/17/© 2017 Elsevier Inc. All rights reserved.

estimated 453,000 incident US cases, and persons over 65 years were most vulnerable (OR-8.7). The estimated annual mortality in the United States was 29,000.[4] Another analysis based on large inpatient centers in 477 acute care hospitals with 71,586 discharges showed CDI was associated with significantly higher mortality rates, increased hospital costs averaging $7286 per case, and a significant increase in readmission rate.[5] These data for CDI incidence, morbidity, and mortality also applied to US intensive care units (ICUs) based on data from 1983 to 2015.[5]

INTENSIVE CARE UNIT ISSUES

Intensive care units have patients with CDI in 3 categories: those with CDI that is incidental to the reason for ICU need, patients who are transferred because of serious CDI such as toxic megacolon, and those who develop CDI while in the ICU. A meta-analysis of 22 reports of CDI among 80,835 ICU patients showed the prevalence of CDI was 2%.[6] The analysis comparing those with CDI versus other patients showed the mortality in the CDI group was significantly higher (32% compared to 24% without CDI; $P = .03$), and the mean length of ICU stay was significantly longer ($P = .003$). It was estimated that a 30% reduction in use of broad-spectrum antibiotics with improved stewardship would result in an estimated 26% reduction in CDI cases.[7]

CLINICAL FEATURES

The major clinical feature is diarrhea that is large in volume, usually watery, and often has a distinctive odor attributed to P-cresol produced by C difficile in the laboratory and in the patient stool.[8] There is usually stool urgency; there may be incontinence, and most patients have abdominal pain or abdominal cramps. Low-grade fever is common, and there is usually leukocytosis. A white blood cell (WBC) count greater than 15,000/mm^3, renal insufficiency, and elevated lactate levels correlate with disease severity and mortality.[9–11] Particularly concerning is ileus or its most serious form toxic megacolon. Imaging shows disease that is usually limited to the colon; small bowel involvement is reported, but rare. Nearly all cases are preceded by the implicated antibiotics, with the highest rates associated with fluoroquinolones, clindamycin, and second-/third-generation cephalosporins.[11] Nevertheless, nearly all antibiotics may cause this complication; those noted, however, account for the vast majority, and the risk is far less with macrolides, tetracyclines, narrow-spectrum beta-lactams, urinary antiseptics, aminoglycosides, and sulfa/trimethoprim.

RISK

The major risks include the antibiotics noted previously and advanced age (especially age >75 years); there is invariably current or recent use of an implicated antibiotic, and most patients have current or recent health care facility exposure. Some studies show up to 75% of CDI patients are colonized by C difficile at admission[10] Less common risks include immunosuppression and achlorhydria. Health care facilities are the major source of C difficile including clinics, long-term care facilities, nursing homes, and prior hospitalization. These CDI patients usually have acquired C difficile from the health care system and are sometimes referred to as health care-associated CDI. Such patients may be identified by a positive polymerase chain reaction (PCR) stool test for toxin B. A prior report shows that this asymptomatic C difficile colonization. These C difficile carriers should not be treated for the carrier state, but, if detected, they should theoretically be regarded as potential sources of transmission meriting infection control; they should not be given antibiotics likely to cause clinical expression of CDI.[10] One review indicated that the CDI risk in *C difficile* carriers compared with noncarriers is 9.[10] Note that this observation with screening of asymptomatic patients is not considered standard practice. There are multiple strain types that are differentiated by ribotyping that is sometimes useful in epidemiologic analyses. Ribotypes do not appear to be different in clinical expression except for ribotype 027 (also called NAP-1) and, to a lesser extent, ribotype 078. These strains often show resistance to macrolides and fluoroquinolones; they may cause more serious disease, and they are common causes of CDI epidemics.[11,12]

TESTING FOR *CLOSTRIDIUM DIFFICILE* INFECTION

There are multiple reviews of the relative merits of different testing methods based on sensitivity, specificity, and cost. Possibly the best review is from Planche and colleagues,[13] who compared different tests using diarrheal stools from 6522 patients with supporting clinical evidence for CDI based on clinical and laboratory correlates including leukocytosis, reduced renal function, and abdominal imaging or colonoscopy showing pseudomembraneous colitis. Laboratory testing policies used varies by detection test using 3 different targets: *C difficile* toxin (EIA, cytotoxin), *C difficile* (GDH, cytotoxin culture), and toxin B gene (PCR). The authors of the review concluded that there were 3 categories: *C difficile* colonization, CDI or *C difficile* negative. Most clinicians do not select the test, but use the test offered by their laboratory, a decision commonly made by available resources, population served, speed of results, as well as sensitivity and specificity. A survey of 711 hospital laboratories[14] indicated about 50% of US laboratories use EIA for toxin detection, where the concern is poor sensitivity with false-negative results, and about one third used PCR that is sensitive, but the concern is false-positive results. The cytotoxin assay is possibly the best test, but use in US laboratories is rare due to cost and inconvenience of maintaining tissue cultures. Virtually all laboratories limit testing to diarrhea stools and limit the number of tests per patient over a specified time frame. Note that there is no test of cure, no gold standard test, and knowing the qualities of the test used is important for interpretation.

TREATMENT

Recommendations for therapy are based on CDI guidance documents from 5 nation/society-specific guideline documents from 5 medical societies representing different graphic areas. All 5 documents are remarkably similar, except only the more recent documents include fidaxomicin, which was introduced in 2011,[15–17] and stool transplant, which was popularized beginning in 2010. The 5 treatment guidelines are summarized in Table 1 of Ref.[15] For mild or moderate disease, the recommendation is either vancomycin given orally or metronidazole given orally or parenterally. For moderately severe disease, the recommendation is oral vancomycin, and for serious disease, the recommendation is combination of oral vancomycin and intravenous metronidazole.[15] More recent guidelines include the more recently introduced fidaxomicin, which has the advantage of a significantly reduced rate of relapse,[16] but is controversial because of cost.[17] A third category is severe and complicated, which often includes patients who cannot take oral medications, limiting options to intravenous metronidazole, although 1 guideline also includes intravenous tigecycline for parenteral therapy. For patients with their first relapse, the recommendation is to repeat the initial treatment; for patients with multiple relapses, the supporting data are sparse, but the 2 guidance documents that address this issue suggest oral vancomycin with taper or oral vancomycin for the standard 10-day treatment followed by oral vancomycin qod.

ROLE OF SURGERY

Surgical intervention is sometimes indicated, primarily for patients with severe CDI combined with selected host factors and laboratory test results. The main host factor is advanced age (>70 years); the most important test results are leukocytosis with WBC greater than 15,000/mL; creatinine elevated to greater than 1.5 x baseline; albumin less than 3 g/d; the clinical triad of abdominal pain, abdominal distension, and diarrhea; or toxic megacolon.[18–22] Surgical consultation is indicated for patients with these findings if they are attributable to CDI. The prior standard procedure was colectomy, but more recently an alternative procedure has been a diverting ileostomy with colonic lavage using vancomycin and metronidazole.[23] The advantage is that the patient still has a colon.

RELAPSING *CLOSTRIDIUM DIFFICILE* INFECTION

The frequency of post-therapy relapses is reported at 20% to 30%.[24] Increased risk of relapse is noted for older patient age, antibiotic exposure during CDI treatment, severe CDI infection, or infection involving the NAP-1 strain. The symptoms are the same as the prior episode, but the severity may be more or less. PCR testing is useful only if negative, and the long-term prognosis is good. A review of 1527 cases of CDI showed a rate of at least one CDI relapse is 20% to 25% for at least 1 relapse; after 2 relapses the risk for another relapse was 38%. For 3 relapses, the rate was 29%, and the rate for 4 or more relapses was 27%.[24] The patient should be warned about this complication and need for care.

STOOL TRANSPLANT

Stool transplant was initially reported in 1980 in a patient with *Staphylococcus aureus* enterocolitis. A review of reports of stool transplant primarily for relapsing CDI was based on a meta-analysis of 18 reports with 611 cases published through 2015.[25] Results showed sustained symptom resolution in 91% of cases, with no reported serious adverse events. The donor source of stool for transplant was usually selected by the patient in initial reports, but more recently there has been a commercial nonprofit source based at Massachusetts Institute of Technology (MIT) (open.biome) that carefully screens donors with an extensive history for conditions possibly related to the microbiome and baseline laboratory tests that includes screening donor stool for resistant organisms.[26] Only 2.8% of applicant donors are selected, and they supply specimens 3 times per week. This group provides stool specimens in frozen state; the group now has a cumulative experience of over 16,000 cases and reports a cure rate of 83%.[25] Using stool capsules for oral consumption is an alternative approach also offered by this group, again using carefully screened donors.[27] Stool transplant is now regarded by many authorities as the method of choice for managing relapsing CDI, especially for patients with multiple relapses.[25] The 2010 Infectious Diseases Society of America (IDSA) CDI guidelines recommend this after the third relapse.[28] As noted, a theoretic concern with stool transplants is long-term outcome following stool replacement, with the theoretic long-term complications attributed to the new colonic microbiome, including obesity, diabetes and the metabolic syndrome.[29] Note that open.biome screens out donors with these conditions, as well as for resistant bacteria in the donor specimens. Additionally, the group is now initiating long-term follow-up of recipients to provide further assurance regarding long-term health outcomes.

PREVENTION

Standard infection control recommendations include

Contact isolation of cases until at least 48 hours after resolution of diarrhea
Preference for chlorine-containing disinfectant to clean patient rooms and equipment
Emphasis on hand hygiene with soap and water
Gown and gloves for patient contact, private room or CDI patient cohorting
Continuation of these precautions until diarrhea has resolved for at least 48 hours

There should be room disinfection of environmental surfaces with a disinfectant containing chlorine at a concentration of at least 1000 ppm or use of an alternative sporicidal agent. This should also be used on dedicated equipment except disposable equipment. There needs to be recognition that the health system is the major source of *C difficile* in most CDI cases, with 2 quite different contributing factors: *C difficile* in the health care environment mandating infection control and antibiotic use mandating antibiotic control. CDI was a major concern in the United Kingdom demanding a response. Analysis using gene sequencing to establish transmission patterns showed patient-to-patient transmission accounted for only about 13% of cases, leading to the conclusion that emphasis was needed on antibiotic control[27,30] and use of electronic databases to identify outbreaks. These efforts led to a vigorous antibiotic stewardship intervention, and the UK health system rates for CDI subsequently decreased by 80%.

FUTURE

CDI is now recognized as a major health care challenge in terms of patient and economic consequences. For the patient, it is a morbid and sometimes a life-threatening iatrogenic complication of antibiotic treatment. In the United States, the provider's institution may face financial penalties since the Centers for Disease Control and Prevention (CDC) now views CDI as an iatrogenic health care-associated complication that may not be reimbursable by the Centers for Medicare and Medicaid Services. This has resulted in substantial incentives for new approaches to prevention and treatment. The result is a substantial portfolio of recommendations for new and better treatment[27], especially for relapsing CDI with stool transplant [28], but also this treatment for a number of other conditions.[29] Gene sequencing has proven especially important for showing the role of antibiotic control.[30] Other promising new treatment options for CDI[31] include bezlotoxumab, which has the advantage of reducing rates of relapse.[31,32] Other new agents that are in the pipeline to address the relapse problem include cadazolid and ridinilazole. There are also 3 vaccines that are currently in phase 3 US Food and Drug Administration trials and a *C difficile* intravenous antibody product in phase 3 testing. Thus, the landscape of products available to clinicians for better tools for treating and preventing CDI is optimistic.

REFERENCES

1. Lawson PA, Citron DM, Tyrrell KL, et al. Reclassification of *Clostridium difficile* as *Clostridioides difficile* (Hall and O'Toole) Prevot 1938. Anaerobe 2016;40:95–9.
2. Bartlett JG, Moon N, Chang TW, et al. Role of *Clostridium difficile* in antibiotic-associated pseudomembraneous colitis. Gastroenterology 1978;75:778–82.
3. Talpaert MJ, Gopal RG, Cooper BS, et al. Impact of guidelines and enhanced antibiotic stewardship on reducing broad-spectrum antibiotic usage and its affect

on the incidence of *Clostridium difficile* infection. Antimicrob Chemother 2011;66: 168–74.

4. Lessa FC, Bamberg WM, Beldavs ZG, et al. Burden of *Clostridium difficile* infection in the United States. N Engl J Med 2015;372:825–34.

5. Magee G, Strauss ME, Thomas SM, et al. Impact of *Clostridium difficile*-associated diarrhea on acute care length of stay and hospital costs and readmission: a multi-center retro spec give study of patients, 2009-2011. Am J Infect Control 2015;43:1148–53.

6. Fridkin S, Baggs J, Fagan R, et al. Vital signs: improving antibiotic use among hospitalized patients. MMWR Morb Mortal Wkly Rep 2014;63:194–200.

7. Karanika S, Paudel S, Zervou FN, et al. Prevalence and clinical outcomes of *Clostridium difficile* infection in the intensive care unit: a systematic review and meta-analysis. Open Forum Infect Dis 2015;3(1):ofv186.

8. Bomers MK, van Agtmael MA, Luik H, et al. Using a dog's superior olfactory sensitivity to identify *Clostridium difficile* in stools and patients: Proof of principle study. BMJ 2012;345:e7396.

9. Aronsson B, Mollby R, Nord CE. Antimicrobiol agents and *Clostridium difficile* in acute enteric disease epidemiological data from Sweden, 1980-82. J Infect Dis 1985;151:476–81.

10. Tschudin-Sutter S, Carroll KC, Tamma PD, et al. Impact of toxigenic *Clostridium difficile* colonization on the risk of subsequent *C. difficile* infection in the intensive care unit patients. Infect Control Hosp Epidemiol 2015;36:1324–9.

11. Wiewicz JT, Lopansri BK, Cheknis A, et al. Fluoroquinolone and macrolide exposure predict *Clostridium difficile* infection with highly fluoroquinolone and macrolide-resistant epidemic *C. difficile* strain BI/NAP1/027. Antimicrobial Agents Chemother 2015;60:418–23.

12. Spigaglia P. Recent advances in the understanding of antibiotic resistance in *Clostridium difficile* infection. Ther Adv Infect Dis 2016;3:23–42.

13. Planche T, Wilcox MH. Diagnostic pitfalls in *Clostridium difficile* infection. Infect Dis Clin North Am 2015;29:63–82.

14. McDonald C. Vital Signs: Preventing *Clostridium difficile* infections. MMWR Morb Mortal Wkly Rep 2012;61:157–62.

15. Feher C, Mensa J. Comparison of current guidelines of five international societies. Infect Dis Ther 2016;5:207–30.

16. Louie T, Mullane KM, Weiss K, et al. Fidaxomicin verses vancomycin for *Clostridium difficile* infection. N Engl J Med 2011;364:422–31.

17. Hartzema AG, Chen C. Is fidaxomicin worth the cost? The verdict is still out! Clin Infect Dis 2014;58:604–5.

18. Ong GKB, Reidy TJ, Huk MD, et al. Clostridium difficile colitis: a clinical review. Am J Surg 2017;213:565–7.

19. Napolitano LM, Edmonson LM. *Clostridium difficile* disease: diagnosis, pathogenesis and treatment update. Surgery 2017. http://dx.doi.org/10.1016/j.surg.2017.01.018.

20. Kassam Z, Zee CH, Hunt RH. Review of the emerging treatment of Clostridium difficile infection with fecal microbiota transplantation and insights into future challenges. Clin Lab Med 2014;34:787–98.

21. Sarelli M, Malangoni MA, Abu-Zidan FM, et al. WSES guidelines for management of *Clostridium difficile* infection in surgical patients. World J Surg 2015;10:38.

22. Butala P, Divino CM. Surgical as PACS of fulminant *Clostridium difficile* colitis. Am J Surg 2010;200:131–5.

23. Neal MD, Alverdy JC, Hall DE, et al. Diverting loop ileostomy and colonic lavage: an alternative to total abdominal colectomy for the treatment of severe, complicated *Clostridium difficile* associated disease. Ann Surg 2011;254:423–9.
24. Deshande A, Pasupuleti V, Thota P, et al. Risk factors for recurrent *Clostridium difficile* infection: a systemic review and meta-analysis. Infect Control Hosp Epidemiol 2015;36:452–60.
25. Cohen SH, Gerding DN, Johnson S, et al. Clinical practice guidelines for *Clostridium difficile* infection in adults: 2010 update by the Society for Healthcare Epidemiology of America (SHEA) and the Infectious diseases society of America (IDSA). Infect Control Hosp Epidemiol 2010;31:431–55.
26. open.biome.
27. Eyre DW, Cule ML, Wilson DJ, et al. Diverse sources of *Clostridium difficile* infection identified on whole-genome sequencing. N Engl J Med 2013;369:1195–205.
28. Youngster I, Russell GH, Pindar C, et al. Oral encapsulated frozen fecal mictobiota transplantation for relapsing Clostridium difficile infection. JAMA 2014; 312:1772–8.
29. Marotz CA, Zarrinpar A. Treating obesity and metabolic syndrome with fecal microbiota transplantation. Yale J Biol Med 2016;89:383–8.
30. Walker AS, Eyre DW, Wyllie DH, et al. Characterization of *Clostridium difficile* hospital ward-based transmission using extensive epidemiological data and molecular typing. PLoS Med 2012;9:1001172.
31. Bartlett J. New antimicrobial agents for patients with *Clostridium difficile* infections. N Engl J Med 2017;376:381–2.
32. Bsseres E, Endres BT, Dotson KM, et al. Novel antibiotics in development to treat *Clostridium difficile* infection. Curr Opin Gastroenterol 2017;33:1–7.

Evaluation and Management of Necrotizing Soft Tissue Infections

Stephanie L. Bonne, MD, FACS[a], Sameer S. Kadri, MD, MS[b],*

KEYWORDS

- Necrotizing fasciitis • Soft tissue infection • Sepsis • Gangrene

KEY POINTS

- Necrotizing soft tissue infections (NSTI) are generally severe and rapidly progressive and accompanied by sepsis, multisystem organ failure, and often death.
- Rapid recognition and early surgical intervention form the mainstay of management of NSTIs. Most cases require more than 1 debridement. Imaging can facilitate diagnosis and the decision to operate should not delay treatment in unequivocal cases; direct exploration remains the gold standard for diagnosis.
- Initial surgical debridement should be promptly performed, preferably at the presenting hospital when adequate surgical infrastructure and personnel exist. Transfer of the patient to a referral center may be necessary for definitive surgical and complex wound care.
- Broad-spectrum empiric antibiotics directed at the likely organisms are essential early in the treatment course but do not substitute surgical management. Antibiotic therapy should be subsequently tailored to the etiologic agent. In cases of documented NSTI due to group A *Streptococcus*, clindamycin should be administered in addition to penicillin.
- There are insufficient data to warrant routine use of adjuvant hyperbaric oxygen. Adjuvant intravenous immunoglobulin is an expensive intervention that is not likely to improve survival or physical quality of life and is best reserved for use on a case-by-case basis.

INTRODUCTION

Necrotizing soft tissue infections (NSTIs) are rapidly progressive skin and soft tissue infections that cause widespread tissue necrosis and are associated with systemic illness.[1] The term NSTI has been increasingly used in lieu of the term necrotizing fasciitis, originally coined by BL Wilson[2] in 1952 to encompass cases in which necrosis

[a] Division of Trauma and Critical Care, Department of Surgery, Rutgers New Jersey Medical School, 185 South Orange Avenue, Newark, NJ 07101, USA; [b] Clinical Epidemiology Section, Department of Critical Care Medicine, National Institutes of Health Clinical Center, 10 Center Drive 10/2C145, Bethesda, MD 20892, USA
* Corresponding author.
E-mail address: Sameer.kadri@nih.gov

Infect Dis Clin N Am 31 (2017) 497–511
http://dx.doi.org/10.1016/j.idc.2017.05.011
0891-5520/17/Published by Elsevier Inc.
id.theclinics.com

extends beyond the fascia and can involve the muscle, skin, and surrounding tissues. The incidence and prevalence of NSTIs varies by season, location, and patient population. It is known from the active surveillance operations of the Centers for Disease Control and Prevention that the incidence of NSTI due to invasive group A streptococcal (GAS) infections in the United States is 0.4 per 100,000.[3] The estimated incidence of all-cause NSTI remains less clear due to wide variability in reporting practices. Despite advances in the care, mortality from NSTI has remained relatively high at 25% to 30% for the past 30 years, and has only recently seen a decrease to just over 20%.[4–8] Case fatality rates remain highest when NSTI is accompanied by shock and/or host factors such as advanced age, comorbidities, or immunocompromised state.[1]

Necrotizing soft tissue infections can be classified based on microbiology, location, or depth of tissue involvement. Giuliano and colleagues[9] originally described 2 distinct microbiologic profiles in NSTI; however, the classification system has evolved over time with the recognition of additional pathogen classes (**Table 1**). Type 1 is the most common infection seen, and describes polymicrobial infections, often including anaerobes. Type 2 infections are monomicrobial and typically involve GAS or, less commonly, *Staphylococcus aureus*. Monomicrobial NSTI can also be caused by *Clostridium* spp and, rarely, by *Vibrio vulnificus* (from exposure to warm coastal seawater or consumption of raw oysters; classified by some as type III), *Aeromonas hydrophila* (from exposure to leech therapy or traumatic lesions in fresh water),[10] and fungi (classified by some as type IV) such as *Apophysomyces* spp. Certain monomicrobial causes have presented as local outbreaks (eg, community-associated methicillin-resistant *Staphylococcus aureus* [MRSA] in Los Angeles)[11] or exhibited geographic clustering (eg, *Klebsiella pneumoniae* among diabetic patients with NSTI in Taiwan).[12] Terminology varies by anatomic site as well. Fournier gangrene is used to describe NSTIs of the perineum, which is generally polymicrobial. Diabetic foot infections are polymicrobial and associated with an anaerobic milieu and compromised microvasculature and can sometimes progress to a necrotizing pattern. Finally, the depth of necrosis can also help classify NSTI, with necrotizing cellulitis describing an infection involving the dermis and subcutaneous tissue, necrotizing fasciitis involving the fascia, and pyomyositis or myonecrosis describing involvement of the muscle fascicle without necessarily having overlying skin infections.

PATHOPHYSIOLOGY

The vicious cycle of fulminant infection, toxin production, cytokine activation, microthrombosis and ischemia, and tissue dysfunction and death, and, in turn, greater dissemination of infection is central to the rapidly progressive necrosis seen in NSTI and differentiates it from that of uncomplicated skin and soft tissue infections (**Fig. 1**).[13] Inoculation may be related to trauma or surgery; injured skeletal muscle cells have demonstrated greater adherence to bacteria.[14] The pathogen first spreads in the tissue, releasing a variety of toxins. In the case of GAS and *S aureus*, these are exotoxins.[15] Toxins mediate an inflammatory change in the walls of the microvasculature that facilitates microvascular thrombosis. Pyrogenic exotoxins act as superantigens that bind to antigen-presenting cells and cause rapid proliferation of T cells, and, in turn, production of cytokines that perpetrate shock and multiorgan failure. This is the mechanism for development of toxic shock syndrome (TSS), which is seen with up to half of the NSTI cases due to GAS[16] and can also be seen in cases due to *S aureus*. All the clinical criteria of TSS, including macular rash and desquamation of palms and soles, are not always present, making TSS difficult to distinguish from septic shock by the bedside; the latter can be associated with all causes of NSTI.

Table 1
Microbiologic classification of necrotizing soft tissue infections

Types of Necrotizing Fasciitis	Cause	Organisms	Clinical Progress	Mortality
Type I (70%–80% of cases)	Polymicrobial or synergistic, often bowel flora–derived	Mixed anaerobes and aerobes	More indolent, better prognosis, easier to recognize	Variable, depends on underlying comorbidities
Type II (20%–30% of cases)	Often monomicrobial-, skin-, or respiratory-derived	Usually A β-hemolytic Streptococcus (GAS), occasionally S aureus	Aggressive, presentation easily missed	>30%, depends on associated myositis
Type III (more common in Asia)	Gram-negative, often marine-related organisms	Vibrio spp	Seafood ingestion or water contamination in wounds	30%–40%
Type IV (Fungal)	Trauma-associated	Candida spp, immunocompromised patients Zygomycetes in immunocompetent patients	Aggressive with rapid extension, especially if immunocompromised	>50%, higher if immunocompromised

Adapted from Morgan MS. Diagnosis and management of necrotising fasciitis: a multiparametric approach. J Hosp Infect 2010;75:249–57.

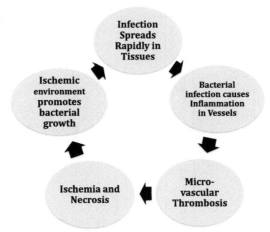

Fig. 1. Vicious cycle of necrotizing soft tissue infection.

Antibiotics penetrate dead and dying tissue poorly and such organism-laden dead tissue represents a perpetual source of infection, underscoring the need for emergent surgical source control in NSTI.

DIAGNOSIS
Clinical Assessment

Nothing replaces early recognition and immediate initiation of treatment of NSTI, which are key to a favorable outcome. Most cases exhibit swelling and erythema but the most consistent finding is pain that is out of proportion to examination findings.[17] However, it can often be difficult to discern a necrotizing process from a simple cellulitis. Patients with NSTI may often present with systemic illness and encephalopathy alone. A thorough examination is valuable when history cannot be easily elicited. Suspicion should be very high in patients with a soft tissue infection who rapidly deteriorate with organ system failure.[18] Additional skin examination findings that should lead to a high index of suspicion include bullae, skin ecchymosis, skin necrosis, and edema outside of the area of erythema, as well as, sometimes, cutaneous anesthesia.[19]

Laboratory Values and Scoring Systems

Laboratory values and imaging have little to add to diagnosis when clinical suspicion of NSTI is high enough to warrant treatment. However, clinical features alone might be poorly sensitive for making a diagnosis of NSTI in equivocal cases. Additionally, the disease is rare enough that some practitioners may have limited experience with these severe infections and supplemental diagnostic assistance may be desirable to those less familiar with NSTI.[20] Notably, laboratory findings of leukocytosis and hyponatremia have been shown to improve sensitivity from clinical examination alone.[21] An admission lactate greater than 6 mmol/L and a serum sodium less than 135 mEq/L have been shown to be independent predictors of in-hospital mortality in those presenting with NSTI.[22] In 2004, Wong and colleagues[23] developed the Laboratory Risk Indicator for Necrotizing Fasciitis (LRINEC) score. White blood cell count, hemoglobin, sodium, glucose, serum creatinine, and serum C-reactive protein are used to score for the likelihood of necrotizing fasciitis. In the original publication, a score of equal to or greater than 6 yielded a positive predictive value of 92% and negative predictive value of 96%, displaying promise for predicting severity of skin and soft tissue infection among patients presenting to emergency care. Although retrospective validation of this scoring system has been attempted in small case-series,[24,25] a recent multicenter prospective evaluation of the LRINEC score has lessened the excitement around this predictive tool; a cut-off of greater or less than 6 in NSTI patients failed to discriminate between those with and without high cytokine levels, septic shock, and death.[26] Furthermore, the LRINEC score can be artificially elevated in other musculoskeletal infections. The Fournier's Gangrene Risk Index, although shown to be a predictor of outcome in retrospective studies, has not shown to be any better than the age-adjusted Charlson comorbidity index and remains of research interest alone.[27] As such, these scoring systems should not be solely relied on for diagnosing or excluding NSTI.

Imaging

Gas in the soft tissues on plain, portable radiographs, when seen, can aid in the diagnosis of NSTI in patients who are too unstable to travel for more advanced radiographic studies (**Fig. 2**). However, for those patients able to undergo computed tomography (CT) scan or MRI, both have been shown to be useful adjuncts for diagnosis when the diagnosis is not certain on clinical evaluation. A CT scan with contrast that demonstrates lack of enhancement of the fascia, along with involvement of the fascia in the infectious process, is more specific for NSTI than air or edema alone (**Fig. 3**).[28] In the case of MRI, imaging finding consistent with a diagnosis of NSTI includes greater thick signal intensity on T2-weighted images and focal nonenhancing

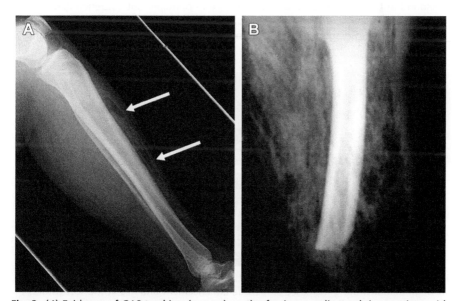

Fig. 2. (*A*) Evidence of GAS tracking (*arrows*) on the fascia on radiograph in a patient with NSTI involving the leg. (*B*) Subcutaneous emphysema on radiograph in a patient with NSTI of the thigh. ([A] *Data from* Chaudhry A, Baker K, Gould E, et al. Necrotizing fasciitis and it's mimics: what radiologists need to know. AJR 2015;204:128–39; and [B] *From* Sarani B, Strong M, Pascual J, et al. Necrotizing fasciitis: current concepts and review of the literature. JACS 2009;208(2):282; with permission.)

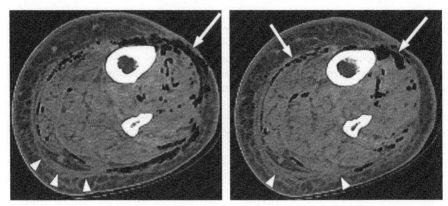

Fig. 3. Two Axial CT Images of the left lower extremity of a patient with necrotizing soft tissue infection, demonstrating edema in the soft tissues (*arrowheads*) and air tracking along the fascial planes (*arrows*). (*From* Chaudhry A, Baker K, Gould E, et al. Necrotizing fasciitis and it's mimics: what radiologists need to know. AJR 2015;204:133; with permission.)

areas of abnormal signal intensity in the deep fascia (**Fig. 4**). This is useful in distinguishing a necrotizing infection from a non-necrotizing infection in the case of nondiagnostic CT and plain radiograph findings, such as soft tissue swelling.[29] However, MRI can be overly sensitive as well as time consuming; it can certainly delay necessary surgical management and should be used with caution. Ultrasound can identify soft tissue abscesses in NSTI. The rapidity and portability of point-of-care ultrasound in the emergency room is attractive in principle but evidence is currently limited to sporadic reports and additional data are needed before it can be thought of as a mainstream diagnostic modality for NSTI.[30]

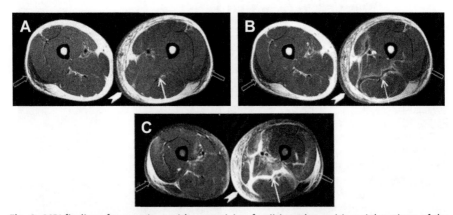

Fig. 4. MRI findings for a patient with necrotizing fasciitis and myositis: axial sections of the left thigh demonstrating increased soft tissue enhancement and gas in the soft tissues. T1 images (*A*) before and (*B*) after contrast injection where thick white arrows show thickening of skin and subcutaneous fat infiltration and with (*C*) Short TI Inversion Recovery (STIR) sequence where thin white arrows show thickening of the deep intermuscular fasciae and hollow arrows show stasis edema. (*Reproduced from* Malghem J, Lecouvet FE, Omoumi P, et al. Necrotizing fasciitis: contribution and limitations of diagnostic imaging. Joint Bone Spine 2013;80(2):146–54; with permission. Copyright © 2013.)

Bedside Exploration and Biopsy

The definitive diagnosis of NSTI is made surgically. A large number of equivocal cases exist in which additional evidence might be needed before the patient is taken for surgery. In such cases, before any formal operation, surgeons can assist in the bedside diagnosis of NSTI by performing a local exploration of the area under local anesthetic. Alternately, surgeons may proceed to the operating room where additional debridement can be immediately performed if NSTI is diagnosed on local exploration. In this case, a small incision is made over the area of maximal suspicion and the overlying soft tissue is divided. The fascia is examined locally for signs of necrosis: dishwater brown fluid or positive finger sign in which a finger inserted along the fascial planes easily dissects the overlying tissue without resistance.[31] Similarly, the underlying muscle tissue can be examined intraoperatively for evidence of necrosis. Electrocautery may be used in anesthetized patients without systemic paralytic therapy in place to demonstrate muscle fiber nonreactivity, which indicates tissue death. High organism density and worse clinics outcome have been suggested; albeit on univariate analyses alone.[1] Use of biopsy for frozen section analysis might aid in unequivocal cases; however, Infectious Disease Society of America (IDSA) guidelines caution against undue reliance due to potential false negatives from sampling error.[32,33]

TREATMENT

Any patient with evidence of septic shock should be treated in the critical care setting. The intensivist should maintain a high clinical suspicion and heighten the level of urgency among members of the care team at the point of initial patient contact so that all aspects of workup and treatment are expedited wherever possible. Once the diagnosis of NSTI is suspected, early consultation with a surgeon is warranted. Even in institutions with immediate surgical capabilities, however, a period of time will be spent evaluating the patient and preparing transport to the operating room, during which delivery of antibiotic therapy and supportive critical care must be expedited. In the case of a patient with systemic illness and shock, resuscitation is performed in a similar manner as is done for septic shock and initial management occurs simultaneous to the search for pathogen and source.

Antibiotic Therapy

Early and aggressive use of antibiotic therapy is essential and should be performed concomitant to the patient undergoing surgical evaluation and treatment. Blood cultures, and if possible, deep tissue, abscess, and/or operative cultures must be obtained promptly because these will help tailor antibiotic therapy. Antibiotic therapy for necrotizing infections in particular has not been studied in randomized controlled trials. Data for antibiotic treatment are extrapolated from proposed therapy for non-necrotizing complicated skin and soft tissue infections.

Initial empirical therapy should encompass a broad-spectrum coverage of polymicrobial infections because about half of these infections will be polymicrobial in nature.[33] This should include a MRSA-active agent, such as vancomycin, daptomycin, linezolid, or ceftaroline, as well as a broad-spectrum agent against gram-negative pathogens, such as piperacillin-tazobactam, ampicillin-sulbactam, ticarcillin-clavulanate, extended-spectrum cephalosporins, or carbapenems. If the selected regimen lacks anaerobic activity, an agent such as metronidazole or clindamycin must be added. More recently, a German study has suggested tigecycline as a possible single-agent therapy in patients previously colonized with resistant bacteria, such as patients who have been recently hospitalized or institutionalized[34]; however, such practice must be guided by local epidemiologic patterns. Similarly, empirical use of fluoroquinolones and ceftriaxone in areas with high prevalence of resistance to these agents among gram-negative bacteria must be avoided. Empirical antifungal therapy is not essential but an appropriate antifungal agent may be added on visual evidence on stains or growth in blood or operative cultures of fungal elements such as *Candida* or *Mucorales* spp.

Animal models have demonstrated greater efficacy with the clindamycin (a lincosamide antibiotic that works by inhibition of ribosomal translocation) compared with β-lactams in GAS infection; these findings were corroborated in 2 small retrospective cohort studies.[35,36] Notably, clindamycin may have multiple advantages over β-lactams, including an effect that is independent of inoculum size or infection stage, as well as potential antitoxin properties. In TSS, clindamycin is thought to mitigate the severity of shock by decreasing toxin production.[37] Although macrolide resistance in GAS remains low in the United States, it tends to be relatively higher among invasive strains of GAS; consequently, penicillins being universally active against GAS could offer coverage in clindamycin-resistant infections. Hence, the Surgical Infection Society and IDSA guidelines both strongly recommend combination therapy with penicillin and clindamycin in NSTI (with or without TSS) due to GAS.[33,38,39] Because the causative pathogen is not usually known up front, it is reasonable to add clindamycin to the empirical regimen for suspected NSTI. Like clindamycin, linezolid is also a protein synthesis inhibitor with potential toxin-inhibiting properties (particularly in the case of *S aureus* infection); however, no clinical studies to date have evaluated the clinical impact of this property of linezolid in NSTI.

After the organisms have been identified in the microbiology laboratory, therapy can usually be tailored further. The absence of growth of MRSA in cultures demonstrates a high negative predictive value and can facilitate discontinuation of the MRSA-active agent. For known or suspected *Vibrio* spp, NSTIs, doxycycline plus a third-generation cephalosporin is recommended, and combination therapy is key when a cell wall–inhibiting agent is used.[40] For known or suspected *Aeromonas* infections, doxycycline is recommended in combination with ciprofloxacin for community-acquired infections or cefepime for leech therapy–acquired infections, which have been reported to be resistant to ciprofloxacin.[41]

No clinical trials have evaluated duration of therapy in NSTI. Guidelines suggest continuation of appropriate antibiotics for a minimum of 48 to 72 hours after resolution of fever and other systemic signs of infection, as well as hemodynamic stabilization. Please refer to IDSA practice guidelines for skin and soft tissue infections for additional details on antibiotic therapy for NSTI.[33]

Surgical Intervention

Although antibiotic therapy, resuscitation and critical care evaluation are necessary in the treatment of patients presenting with NSTIs, the mainstay of therapy remains surgical treatment. **Fig. 5** shows a proposed management pathway in NSTI. Multiple large studies cite the need for early and aggressive debridement in NSTIs, and claim it as the single most important treatment intervention for this disease process, although no randomized controlled trial has studied the timing or extent of surgical therapy or clearly defined an adequate debridement.[42–45] Delay in the identification or early surgical management of these infections clearly increases mortality.[45] In addition, recent data suggest that delay not only increases mortality but, in survivors, also increases the number of subsequent operations needed to control the infection.[46] Increased number of operations may increase the total tissue loss from the disease process because more tissue is removed with each operation and, therefore, limit functional recovery because more muscle and, possibly, critical structures such as nerves are

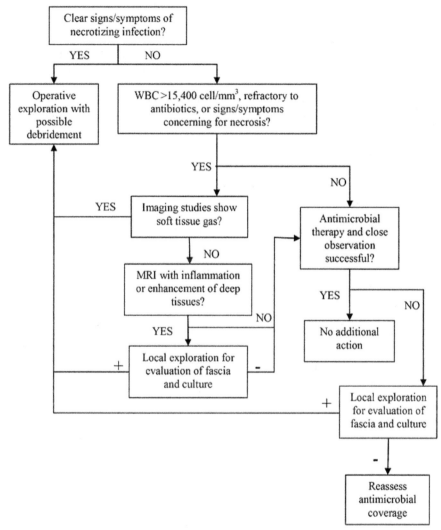

Fig. 5. Management pathway in NSTI. WBC, white blood cell. (*From* Burnham JP, Kriby JP, Kollef MH. Diagnosis and management of skin and soft tissue infections in the intensive care unit: a review. Intensive Care Med 2016;42:1904; with permission.)

sacrificed. There is also associated increased cost with each subsequent operation. Early identification and aggressive treatment, therefore, remains critical in the treatment of these infections.[47] Time to surgical debridement has been demonstrated as an independent predictor of improved outcome in large studies.[18,42] In another study, the presence of a 24-hour in-house emergency general surgical team provided both the expertise and expeditious treatment needed to reduce time to operation and improve mortality.[48] Although this was an isolated single-center experience, it underscores the importance of early surgical evaluation and advocates for widespread emergency surgical capability or early transfer to a facility with these capabilities.

Despite being a mainstay of therapy for this infection, no study has defined what an adequate debridement is, although typical training dictates that all necrotic tissue should be removed. Debridement, therefore, remains at the discretion of the operating surgeon.[43] Many studies refer to aggressive debridement without objectively quantifying the term. It is, however, well demonstrated that wounds should be frequently re-evaluated, typically with re-exploration in the operating room within 24 to 48 hours of the initial debridement procedure. The return to the operating room is intended for re-evaluation of the wound, debridement of any further necrotic tissue, confirming the absence of progression, and to facilitate dressing changes. The average number of debridement procedures is 3 to 4 before further dressing changes are performed at the bedside.[18,42,46]

In the case of wide or disfiguring debridements, involvement of additional teams, including urology for perineal wounds or wounds involving the penis or scrotum, plastic surgery for complex reconstruction or muscle flap reconstruction, or orthopedics for bony involvement, may be necessary. In the case of perineal wounds, it may be necessary to divert the fecal stream away from the area of contamination with a loop colostomy.[49] Amputations may be necessary in the case of diabetic foot infections or larger scale debridements of entire muscle compartments, resulting in a nonfunctioning limb. Reconstruction with rotational flaps or skin graft techniques may be necessary and warrant early intervention and comanagement with plastic surgery. Widespread use of vacuum-assisted closure devices provides consistent and easy nursing care, suctioning of soft tissue edema, and promoting granulation tissue.[50] Newer vacuum-assisted closure products are accompanied by continuous wound irrigation, which may be beneficial in wounds from debridement of NSTI.[51] Negative pressure dressings can provide dermatotraction to limit the wound size and facilitate closure.[52] In the case of complex and repeated reconstructive surgeries, rehabilitation, physical therapy, or occupational therapy may be necessary and treatment courses can be significantly life-altering and prolonged.

The impact of early transfer versus on-site initial debridement in NSTI has not been systematically investigated in a clinical trial and, as such, is difficult to decipher retrospectively. Initial resuscitation, initial debridement (when available), and control of the infectious process must be prioritized at the presenting hospital. Often, however, the decision of when to operate and when to transfer is complex and must be made carefully, taking into account clinical severity and institutional capabilities. Institutional factors that might prompt transfer include the lack of an intensive care unit; the lack of availability of advanced services, such as continuous renal replacement therapy, large volume blood transfusion, or on-call surgical staff; and the need for complex reconstruction techniques that may not be available at certain hospitals.

Adjuvant Therapies

The 2 most common adjunctive medical treatments discussed for NSTIs include intravenous immune globulin and hyperbaric oxygen. Intravenous immunoglobulin has been suggested as a treatment of superantigen-mediated TSS due to streptococcal[53] or staphylococcal necrotizing fasciitis.[54] The proposed mechanism of action is that IVIG binds and inactivates circulating superantigens, thereby blunting the superantigen-mediated cytokine cascade. Initial retrospective studies demonstrated some promise but a randomized controlled trial on the subject was terminated early and lacked sufficient power to detect a survival benefit.[55] A subsequent pediatric study also demonstrated no benefit of IVIG therapy.[56] Additionally, the cost associated with the treatment is high. In 2016, Kadri and colleagues[57] reported findings of a propensity-matched analysis of administrative data from 130 US hospitals evaluating the role of adjunctive IVIG in NSTI and validated administrative data algorithms against clinical data from 4 hospitals. There was no clinical benefit to IVIG therapy observed, regardless of timing of treatment. Also, not surprisingly, IVIG was found to be used rather sporadically at 4%. In 2017, the Immunoglobulin G for Patients with Necrotizing Soft Tissue Infection (INSTINCT) study, a Danish multicenter randomized controlled trial also evaluating the adjunctive potential of 3 days of IVIG therapy in NSTI found no benefit of the same on physical functioning or survival at 6-months.[58] Plasmapheresis, in principle, could remove circulating inflammatory mediators and potentially decrease the host's intrinsic inflammatory response, lessening the severity of vasodilatory shock. However, the data supporting this strategy remain anecdotal.[59]

Hyperbaric oxygen has been proposed as an adjunctive therapy after surgical debridement for NSTI.[60] The fascia is known to be a relatively hypoxic environment owing to its tenuous blood supply when compared with surrounding muscle or skin. By increasing plasma dissolved oxygen concentration, hyperbaric oxygen is believed to potentially enhance oxygen delivery to hypoxic tissues surrounding areas of necrosis, directly killing anaerobic bacteria and improving leukocyte activity.[61] This proposed mechanism has led to a series of retrospective studies, with some showing decreased mortality and others showing no effect.[60,62] These studies are not compelling to recommend hyperbaric therapy. Furthermore, the greatest barrier to practical use of this modality in NSTI is the limited number of centers nationwide with hyperbaric chambers where critically ill patients can be adequately monitored. In summary, despite theoretic benefits, no prospective literature exists to support use as adjuvant therapy and society guidelines to do not recommend routine use in these infections.[17]

SUMMARY

In summary, NSTI remains a disease with high morbidity and mortality, despite improvements in care. In the past several decades, understanding of this disease process has improved such that it is known that early diagnosis, along with rapid aggressive treatment with broad spectrum antimicrobial treatment and wide surgical debridement, are necessary to effectively treat this disease process. Adjunctive therapies have been explored and found to be largely ineffective and are not routinely recommended. More recently, differences in the timing of antibiotic therapy administration has been observed between high-volume and low-volume centers for the treatment of necrotizing fasciitis, and suggests that differences in care may exist between centers with high-volume care of this disease.[1] If indeed, patients must be identified early, treated expeditiously, and supported with the best available critical care, then perhaps further advances in the care of this disease will be less about finding a better treatment modality. It may be that improving the systems that bring patients to the attention and care of appropriate clinicians will be the intervention that moves the needle on the burden of this disease.

REFERENCES

1. Faraklas I, Yang D, Eggerstedt M, et al. A multi-center review of care patterns and outcomes in necrotizing soft tissue infections. Surg Infect (Larchmt) 2016;17(6): 773–8.
2. Wilson B. Necrotizing fasciitis. Am Surg 1952;18:416–31.
3. Nelson GE, Pondo T, Toews KA, et al. Epidemiology of invasive group A streptococcal infections in the United States, 2005-2012. Clin Infect Dis 2016;63(4): 478–86.
4. Yilmazlar T, Ozturk E, Alsoy A, et al. Necrotizing soft tissue infections: APACHE II score, dissemination, and survival. World J Surg 2007;31:1858–62.
5. Miller AT, Saadai P, Greenstein A, et al. Postprocedural necrotizing fasciitis: A 10-year retrospective review. Am Surg 2008;74:405–9.

6. Lee TC, Carrick MM, Scott BG, et al. Incidence and clinical characteristics of methicillin-resistant *Staphylococcus aureus* necrotizing fasciitis in a large urban hospital. Am J Surg 2007;194:809–12.

7. Hefny AF, Eid HO, Al Hussona M, et al. Necrotizing fasciitis: a challenging diagnosis. Eur J Emerg Med 2007;14:50–2.

8. Childers BJ, Potyondy LD, Nachreiner R, et al. Necrotizing fasciitis: a fourteen-year retrospective study of 163 consecutive patients. Am Surg 2002;68:109–16.

9. Giuliano A, Lewis F, Hadley K, et al. Bacteriology of necrotizing fasciitis. Am J Surg 1977;134:52–7.

10. Sartor C, Limouzin-Perotti F, Legré R, et al. Nosocomial infections with *Aeromonas hydrophila* from leeches. Clin Infect Dis 2002;35(1):E1–5.

11. Miller LG, Perdreau-Remington F, Rieg G, et al. Necrotizing fasciitis caused by community-associated methicillin-resistant *Staphylococcus aureus* in Los Angeles. N Engl J Med 2005;352(14):1445–53.

12. Cheng NC, Yu YC, Tai HC, et al. Recent trend of necrotizing fasciitis in Taiwan: focus on monomicrobial *Klebsiella pneumonia* necrotizing fasciitis. Clin Infect Dis 2012;55(7):930–9.

13. Anaya DA, McMahon K, Nathens AB, et al. Predictors of mortality and limb loss in necrotizing soft tissue infections. Arch Surg 2005;140(2):151–7.

14. Bryant AE, Bayer CR, Huntinton JD, et al. Group A streptococcal myonecrosis: increased vimentin expression after skeletal-muscle injury mediates the binding of *Streptococcus pyogenes*. J Infect Dis 2006;193(12):1685–92.

15. Bohach GA, Fast DJ, Nelson RD, et al. Staphylococcal and streptococcal pyrogenic toxins involved in toxic shock syndrome and related illnesses. Crit Rev Microbiol 1990;17:251–72.

16. Darenberg J, Luca-Harari B, Jasir A, et al. Molecular and clinical characteristics of invasive group A streptococcal infection in Sweden. Clin Infect Dis 2007;45(4):450–8.

17. Stevens DL, Bisno AL, Chambers HF, et al. Practice guidelines for the diagnosis and management of skin and soft-tissue infections. Clin Infect Dis 2005;41:1373–406.

18. Elliott DC, Kufera JA, Myers RA. Necrotizing soft tissue infections: risk factors for mortality and strategies for management. Ann Surg 1996;224:672–83.

19. Wall DB, de Virgilio C, Black S, et al. Objective criteria may assist in distinguishing necrotizing fasciitis from nonnecrotizing soft tissue infection. Am J Surg 2000;179:17–21.

20. Anaya DA, Dellinger EP. Necrotizing soft-tissue infection: diagnosis and management. Clin Infect Dis 2007;44:705–10.

21. Chan T, Yaghoubian A, Rosing D, et al. Low sensitivity of physical examination findings in necrotizing soft tissue infection is improved with laboratory values: a prospective study. Am J Surg 2008;196(6):926–30.

22. Yaghoubian A, de Virgilio C, Dauphine C, et al. Use of admission serum lactate and sodium levels to predict mortality in necrotizing soft-tissue infections. Arch Surg 2007;142(9):840–6.

23. Wong CH, Khin LW, Heng KS, et al. The LRINEC (Laboratory Risk Indicator for Necrotizing Fasciitis) score: a tool for distinguishing necrotizing fasciitis from other soft tissue infections. Crit Care Med 2004;32(7):1535–41.

24. Kincius M, Telksnys T, Trumbeckas D, et al. Evaluation of LRINEC scale feasibility for predicting outcomes of Fournier gangrene. Surg Infect (Larchmt) 2016;17(4):448–53.

25. Chao WN, Tsai SJ, Tsai CF, et al. The laboratory risk indicator for necrotizing fasciitis score for discernment of necrotizing fasciitis originated from *Vibrio vulnificus* infections. J Trauma Acute Care Surg 2012;73(6):1576–82.

26. Hansen MB, Rasmussen LS, Svensson M, et al. Association between cytokine response, the LRINEC score and outcome in patients with necrotizing soft tissue infection: a multicentre, prospective study. Sci Rep 2017;7:42179.

27. Roghmann F, von Bodman C, Loppenberg B, et al. Is there a need for the Fournier's gangrene severity index? Comparison of scoring systems for outcome prediction in patients with Fournier's gangrene. BJU Int 2012;110(9):1359–65.

28. Carbonetti F, Cremona A, Carusi V, et al. The role of contrast enhanced computed tomography in the diagnosis of necrotizing fasciitis and comparison with the laboratory risk indicator for necrotizing fasciitis (LRINEC). Radiol Med 2016;121(2):106–21.

29. Kim KT, Kim YJ, Won Lee J, et al. Can necrotizing infectious fasciitis be differentiated from nonnecrotizing infectious fasciitis with MR imaging? Radiology 2011;259(3):816–24.

30. Kehrl T. Point-of-care ultrasound diagnosis of necrotizing fasciitis missed by computed tomography and magnetic resonance imaging. J Emerg Med 2014;47(2):172–5.

31. Green RJ, Dafoe DC, Raffin TA. Necrotizing fasciitis. Chest 1996;110:219–29.

32. Hietbrink F, Bode LG, Riddez L, et al. Triple diagnostics for early detection of ambivalent necrotizing fasciitis. World J Emerg Surg 2016;11:51.

33. Stevens DL, Bisno AL, Chambers HF, et al. Practice guidelines for the diagnosis and management of skin and soft tissue infections: 2014 update by the Infectious Diseases Society of America. Clin Infect Dis 2014;59:147–59.

34. Eckmann C, Heizmann W, Bodmann KF, et al. Tigecycline in the treatment of necrotizing soft tissue infections due to multiresistant bacteria. Surg Infect (Larchmt) 2015;16:618–25.

35. Zimbelman J, Palmer A, Todd J. Improved outcome of clindamycin compared with beta-lactam antibiotic treatment for invasive *Streptococcus pyogenes* infection. Pedatr Infect Dis J 1999;18(12):1096–100.

36. Mulla ZD, Leaverton PE, Wiersma ST. Invasive group A Streptococcal infections in Florida. South Med J 2003;96(10):968–73.

37. Bernardo K, Pakulat N, Fleer S, et al. Subinhibitory concentrations of linezolid reduce *Staphylococcus aureus* virulence factor expression. Antimicrob Agents Chemother 2004;48:546–55.

38. Gemmell CG, Ford CW. Virulence factor expression by gram-positive cocci exposed to subinhibitory concentrations of linezolid. J Antimicrob Chemother 2002;50:665–72.

39. May AK, Stafford RE, Bulger EM, et al, Surgical Infection Society. Treatment of complicated skin and soft tissue infections. Surg Infect (Larchmt) 2009;10(5):467–99.

40. Zanetti S, Spanu T, Deriu A, et al. In vitro susceptibility of *Vibrio* spp. isolated from the environment. Int J Antimicrob Agents 2001;17:407–9.

41. Aravena-Román M, Inglis TJ, Henderson B, et al. Antimicrobial susceptibilities of *Aeromonas* strains isolated from clinical and environmental sources to 26 antimicrobial agents. Antimicrob Agents Chemother 2012;56(2):1110–2.

42. McHenry CR, Piotrowski JJ, Petrinic D, et al. Determinants of mortality for necrotizing soft-tissue infections. Ann Surg 1995;221:558–63.

43. Sudarsky LA, Laschinger JC, Coppa GF, et al. Improved results from a standardized approach in treating patients with necrotizing fasciitis. Ann Surg 1987;206: 661–5.
44. Tillou A, St Hill CR, Brown C, et al. Necrotizing soft tissue infections: improved outcomes with modern care. Am Surg 2004;70:841–4.
45. Bilton BD, Zibari GB, McMillan RW, et al. Aggressive surgical management of necrotizing fasciitis serves to decrease mortality: a retrospective study. Am Surg 1998;64:397–400.
46. Kobayashi L, Konstantinidis A, Shackelford S, et al. Necrotizing soft tissue infections: delayed surgical treatment is associated with increased number of surgical debridements and morbidity. J Trauma 2011;71(5):1400–5.
47. Sartelli M, Malangoni MA, May AK, et al. World Society of Emergency Surgery (WSES) guidelines for the management of skin and soft tissue infections. World J Emerg Surg 2014;9:57.
48. Gunter OL, Guillamondegui OD, May AK, et al. Outcome of necrotizing skin and soft tissue infections. Surg Infect 2008;9:443–50.
49. Kilic A, Aksoy Y, Kilic L. Fournier's gangrene: etiology, treatment, and complications. Ann Plast Surg 2001;47:523–7.
50. Czymek R, Schmidt A, Eckmann C, et al. Fournier's gangrene: vacuum-assisted closure versus conventional dressings. Am J Surg 2009;197:168–76.
51. Kiyokawa K, Takahashi N, Rikimaru H, et al. New continuous negative-pressure and irrigation treatment for infected wounds and intractable ulcers. Plast Reconstr Surg 2007;120(5):1257–65.
52. Lee JY, Jung H, Kwon H, et al. Extended negative pressure wound therapy-assisted dermatotraction for the closure of large open fasciotomy wounds in necrotizing faciitis patients. World J Emerg Surg 2014;9:29–39.
53. Linnér A, Darenberg J, Sjölin J, et al. Clinical efficacy of polyspecific intravenous immunoglobulin therapy in patients with streptococcal toxic shock syndrome: a comparative observational study. Clin Infect Dis 2014;59(6): 851–7.
54. Darenberg J, Söderquist B, Normark BH, et al. Differences in potency of intravenous polyspecific immunoglobulin G against streptococcal and staphylococcal superantigens: implications for therapy of toxic shock syndrome. Clin Infect Dis 2004;38(6):836–42.
55. Darenberg J, Ihendyane N, Sjolin J, et al. Intravenous immunoglobulin G therapy in streptococcal toxic shock syndrome: a European randomized, double-blind, placebo-controlled trial. Clin Infect Dis 2003;37:333–40.
56. Shah SS, Hall M, Srivastava R, et al. Intravenous immunoglobulin in children with streptococcal toxic shock syndrome. Clin Infect Dis 2009;49:1369–76.
57. Kadri SS, Swihart BJ, Bonne SL, et al. Impact of intravenous immunoglobulin on survival in necrotizing fasciitis with vasopressor-dependent shock: a propensity-score matched analysis from 130 US hospitals. Clin Infect Dis 2016;64(7): 877–85.
58. Madsen MB, Hjortrup PB, Hansen MB, et al. Immunoglobulin G for patients with necrotizing soft tissue infection (INSTINCT): a randomized, blinded, placebo-controlled trial. Intensive Care Med 2017. [Epub ahead of print].
59. Kyles DM, Baltimore J. Adjunctive use of plasmapheresis and intravenous immunoglobulin therapy in sepsis: A case report. Am J Crit Care 2005;14:109–12.
60. Shupak A, Shoshani O, Goldenberg I, et al. Necrotizing fasciitis: An indication for hyperbaric oxygenation therapy? Surgery 1995;118:873–8.

61. Jallali N, Withey S, Butler PE. Hyperbaric oxygen as adjuvant therapy in the management of necrotizing fasciitis. Am J Surg 2005;189:462–6.
62. Riseman JA, Zamboni WA, Curtis A, et al. Hyperbaric oxygen therapy for necrotizing fasciitis reduces mortality and the need for debridements. Surgery 1990; 108:847–50.

Antimicrobial Stewardship Approaches in the Intensive Care Unit

Sarah B. Doernberg, MD, MAS[a],*, Henry F. Chambers, MD[b]

KEYWORDS

- Antimicrobial stewardship • Antibacterial resistance • Rapid diagnostics
- *Clostridium difficile* infection • Prospective audit and feedback
- Formulary restriction • Computerized decision support

KEY POINTS

- Antibiotic resistance is a major and growing problem, and antimicrobials are a limited resource. Antimicrobial stewardship is an approach to improving and monitoring the use of existing antimicrobials.
- The intensive care unit (ICU) is a unique and high-stakes setting for antimicrobial use that presents distinct challenges for antimicrobial stewardship programs. This article outlines approaches to antimicrobial stewardship with a focus on the ICU setting.
- Opportunities for antimicrobial stewardship exist during the diagnosis, empirical treatment, and definitive antimicrobial choice. General approaches and ICU-specific application are discussed.
- Both process and outcome measures should be monitored as antimicrobial stewardship initiatives are implemented in the ICU to demonstrate effectiveness and ensure safety.

CASE PRESENTATIONS

- A 75-year-old man who underwent a Whipple procedure for pancreatic cancer 1 month prior with a rocky postoperative course, including respiratory failure, shock, upper gastrointestinal bleed, and surgical site infection, develops a new fever, need for reintubation, and pressor requirement. Blood and urine cultures are negative and chest radiograph demonstrates bilateral infiltrates, stable

Disclosure Statement: SBD has received research funding from Merck, Genentech, Cerexa, and Cubist Pharmaceuticals and serves as a consultant to Actelion. HFC has received grant support from Allergan and Genentech.
[a] Division of Infectious Diseases, Department of Medicine, University of California, 513 Parnassus Avenue, Box 0654, San Francisco, CA 94143, USA; [b] Division of Infectious Diseases, Department of Medicine, Zuckerberg San Francisco General Hospital, University of California, Room 3400, Building 30, 1001 Potrero Avenue, San Francisco, CA 94110, USA
* Corresponding author.
E-mail address: sarah.doernberg@ucsf.edu

from prior. How should this patient's antibiotics be managed initially? What tests are useful to help direct therapy? What antibiotic stewardship strategies are helpful in this situation?

- A 19-year-old trauma patient is admitted with multiple fractures and a subarachnoid hemorrhage, now has a fever 4 days after admission. How does one determine whether this patient has an infectious cause for fever? Does this patient need antibiotics?
- A 60-year-old lung transplant recipient is admitted from the community with septic shock. How can one rapidly determine the cause? When is it safe to deescalate antibiotics? When can antibiotics be stopped?

BACKGROUND

More than 2 million illnesses and 23,000 deaths occur each year in the United States due to infections caused by antimicrobial-resistant pathogens, a large burden of which occur in the intensive care unit (ICU) setting.[1,2] Since the discovery of penicillin, there has been a clear temporal relationship between the introduction of antibiotics into clinical practice and development of resistance.[3] Though the antibiotic pipeline has improved in recent years, new drugs have not kept pace with threatening antibiotic-resistant organisms.[4–6] Antimicrobial stewardship has emerged as a strategy to preserve existing drugs, as well as newly developed drugs, so that these remain effective.

Antimicrobial stewardship refers to an organized program designed to monitor, improve, and measure the responsible use of antibiotics.[7] Though there are many approaches to antimicrobial stewardship, fundamental strategies include development and implementation of facility-specific treatment guidelines, restriction of certain types of high-risk antibiotics, and review of antibiotic therapy by an infectious disease (ID) expert (physician or pharmacist) with feedback to providers.[8] These programs are often led by an interdisciplinary team composed of an ID and/or stewardship-trained physician and pharmacist, who oversee the core actions, monitor antibiotic use, and provide education for their facility in conjunction with key stakeholders, including clinicians, the microbiology laboratory, hospital infection control, information technology (IT), quality groups, and executive leadership. First described as far back as the 1970s, antimicrobial stewardship has grown immensely in past years due to a combination of increasing attention to patient safety, increasing reports of antibiotic resistance, and regulatory mandates.[9–12] The underlying goal for stewardship programs is to improve clinical outcomes in individual patients, through improved treatment of infection and prevention of adverse events, while limiting selective pressure for antimicrobial resistance for the population as a whole and, to the extent possible, decreasing costs.

The ICU is a unique and high-stakes setting for antimicrobial use. Antimicrobial resistance rates are high, resulting in poor clinical outcomes and high cost.[2,13] Inadequate initial antimicrobial therapy in the ICU setting is associated with worse outcomes, which given the prevalence of antimicrobial resistance often results in use of very broad-spectrum agents in critically ill patients, even when risk factors for resistance are not present.[14–17] On the flip side, inappropriate antimicrobial therapy accounts for approximately 30% of prescriptions in the ICU setting, most frequently for treatment of colonization or contamination, treatment of noninfectious or viral infections, or too-long or too-broad treatment.[18,19] The combination of the acuity of illness in the ICU setting mixed with the high stakes of inadequate initial therapy can push providers to use antibiotics in inappropriate ways, such as treatment of community-acquired infections or organisms with very low likelihood of resistance with overly broad-spectrum agents.[20]

The goal of this review article is to provide an overview of strategies and opportunities for stewardship in the ICU setting, from the diagnosis and empirical therapy for suspected infection to management of confirmed and documented infection. Although it touches on core elements of stewardship in general, the focus is on applications specific to the ICU setting.

GENERAL ANTIMICROBIAL STEWARDSHIP APPROACHES

Basic elements of antimicrobial stewardship programs (ASPs) include having a dedicated institutional policy, an interdisciplinary team, members (ideally both MD and PharmD degrees) with training in antimicrobial stewardship or ID, and monitoring and reporting of activities (**Fig. 1**). Core actions of ASPs include[7,8]

- Facility-specific guidelines based on national guidelines, local antibiogram, and formulary availability. These can be for particular syndromes such as pneumonia, individual infections such as *Clostridium difficile*, or based on certain antimicrobials such as guidance on appropriate vancomycin use.
- Prior authorization or restricted formulary (eg, restrictive program): Requirement that approval is given by the ASP team before release of an antimicrobial. Restricted agents are generally chosen based on spectrum, cost, and risks of side effects such as nephrotoxicity.
- Prospective audit and feedback (PAF; eg, persuasive program): Review of patients on antimicrobials by the ASP with feedback to providers recommending changes or discontinuation if appropriate. For larger facilities where comprehensive review is impractical, criteria for review can include specific units, certain targeted antimicrobials, or selected diagnoses.
- Automatic stop orders: Having a set date for discontinuation of antimicrobials that would require an additional order for the drug to be continued.

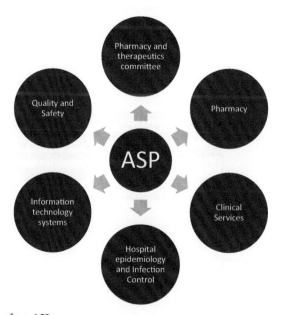

Fig. 1. Structure of an ASP.

- Antibiotic time-out: A prompt to providers to review antimicrobial use at a certain time point after initiation (generally 48 hours) to assess diagnostic test results, need for ongoing treatment, and appropriate choice of agent.
- Automatic pharmacy interventions to improve antibiotic use and safety: Interventions include intravenous to oral conversions, dose adjustment for renal dysfunction, therapeutic drug monitoring, pharmacodynamic or pharmacokinetic optimization, and notification of duplicative agents or agents with drug interactions.
- Education to providers on antimicrobial use and stewardship principles.
- Though not generally considered a core stewardship activity, embedding an ASP physician or pharmacist on rounds or requiring routine consultation in ICU patients started on antimicrobials are other approaches that have been reported in the literature.[21–23]
- Integration of IT into these activities or use of IT to aid with stewardship is another emerging field that is likely to gain increasing attention.

These approaches to stewardship can be tailored to the institution and the phase of care, and data of varying quality exist to support each approach. See later discussion of application of these general approaches to the ICU setting. This discussion is framed around the natural phases of suspected infection, from diagnostic testing to empirical therapy to definitive therapy (**Fig. 2**).

DIAGNOSIS

As a corollary to the common use of inappropriate antimicrobial therapy in the ICU setting for noninfectious or nonbacterial syndromes, or treatment of colonization or contamination, more accurate and timely diagnosis of infection should result in improved antimicrobial use.[18,19] Goals of diagnostics for infection include

- Establishing an infection as the cause of the presenting syndrome; discrimination of bacterial infection from noninfectious syndrome
- Discrimination of bacterial from nonbacterial infections
- Rapidly identifying a microbial pathogen, if present, to direct therapy
- Providing timely information about drug susceptibility of the pathogen.

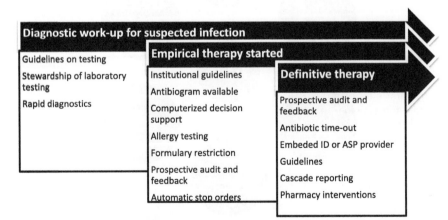

Fig. 2. Opportunities for antimicrobial stewardship interventions.

Currently available approaches that fulfill some of these goals include markers of bacterial infection, including biomarkers such as procalcitonin, and characterization of the host immune response, as well as rapid identification of bacteria or other pathogens from clinical samples.

Host Response to Infection

For a deeper discussion of procalcitonin in the ICU setting. (See David N. Gilbert's article, "Role of Procalcitonin in the Management of Infected ICU Patients," in this issue.) The bottom line for this biomarker is that it generally does not decrease initiation of antibiotics in the ICU but can help with de-escalation and discontinuation of therapy.[24,25] Identification of a host immune genetic expression (eg, transcriptome) to identify specific responses to bacterial infections has been another recent promising focus of investigation, though the application of these classifiers to clinical care needs further study.[26–29] In particular, whether the good but imperfect sensitivity will be enough to confidently allow for discontinuation of antimicrobials in the critically ill and improve outcomes in a real-world setting remains unclear. As precision medicine and molecular diagnostics are introduced into clinical practice, there will likely be refinements and advances in use of host biomarkers and protein and gene expression to discriminate bacterial infections from nonbacterial infections and noninfectious syndromes.

Discussion of utility of combinations of clinical markers or scoring systems (eg, clinical pulmonary infection score [CPIS]) for accurate diagnosis of infection is beyond the scope of this article, but there is significant literature regarding this topic.[30–34] For instance, the CPIS has been studied as a tool for antimicrobial stewardship in the setting of suspected ventilator-associated infection (VAP) and was shown to decrease antibiotic duration by more than 6 days without adverse clinical consequences.[35] Commentators note, however, that in the absence of a CPIS scoring system, clinical judgment of patients with suspected VAP by the ASP provider might accomplish the same outcomes.[33]

The Role of Traditional Microbiology Testing

Before launching into further discussion of advanced molecular methods for diagnosis of microbes, a review of the utility of traditional clinical laboratory and microbiology testing is important. Traditional testing includes

- Gram stain and culture of various specimen sites
- Urinalysis (UA) and urine microscopy
- Cellular analysis of bodily fluids (eg, bronchoalveolar lavage fluid, cerebrospinal fluid, ascitic fluid)
- In vitro drug susceptibility testing through disk diffusion testing, antimicrobial gradient methods, or broth microdilution, including automated systems.

The first step of analysis of a clinical culture is performance of a Gram stain to identify the staining pattern and shape of the bacteria, if present, which can help to direct therapy. Particularly from respiratory specimens, Gram stains have the potential to aid in decision-making about antibiotic therapy. VAP is a good example of the utility of a negative Gram stain. Without a gold standard, VAP is a notoriously difficult diagnosis to make.[36] Although a positive respiratory Gram stain or culture needs to be interpreted with caution given the strong possibility of colonization, a negative Gram stain from an invasively obtained sputum culture was found to have a negative predictive value of 91% in the setting of a VAP prevalence of 20% to 30% and thus can be useful in the decision to stop antibiotics.[37] A positive

Gram stain, on the other hand, has only fair concordance with culture and poor positive predictive value, making this a poor test to use for clinical decision-making in general.[37,38]

Identification of a pathogen from a clinical specimen from the ICU can take between 48 and 96 hours, and susceptibility testing generally takes another 48 to 72 hours. Thus, by the time full susceptibility is available, patients have often been on empirical therapy for several days. In a multicenter point prevalence study of empirical antimicrobial use in the ICU, 50% of subjects were still on empirical therapy (ie, did not meet definitions for confirmed infection with directed therapy) at 72 hours, reflecting at least in part the delay in confirmation of infection.[39] In another multicenter study of subjects in the ICU with suspected nosocomial infections, antibiotics were continued for at least 72 hours in 69% of subjects and 5 days in 59% of subjects with negative cultures.[40] Despite the trends suggesting that prolonged empirical therapy is common, small studies suggest that stopping antibiotics in ICU patients with suspected pneumonia and negative cultures, even at 24 to 48 hours, can be safe.[41,42]

A negative UA can be useful in the decision not to send a urine culture and/or treat for possible urinary tract infection (UTI).[43] Although the UA has a poor positive predictive value for true UTI, especially in catheterized patients, a negative UA has been shown to have 100% negative predictive value in the febrile trauma ICU patient, though the utility of a negative UA is controversial in some populations.[44,45] Epstein and colleagues[46] report an interrupted time-series analysis of an ICU intervention at their institution that mandated a positive UA (defined as >10 white blood cells per high-powered field) before urine culture performance, though oncology and transplant patients were excluded and providers could override. Although they did not examine antimicrobial use, they did find a significant decrease in urine culture rate, which could reduce inappropriate treatment of asymptomatic bacteriuria. Further studies are needed to determine whether decreasing reporting of positive urine cultures in the setting of likely asymptomatic bacteriuria (eg, with negative UA) affects antibiotic use.

The way in which microbiology tests are reported can also affect antimicrobial use. One common approach, known as cascade or selective reporting, involves releasing susceptibility information for broad-spectrum antibiotics to clinicians only when there is resistance to more narrow-spectrum agents. The Infectious Diseases Society of America (IDSA) supports this practice, and the Clinical and Laboratory Standards Institute provides guidance on how to actually perform the reporting.[7] There are limited data supporting use of cascade reporting in the inpatient setting. In 1 health system that implemented cascade reporting for Enterobacteriaceae, there was a decrease in the use of anti-pseudomonal beta-lactams for definitive treatment of cefazolin-susceptible organisms isolated from blood cultures from 26% to 0% of cases in a population made up of 23% ICU patients.[47] Interestingly, this improvement in appropriate de-escalation occurred in the setting of a very high rate of ID consultation: 81% in the baseline group. At another hospital implementing cascade reporting for gram-negative bacilli, there were notable decreases in resistance of *Enterobacter* and *Proteus* species to third-generation cephalosporins coupled with changes in antimicrobial usage and decreased *C difficile* rates, though resistance to other antibiotics paradoxically increased over time.[48] Still another group reported inappropriate use of rifamycins for primary treatment of staphylococcal infections after their laboratory began reporting susceptibilities to these drugs routinely, underscoring the importance of continued surveillance for unintended consequences of changes in laboratory reporting.[49]

Coupling of antimicrobial stewardship interventions to specific culture results has also been shown to improve antimicrobial use and clinical outcomes.[7] Several studies examining routine antimicrobial stewardship program (ASP) review of positive blood cultures coupled with bundled interventions have demonstrated improvements in appropriate antibiotic use as well as clinical benefit, including decreased mortality.[50–52] These studies highlight the importance of expert guidance in treatment of serious infectious syndromes, many of which are managed in the ICU setting.

Rapid Microbial Identification and Susceptibility Testing

Because the turnaround time for traditional microbiology testing is on the order of days, there has been significant interest in and focus on more rapid diagnostic testing for pathogen identification and drug susceptibility information. More rapid information can lead to more rapid and appropriate antibiotic decisions, which can result in improved clinical outcomes and decreased antibiotic use. In recent years, many rapid test methods have emerged, including[53]

- Nucleic acid amplification tests, such as multiplex polymerase chain reaction (PCR) for respiratory viruses and real-time PCR to detect genes for vancomycin-resistant enterococci (VRE), methicillin-resistant *Staphylococcus aureus* (MRSA), and beta-lactamase producing gram-negative rods from positive cultures
- Latex agglutination testing for penicillin-binding protein 2a for detection of MRSA directly from culture
- Matrix-associated laser desorption or ionization time-of-flight mass spectrometry, which can rapidly identify organisms and also may be able to detect resistance
- Rapid detection of bacterial cell lysis after incubation with an antibiotic
- Whole-genome sequencing.

The IDSA recommends use of rapid diagnostic testing in combination with support in interpretation by an ASP and use of rapid viral testing for respiratory pathogens.[7] (See James M. Walter and Richard G. Wunderink's article, "Severe Respiratory Viral Infections: New Evidence and Changing Paradigms," in this issue.) Several studies have demonstrated that antimicrobial stewardship enhances the benefits of rapid diagnostics. For instance, in a study of rapid multiplex PCR testing of positive blood cultures, Banerjee and colleagues[54] demonstrated that 24% of subjects in the rapid testing plus stewardship arm had de-escalation of therapy compared with only 15% in the rapid testing alone group and 12% in the control group. Interestingly, the involvement of the stewardship team mainly affected time to de-escalation, whereas the results of the multiplex PCR affected time to appropriate escalation regardless of whether the subject was in the stewardship arm or not. It is possible that having the stewardship team support to de-escalate in addition to the rapid test results provided more confidence for the providers facing complex clinical scenarios. This may be even more important in critically ill ICU patients for whom providers may be reticent to narrow antimicrobials, even when an organism has been identified and susceptibilities reported. Several other observational studies have shown clinical benefit of rapid diagnostics for assorted infections combined with antimicrobial stewardship to varying degrees, though these studies are uncontrolled so that the degree of impact of adding stewardship is difficult to quantify.[55–62] Further research is needed to quantify the benefit of rapid testing in the ICU setting and the degree to which stewardship programs are needed to assist with interpretation and management based on the results.

Diagnostic Testing Take-Home Points

- Accurate identification of bacterial infection and rapid identification and susceptibility testing can improve antibiotic use and clinical outcomes.
- Negative test results can assist providers with stopping antibiotics when no alternative infections have been identified.
- Cascade reporting of antibiotics may improve appropriate selection of antibiotics for documented bacterial infections.
- ASPs are important adjuncts to help providers with interpretation of rapid identification and susceptibility technologies, particularly in de-escalation of antibiotics.

EMPIRICAL THERAPY

While awaiting results of a work-up for a suspected infection, antimicrobial therapy will likely be administered to the ICU patient. Because inadequate empirical antibiotic therapy, or empirical antibiotics that do not cover the ultimate identified pathogen, accounts for an estimated 39% to 51% of excess mortality in ICU patients with various infectious syndromes, initiation of broad empirical therapy in a patient with high suspicion for infection is appropriate.[15,16,63,64] However, de-escalation can be initiated promptly after a specific diagnosis is made and empirical therapy should only last for 48 to 72 hours. Conversely, overly broad therapy should not be encouraged given the well-documented adverse effects of antibiotics.[65–69]

In general, goals for empirical therapy in the ICU setting include

- Assurance of a high probability of covering commonly recovered organisms for the patient population being treated based on local microbiology
- Promoting timely delivery of antibiotics
- Avoidance of overly broad antibiotics or redundant spectra of activity
- Selection of antimicrobials that are effective at the site of suspected infection (eg, peritoneum, cerebrospinal fluid).

The next sections cover antimicrobial stewardship approaches to guide empirical therapy selection.

Guidelines

Because empirical therapy is, by definition, therapy given without specific knowledge of the infectious organism, guidelines can be an effective method to influence antibiotic choice.[7,70] Recently updated consensus guidelines for empirical antibiotic therapy in specific syndromes relevant to the ICU setting include those for complicated intra-abdominal infections, hospital-acquired pneumonia or VAP, and skin or soft tissue infections.[71–73] These can and should be adapted to each institution based on local antibiograms, patient population, and drug availability. Most studies examining the effectiveness of guideline implementation have been single-center, pre-post analysis, and often are coupled with a concomitant educational campaign. For instance, Worrall and colleagues[74] reported improvements in appropriateness of empirical antibiotics and therapy de-escalation along with decreased duration of antibiotics after implementation of a pneumonia guideline in their trauma ICU. Though not statistically significant on uncontrolled analyses, in a multivariate analysis controlling for severity of illness and isolation of MRSA or *Pseudomonas aeruginosa*, the investigators reported decreased hospital and ICU length-of-stay and ventilator days after guideline implementation. Others have reported that implementation of a guideline for VAP management focusing on quantitative bronchoscopy, local antibiograms, and appropriate duration of therapy resulted in improvements in appropriate therapy and 1.3 days shorter duration of therapy without changes in mortality.[75] Yet another group implementing a VAP guideline in the medical ICU that focused on very broad initial coverage with focused de-escalation reported statistically significant increases in appropriate empirical therapy with decreased duration of total therapy from 14.8 to 8.6 days on average without changes in clinical outcomes.[76] The investigators also reported significantly fewer secondary VAPs, although changes in antimicrobial susceptibility or whether de-escalation occurred after initial broad-spectrum empirical coverage were not described.

Choice of empirical antibiotic regimen is easier when a specific infectious syndrome is presumed than when the source of a suspected infection is unclear. Much attention has been placed recently on the definitions of sepsis, with a main goal of early recognition and treatment.[77–79] These definitions and guidelines rightly emphasize sensitive definitions for sepsis with aggressive early antimicrobial therapy, and the Centers for Medicaid and Medicare Services has recently made management of sepsis a core measure.[80,81] Given this mandate, resultant initial antibiotic management often is very broad. Because of evidence supporting the importance of adequate initial antibiotic therapy, there has been interest in whether addition of empirical antifungal agents and/or additional antibacterial agents to cover resistant gram-negative rods results in better clinical outcomes. Two recent studies on use of empirical antifungals in the ICU setting help to clarify appropriateness of these agents when diagnosis is uncertain.[82,83] The Empirical Antifungal Treatment in ICUs (EMPIRICUS) study was a multicenter, randomized, blinded study of empirical micafungin treatment of patients in the ICU colonized with candida but without clear focus of fungal infection who had unresolved sepsis despite broad-spectrum antibiotics.[83] In this population of nonimmunocompromised but critically ill patients, there were no significant differences in mortality detected, even in those patients with the highest suspicion for candidal infection. Another recent study showed no benefit of early empirical therapy for patients with suspected candida peritonitis compared with those who had antifungals started only when fungal peritonitis was confirmed, though delay in systemic antifungals for 6 or more days may lead to worse outcomes.[82] Taken together, these 2 studies suggest that routine empirical antifungal therapy in the ICU setting is not beneficial, even in high-risk populations with sepsis, especially as diagnostics become more rapid and lead to fewer delays in identification of patients with fungal infection.

Computerized Decision Support to Assist with Empirical Antibiotic Choice

In addition to evidence-based guidelines for specific syndromes, computerized decision support (CDS) at the time of initiation of empirical antibiotic initiation can be another tool to support appropriate antibiotic choice.[7] For example, in a multicenter, cluster, randomized trial of a sophisticated CDS tool guiding selection of empirical antibiotics in patients with suspected infection, wards with CDS trended toward having higher rates of appropriate antibiotic usage.[84] In those subjects whose providers followed the CDS advice, the odds of having appropriate antibiotics started were 3.4-fold higher than control subjects (95% confidence interval, 2.3–5.1, in a model accounting for location and clustering). This type of decision support can also be used by antimicrobial stewardship teams to provide advice and feedback to providers, such as dual coverage of gram-negative organisms.[85] Though relatively inexpensive to implement, a limitation to the use of decision support or electronic checklists is alert fatigue.[86]

Formulary Restriction

Requiring prior authorization for release of certain antimicrobials is a proven strategy to limit initiation of unnecessary or inappropriate broad-spectrum antibiotic use safely.[87,88] Benefits include decreased resistance and lower costs. Though most studies of formulary restriction have focused on institutions as a whole, several have concentrated on critical care specifically. For instance, Lewis and colleagues[89] report on the impact of implementation of ciprofloxacin restriction in the intermediate and ICU units of a large tertiary care center. They found that significant decreases in ciprofloxacin usage were associated with significant decreases in percentages and rates of both ciprofloxacin and carbapenem-resistant isolates of *P aeruginosa*. Additionally, they observed a concomitant increase in use of carbapenems, highlighting the importance of monitoring countermeasures when implementing selected antimicrobial restrictions. In fact, after restriction of cephalosporins, 1 institution reported an increase in imipenem use, which was associated with a 69% increase in imipenem-resistant *P aeruginosa* isolates.[90] Though these 2 institutions enacted focused restrictions in response to outbreaks of organisms resistant to particular antibiotics, many institutions introduce formulary restrictions for a broader list of antimicrobials. White and colleagues[87] reported that on implementation of a program to restrict antipseudomonal agents from multiple classes, use of nonrestricted antibiotics increased concomitantly to a decrease in the restricted antibiotics, but the nonrestricted agents were all narrower spectrum. As a result, significant improvements in gram-negative bacterial susceptibilities were noted, including 18% decreases each in ceftazidime-resistant *Escherichia coli* and imipenem-resistant *P aeruginosa*, specifically in the ICU.

Drawbacks of formulary restriction with prior authorization include[7]

- Shift to nonrestricted antibiotic use and resultant downstream effects
- Focus on empirical use when there are often limited microbiological and clinical data available
- Concern for limits on prescriber autonomy
- Potential delays in therapy
- Variation in approval practice based on approver background and information provided by the prescriber
- Need for on-call approver
- Prescriber manipulation and gaming of information presented to the approver or bypass of the system (eg, learning the approval codes).

Because both restricted formulary with prior authorization and PAF are resource-intensive interventions for the ASP, these 2 approaches have been compared in several studies.[91–93] Tamma and colleagues[91] performed a crossover trial comparing the 2 approaches with several internal medicine teams and found that the formulary restriction with prior authorization group had a median of 2 days more antibiotic therapy compared with the PAF group. However, Mehta and colleagues[92] reported opposite results from an interrupted time series study after their ASP moved from a restricted formulary to use of PAF. Tamma and colleagues[91] posited that these differences may have been due to unmeasured temporal trends, the limited scope of the PAF in the latter study, and unaccounted for outpatient prescriptions.[91] In a Cochrane Database of Systematic Reviews assessment of antimicrobial stewardship approaches, there was benefit of both restrictive and persuasive (enabling) interventions, which often were reported together.[93] It should be noted that restrictive interventions included cascade reporting, automatic stop orders, and therapeutic substitution, whereas persuasive interventions included education and reminders, which are known to have limited effectiveness.[7] Taken together, these findings highlight the importance for multiple interventions to improve antimicrobial prescribing.

Allergy Testing

Being labeled as having a penicillin allergy has been linked to poor clinical outcomes, including longer lengths of stay, more readmissions, and higher rates of *C difficile* infection, MRSA, andVRE compared with matched controls.[94,95] In patients with a beta-lactam allergy and gram-negative bacteremia, those patients receiving a non–beta-lactam antibiotic had a 17% increase in risk of inappropriate antibiotics, as well as an 11% increased risk of clinical failure.[96] In contrast there are only approximately 150 deaths from drug-induced anaphylaxis annually in the United States.[97] Because between 8% and 12% of patients report a penicillin allergy and antibiotic use in the hospital is so common, the risks of mislabeling have a huge impact.[98]

Penicillin skin testing and then rechallenge is safe in the ICU and results in clearance of the allergy in most patients, with change in antibiotic management in 48% to 88% of patients.[99,100] The corollary to this is expected to be decreased antibiotic resistance, failure, and costs, though these warrant further study. In addition to skin testing, partnership between ID, pharmacy, and allergists can improve appropriate use of beta-lactam antibiotics in patients with reported beta-lactam allergies. Though not specifically implemented in the ICU setting, King and colleagues[101] report on a bundled guideline and educational intervention aimed at encouraging test doses and appropriate use of beta-lactams in patients with low likelihood of cross-reactivity. Without any increases in antibiotic adverse events, the investigators observed a 31% decrease in vancomycin and 12% decrease in fluoroquinolone use with a concomitant increase in use of beta-lactam antibiotics. An approach of elucidating penicillin allergy history combined with the option for skin testing and/or graded challenge would likely improve appropriate use of beta-lactams with downstream clinical and microbiological benefit.[7,102]

Antimicrobial Stewardship Strategies to Guide Empirical Therapy Take-Home Points

- Appropriate antibiotic therapy improves outcomes, but use of overly broad spectrum agents carries risk of resistance, adverse events, and *C difficile* infection
- Approaches to improve choice of empirical therapy include
  - Local guideline development and implementation
  - CDS at the time of prescription
  - Formulary restriction with prior authorization
  - Beta-lactam allergy pathways, including skin testing, graded challenge, and multidisciplinary evaluation.

DEFINITIVE THERAPY

Once the patient has been stabilized with empirical antimicrobials and diagnostic testing results return, a clinical and/or microbiological diagnosis often, though not always, can be made. At this point, goals of therapy become

- Choosing the narrowest and most potent agent for identifying the syndrome and microbes and treating for minimal effectiveness
- Optimizing pharmacodynamics and pharmacokinetics
- Avoiding adverse consequences of antimicrobial use while ensuring cure of infection.

Prospective Audit and Feedback

In addition to having a restricted formulary with requirement for prior authorization of certain antimicrobials, PAF is among the foundations of most ASPs. PAF entails review of patients on antimicrobials by the ASP pharmacist or physician, with feedback to prescribers on appropriate choice, dose, and/or duration. Depending on the goals, resources, and size of the ASP, the patients reviewed may range from a comprehensive list of all patients on antimicrobials to targeting specific populations (eg, patients in certain units), conditions (eg, positive blood cultures), or drugs (eg, broad-spectrum agents). PAF can be complementary to facility-specific treatment guidelines, reinforcing knowledge about and adherence to these guidelines.

In the ICU setting, PAF has been shown to decrease utilization of inappropriate broad-spectrum antibiotics, rates of bacterial resistance, and *C difficile* infections while maintaining similar mortality and length-of-stay outcomes.[103,104] Because PAF occurs after antimicrobials are started, benefits include having additional clinical information on response to treatment, work-up for source of infection, and laboratory results. In addition, data suggest that there is an educational component to PAF with 1 study suggesting transfer of similar decrease in antimicrobial utilization on other units staffed by the same physicians as the sole unit where PAF was performed but not on units without overlap in staffing.[105]

Drawbacks to PAF include[7]

- Resource-intensive: Can require a significant amount of time to review targeted patients.[106] Computerized tools can help with this process but are costly.[85]
- For patients doing poorly, providers may be disinclined to deescalate, whereas for patients responding to current therapy, providers may opt to continue the successful therapy.
- Choice to follow recommendations is optional.
- Success of the program depends on who and how the feedback is delivered.[107–110]

Antibiotic Time-Out

Given the resource-intensive nature of PAF programs, there has been a push to identify methods by which prescribers could be prompted to perform their own PAF, otherwise known as an antibiotic time-out, at 48 to 72 hours after initiating antibiotics.[7,8] In the ICU setting, approach to a time-out has mainly been use of checklists along with a prompt if the items on the checklist were not addressed.[111,112] Compared with patients whose physicians had a checklist embedded in the electronic medical record without prompting, Weiss and colleagues[111] found that those with in-person prompting to address antibiotic use had a 7% decrease in the proportion of days in which empirical antibiotics were administered, and they even noted a risk-adjusted increase in mortality for each additional day of empirical antibiotics. The marginal benefit of having an unprompted checklist in the ICU is unclear.

Infectious Disease Physician Embedding Within the Intensive Care Unit Rounding Structure

Though resource intensive, routine ASP or ID rounding on ICU patients with suspected or documented infections can improve clinical outcomes and decrease inappropriate or unnecessary antimicrobial use.[21–23] For instance, Gilbert[22] reported on outcomes associated with routine inclusion of an ID physician on ICU multidisciplinary rounds in a 23-bed ICU in a community teaching hospital. When compared with days when the ID physician was not present, there was a significant difference of 0.35 decreased days of antibiotic therapy per patient between the start and end of rounds. Similarly,

Cairns and colleagues[21] describe daily ICU-ASP rounds at their tertiary care center with a 45-bed ICU, which were timed to directly follow the standard ICU ward rounds. Though they do not report antibiotic use before their intervention, there was a high acceptance rate of recommendations for antibiotic change, including discontinuing antibiotics 36% of the time and de-escalation 12% of the time when antibiotic decisions were made. Likewise, Butt and colleagues[23] implemented a program in a noncardiac ICU at a large tertiary care hospital in Abu Dhabi, UAE, which involved dedicated ASP rounds daily and presence at the ICU work rounds at least weekly. Though not statistically significant, there were numerical decreases in antibiotic cost per patient, length-of-hospital and ICU stay, and mortality after this intervention started. The impact of routine ID physician consultation in the ICU has also been assessed with similar results.[113–115]

Studies of Duration

Many of the interventions described above, including guideline development, PAF, antibiotic time-outs, use of biomarkers, and negative predictive value of negative testing, can result in a significantly shorter duration of antibiotic exposure. In general, studies of various infectious syndromes treated in the ICU, including VAP, pyelonephritis, and intraabdominal infection, have all demonstrated that shorter duration of therapy is safe and decreases antibiotic exposure.[116–119] As ASPs develop approaches to definitive therapy, knowledge of these types of studies can be useful in implementing programs aimed to give the shortest effective duration of therapy.

Dosing Strategies

Due to altered hemodynamics, fluid balance, and organ function, as well as frequent use of organ replacement therapies, antibiotic dosing in the ICU is challenging.[120] Among the low-hanging fruits of ASPs are programs aimed at improving dosing strategies for various antibiotics. In the ideal situation, these strategies (generally pharmacy run) improve clinical outcomes by optimizing pharmacookinetic properties but, at the least, they can decrease antibiotic costs without affecting overall clinical outcomes.[121,122] In addition to global benefit from having pharmacists review patients in the ICU on antibiotics, specific interventions aimed at drugs with narrow therapeutic window have proven beneficial. For instance, in the time when aminoglycosides were frequently chosen as primary therapy for gram-negative infections, several studies showed clinical benefit or decreased adverse events related to pharmacist-directed dosing, though these results were not always reproducible.[123–125] Similar programs for vancomycin dose monitoring and adjustment have generally found improved target attainment, decreased adverse events, and lower costs while maintaining comparable clinical endpoints.[126,127]

Recent data suggest that beta-lactam dosing may be inadequate in many ICU patients.[128] Based on pharmacodynamic principles, extended-infusion or continuous-infusion strategies for beta-lactam antibiotics have been studied with the goals of improving outcomes and decreasing costs, though a recent large multicenter, randomized, controlled trial did not find clinical benefit.[129–132] Regardless, it can be a cost-saving measure because the dosing strategies often result in lower overall dosing of the beta-lactam antibiotic.[7]

Antimicrobial Stewardship Strategies to Guide Definitive Therapy Take-Home Points

- PAF is a mainstay of tailoring therapy for definitive management of infection.
- Other less resource-intensive but still effective approaches include CDS and clinician self-stewardship via antibiotic time-outs.

- Strategies to improve antibiotic dosing in this complex population are also important and can be easy wins for an ASP.
- Attention to duration of therapy, whether via PAF or guideline development, may be a way to decrease unnecessary antimicrobials in the ICU setting.

DEMONSTRATING EFFECTIVENESS

As with any quality improvement program, ASPs must track outcomes to focus efforts, demonstrate successes, and ensure no unexpected countermeasures. In general, ASPs should monitor both process and outcome measures.[7] This includes measures of antimicrobial usage (eg, days of therapy) normalized to census, costs, antibiotic resistance, uptake of recommendations, and clinical outcomes such as adverse events, secondary infections, mortality, and length-of-stay.

SUMMARY

Antimicrobial stewardship in the ICU setting can improve quality of care and decrease antimicrobial resistance without compromising patient outcomes. Though low-level evidence supports individual aspects of stewardship, there is little information about which particular interventions have the most impact.[133] Two structured reviews of antimicrobial stewardship in the ICU setting have found modest benefit, though studies tend to be small and uncontrolled, with lack of emphasis on patient-centered outcomes, as previously noted.[113,134] Individual institutions need to consider their own needs, resources, and priorities when designing an ASP, and it is critical to monitor outcomes and adjust interventions. Further high-quality research is needed to define which bundles of interventions might lead to the best outcomes without requiring overly onerous resources.

REFERENCES

1. Antibiotic/antimicrobial resistance. Available at: https://www.cdc.gov/drug resistance/about.html. Accessed March 14, 2017.
2. Carlet J, Ben Ali A, Chalfine A. Epidemiology and control of antibiotic resistance in the intensive care unit. Curr Opin Infect Dis 2004;17(4):309–16.
3. Palumbi SR. Humans as the world's greatest evolutionary force. Science 2001; 293(5536):1786–90.
4. The critical need for new antibiotics. Available at: http://www.pewtrusts.org/en/multimedia/data-visualizations/2016/the-critical-need-for-new-antibiotics. Accessed December 1, 2016.
5. World Health Organization. Global priority list of antibiotic-resistant bacteria to guide research, discovery, and development of new antibiotics. 2017. Available at: http://www.who.int/medicines/publications/WHO-PPL-Short_Summary_25Feb-ET_NM_WHO.pdf?ua=1.
6. Centers for Disease Control and Prevention (CDC). Antibiotic resistance threats in the United States, 2013. 2013. Available at: https://www.cdc.gov/drugresistance/threat-report-2013/pdf/ar-threats-2013-508.pdf.
7. Barlam TF, Cosgrove SE, Abbo LM, et al. Implementing an antibiotic stewardship program: guidelines by the Infectious Diseases Society of America and the Society for Healthcare Epidemiology of America. Clin Infect Dis 2016; 62(10):e51–77.

8. Core elements of hospital antibiotic stewardship programs. Available at: https://www.cdc.gov/getsmart/healthcare/implementation/core-elements.html. Accessed March 14, 2017.

9. McGowan JE Jr, Finland M. Effects of monitoring the usage of antibiotics: an interhospital comparison. South Med J 1976;69(2):193–5.

10. McGowan JE, Finland M. Usage of antibiotics in a general hospital: Effect of requiring justification. J Infect Dis 1974;130(2):165–8.

11. California senate bill 1311. 2014;1311.

12. Center for Medicare and Medicaid Services. Medicare and Medicaid programs; hospital and critical access hospital (CAH) changes to promote innovation, flexibility, and improvement in patient care; proposed rule. Fed Regist 2016. 42 CFR Parts 482 and 485(81 FR 39447). p. 39448–80.

13. Roberts RR, Hota B, Ahmad I, et al. Hospital and societal costs of antimicrobial-resistant infections in a Chicago teaching hospital: implications for antibiotic stewardship. Clin Infect Dis 2009;49(8):1175–84.

14. Hyle EP, Lipworth AD, Zaoutis TE, et al. Impact of inadequate initial antimicrobial therapy on mortality in infections due to extended-spectrum beta-lactamase-producing enterobacteriaceae: variability by site of infection. Arch Intern Med 2005;165(12):1375–80.

15. Leone M, Bourgoin A, Cambon S, et al. Empirical antimicrobial therapy of septic shock patients: adequacy and impact on the outcome. Crit Care Med 2003; 31(2):462–7.

16. Kollef MH, Sherman G, Ward S, et al. Inadequate antimicrobial treatment of infections: a risk factor for hospital mortality among critically ill patients. Chest 1999;115(2):462–74.

17. Tumbarello M, Sanguinetti M, Montuori E, et al. Predictors of mortality in patients with bloodstream infections caused by extended-spectrum-{beta}-lactamase-producing Enterobacteriaceae: importance of inadequate initial antimicrobial treatment. Antimicrob Agents Chemother 2007;51(6):1987–94.

18. Cusini A, Rampini SK, Bansal V, et al. Different patterns of inappropriate antimicrobial use in surgical and medical units at a tertiary care hospital in Switzerland: a prevalence survey. PLoS One 2010;5(11):e14011.

19. Hecker MT, Aron DC, Patel NP, et al. Unnecessary use of antimicrobials in hospitalized patients: current patterns of misuse with an emphasis on the antianaerobic spectrum of activity. Arch Intern Med 2003;163(8):972–8.

20. Metlay JP, Shea JA, Asch DA. Antibiotic prescribing decisions of generalists and infectious disease specialists: thresholds for adopting new drug therapies. Med Decis Making 2002;22(6):498–505.

21. Cairns KA, Bortz HD, Le A, et al. ICU antimicrobial stewardship (AMS) rounds: the daily activities of an AMS service. Int J Antimicrob Agents 2016;48(5):575–6.

22. Gilbert DN. Influence of an infectious diseases specialist on ICU multidisciplinary rounds. Crit Care Res Pract 2014;2014:307817.

23. Butt AA, Al Kaabi N, Khan T, et al. Impact of infectious diseases team consultation on antimicrobial use, length of stay and mortality. Am J Med Sci 2015; 350(3):191–4.

24. Balk RA, Kadri SS, Cao Z, et al. Effect of procalcitonin testing on healthcare utilization and costs in critically ill patients in the United States. Chest 2017;151(1): 23–33.

25. Schuetz P, Raad I, Amin DN. Using procalcitonin-guided algorithms to improve antimicrobial therapy in ICU patients with respiratory infections and sepsis. Curr Opin Crit Care 2013;19(5):453–60.

26. Langley RJ, Tipper JL, Bruse S, et al. Integrative "Omic" analysis of experimental bacteremia identifies a metabolic signature that distinguishes human sepsis from systemic inflammatory response syndromes. Am J Respir Crit Care Med 2014;190(4):445–55.

27. Maslove DM, Tang BM, McLean AS. Identification of sepsis subtypes in critically ill adults using gene expression profiling. Crit Care 2012;16(5):R183.

28. McHugh L, Seldon TA, Brandon RA, et al. A molecular host response assay to discriminate between sepsis and infection-negative systemic inflammation in critically ill patients: discovery and validation in independent cohorts. PLoS Med 2015;12(12):e1001916.

29. Zaas AK, Burke T, Chen M, et al. A host-based RT-PCR gene expression signature to identify acute respiratory viral infection. Sci Transl Med 2013;5(203):203ra126.

30. Fabregas N, Ewig S, Torres A, et al. Clinical diagnosis of ventilator associated pneumonia revisited: comparative validation using immediate post-mortem lung biopsies. Thorax 1999;54(10):867–73.

31. Klompas M. Does this patient have ventilator-associated pneumonia? JAMA 2007;297(14):1583–93.

32. Pugin J, Auckenthaler R, Mili N, et al. Diagnosis of ventilator-associated pneumonia by bacteriologic analysis of bronchoscopic and nonbronchoscopic "blind" bronchoalveolar lavage fluid. Am Rev Respir Dis 1991;143(5 Pt 1):1121–9.

33. Zilberberg MD, Shorr AF. Ventilator-associated pneumonia: the clinical pulmonary infection score as a surrogate for diagnostics and outcome. Clin Infect Dis 2010;51(Suppl 1):S131–5.

34. Fartoukh M, Maitre B, Honore S, et al. Diagnosing pneumonia during mechanical ventilation: the clinical pulmonary infection score revisited. Am J Respir Crit Care Med 2003;168(2):173–9.

35. Singh N, Rogers P, Atwood CW, et al. Short-course empiric antibiotic therapy for patients with pulmonary infiltrates in the intensive care unit. A proposed solution for indiscriminate antibiotic prescription. Am J Respir Crit Care Med 2000;162(2 Pt 1):505–11.

36. Tejerina E, Esteban A, Fernández-Segoviano P, et al. Accuracy of clinical definitions of ventilator-associated pneumonia: comparison with autopsy findings. J Crit Care 2010;25(1):62–8.

37. O'Horo JC, Thompson D, Safdar N. Is the gram stain useful in the microbiologic diagnosis of VAP? A meta-analysis. Clin Infect Dis 2012;55(4):551–61.

38. Albert M, Friedrich JO, Adhikari NKJ, et al. Utility of gram stain in the clinical management of suspected ventilator-associated pneumonia: secondary analysis of a multicenter randomized trial. J Crit Care 2008;23(1):74–81.

39. Thomas Z, Bandali F, Sankaranarayanan J, et al, Critical Care Pharmacotherapy Trials Network. A multicenter evaluation of prolonged empiric antibiotic therapy in adult ICUs in the United States. Crit Care Med 2015;43(12):2527–34.

40. Aarts MW, Brun-Buisson C, Cook DJ, et al. Antibiotic management of suspected nosocomial ICU-acquired infection: does prolonged empiric therapy improve outcome? Intensive Care Med 2007;33(8):1369–78.

41. Raman K, Nailor MD, Nicolau DP, et al. Early antibiotic discontinuation in patients with clinically suspected ventilator-associated pneumonia and negative quantitative bronchoscopy cultures. Crit Care Med 2013;41(7):1656–63.

42. Swanson JM, Wood GC, Croce MA, et al. Utility of preliminary bronchoalveolar lavage results in suspected ventilator-associated pneumonia. J Trauma 2008;65(6):1271–7.

43. Humphries RM, Dien Bard J. Point-counterpoint: reflex cultures reduce laboratory workload and improve antimicrobial stewardship in patients suspected of having urinary tract infections. J Clin Microbiol 2016;54(2):254–8.
44. Stovall RT, Haenal JB, Jenkins TC, et al. A negative urinalysis rules out catheter-associated urinary tract infection in trauma patients in the intensive care unit. J Am Coll Surg 2013;217(1):162–6.
45. Bachur R, Harper MB. Reliability of the urinalysis for predicting urinary tract infections in young febrile children. Arch Pediatr Adolesc Med 2001;155(1):60–5.
46. Epstein L, Edwards JR, Halpin AL, et al. Evaluation of a novel intervention to reduce unnecessary urine cultures in intensive care units at a tertiary care hospital in Maryland, 2011-2014. Infect Control Hosp Epidemiol 2016;37(5):606–9.
47. Johnson LS, Patel D, King EA, et al. Impact of microbiology cascade reporting on antibiotic de-escalation in cefazolin-susceptible gram-negative bacteremia. Eur J Clin Microbiol Infect Dis 2016;35(7):1151–7.
48. Al-Tawfiq JA, Momattin H, Al-Habboubi F, et al. Restrictive reporting of selected antimicrobial susceptibilities influences clinical prescribing. J Infect Public Health 2015;8(3):234–41.
49. Steffee CH, Morrell RM, Wasilauskas BL. Clinical use of rifampicin during routine reporting of rifampicin susceptibilities: a lesson in selective reporting of antimicrobial susceptibility data. J Antimicrob Chemother 1997;40(4):595–8.
50. Antworth A, Collins CD, Kunapuli A, et al. Impact of an antimicrobial stewardship program comprehensive care bundle on management of candidemia. Pharmacotherapy 2013;33(2):137–43.
51. Borde JP, Batin N, Rieg S, et al. Adherence to an antibiotic stewardship bundle targeting staphylococcus aureus blood stream infections at a 200-bed community hospital. Infection 2014;42(4):713–9.
52. Pogue JM, Mynatt RP, Marchaim D, et al. Automated alerts coupled with antimicrobial stewardship intervention lead to decreases in length of stay in patients with gram-negative bacteremia. Infect Control Hosp Epidemiol 2014;35(2):132–8.
53. Pulido MR, Garcia-Quintanilla M, Martin-Pena R, et al. Progress on the development of rapid methods for antimicrobial susceptibility testing. J Antimicrob Chemother 2013;68(12):2710–7.
54. Banerjee R, Teng CB, Cunningham SA, et al. Randomized trial of rapid multiplex polymerase chain reaction-based blood culture identification and susceptibility testing. Clin Infect Dis 2015;61(7):1071–80.
55. Huang AM, Newton D, Kunapuli A, et al. Impact of rapid organism identification via matrix-assisted laser desorption/ionization time-of-flight combined with antimicrobial stewardship team intervention in adult patients with bacteremia and candidemia. Clin Infect Dis 2013;57(9):1237–45.
56. Forrest GN, Mehta S, Weekes E, et al. Impact of rapid in situ hybridization testing on coagulase-negative staphylococci positive blood cultures. J Antimicrob Chemother 2006;58(1):154–8.
57. Forrest GN, Roghmann MC, Toombs LS, et al. Peptide nucleic acid fluorescent in situ hybridization for hospital-acquired enterococcal bacteremia: delivering earlier effective antimicrobial therapy. Antimicrob Agents Chemother 2008; 52(10):3558–63.
58. Forrest GN, Mankes K, Jabra-Rizk MA, et al. Peptide nucleic acid fluorescence in situ hybridization-based identification of candida albicans and its impact on mortality and antifungal therapy costs. J Clin Microbiol 2006;44(9):3381–3.
59. Bauer KA, West JE, Balada-Llasat JM, et al. An antimicrobial stewardship program's impact with rapid polymerase chain reaction methicillin-resistant

Staphylococcus aureus/S. aureus blood culture test in patients with *S. aureus* bacteremia. Clin Infect Dis 2010;51(9):1074–80.

60. Perez KK, Olsen RJ, Musick WL, et al. Integrating rapid diagnostics and antimicrobial stewardship improves outcomes in patients with antibiotic-resistant gram-negative bacteremia. J Infect 2014;69(3):216–25.

61. Perez KK, Olsen RJ, Musick WL, et al. Integrating rapid pathogen identification and antimicrobial stewardship significantly decreases hospital costs. Arch Pathol Lab Med 2013;137(9):1247–54.

62. Carver PL, Lin SW, DePestel DD, et al. Impact of mecA gene testing and intervention by infectious disease clinical pharmacists on time to optimal antimicrobial therapy for *Staphylococcus aureus* bacteremia at a university hospital. J Clin Microbiol 2008;46(7):2381–3.

63. Luna CM, Vujacich P, Niederman MS, et al. Impact of BAL data on the therapy and outcome of ventilator-associated pneumonia. Chest 1997;111(3):676–85.

64. Ibrahim EH, Sherman G, Ward S, et al. The influence of inadequate antimicrobial treatment of bloodstream infections on patient outcomes in the ICU setting. Chest 2000;118(1):146–55.

65. Baxter R, Ray G, Fireman B. Case-control study of antibiotic use and subsequent *Clostridium difficile*–associated diarrhea in hospitalized patients. Infect Control Hosp Epidemiol 2008;29(1):44–50.

66. Brown K, Valenta K, Fisman D, et al. Hospital ward antibiotic prescribing and the risks of *Clostridium difficile* infection. JAMA Intern Med 2015;175(4):626–33.

67. Freedberg DE, Salmasian H, Cohen B, et al. Receipt of antibiotics in hospitalized patients and risk for *Clostridium difficile* infection in subsequent patients who occupy the same bed. JAMA Intern Med 2016;176(12):1801–8.

68. Sanden L, Paul M, Leibovici L, et al. Quantifying the associations between antibiotic exposure and resistance - a step towards personalised antibiograms. Eur J Clin Microbiol Infect Dis 2016;35(12):1989–96.

69. Ray WA, Murray KT, Hall K, et al. Azithromycin and the risk of cardiovascular death. N Engl J Med 2012;366(20):1881–90.

70. Davey P, Brown E, Fenelon L, et al. Interventions to improve antibiotic prescribing practices for hospital inpatients. Cochrane Database Syst Rev 2005;(4):CD003543.

71. Stevens DL, Bisno AL, Chambers HF, et al. Practice guidelines for the diagnosis and management of skin and soft tissue infections: 2014 update by the Infectious Diseases Society of America. Clin Infect Dis 2014;59(2):e10–52.

72. Solomkin JS, Mazuski JE, Bradley JS, et al. Diagnosis and management of complicated intra-abdominal infection in adults and children: guidelines by the Surgical Infection Society and the Infectious Diseases Society of America. Clin Infect Dis 2010;50(2):133–64.

73. Kalil AC, Metersky ML, Klompas M, et al. Management of adults with hospital-acquired and ventilator-associated pneumonia: 2016 clinical practice guidelines by the Infectious Diseases Society of America and the American Thoracic Society. Clin Infect Dis 2016;63(5):e61–111.

74. Worrall CL, Anger BP, Simpson KN, et al. Impact of a hospital-acquired/ventilator-associated/healthcare-associated pneumonia practice guideline on outcomes in surgical trauma patients. J Trauma 2010;68(2):382–6.

75. Dellit TH, Chan JD, Skerrett SJ, et al. Development of a guideline for the management of ventilator-associated pneumonia based on local microbiologic findings and impact of the guideline on antimicrobial use practices. Infect Control Hosp Epidemiol 2008;29(6):525–33.

76. Ibrahim EH, Ward S, Sherman G, et al. Experience with a clinical guideline for the treatment of ventilator-associated pneumonia. Crit Care Med 2001;29(6): 1109–15.

77. Dellinger RP, Levy MM, Rhodes A, et al. Surviving sepsis campaign: international guidelines for management of severe sepsis and septic shock: 2012. Crit Care Med 2013;41(2):580–637.

78. Shankar-Hari M, Phillips GS, Levy ML, et al. Developing a new definition and assessing new clinical criteria for septic shock: for the third international consensus definitions for sepsis and septic shock (sepsis-3). JAMA 2016; 315(8):775–87.

79. Singer M, Deutschman CS, Seymour CW, et al. The Third International Consensus Definitions for Sepsis and Septic Shock (Sepsis-3). JAMA 2016; 315(8):801–10.

80. Faust JS, Weingart SD. The past, present, and future of the centers for Medicare and Medicaid services quality measure SEP-1: the early management bundle for severe sepsis/septic shock. Emerg Med Clin North Am 2017;35(1):219–31.

81. CMS to improve quality of care during hospital inpatient stays. Available at: https://www.cms.gov/newsroom/mediareleasedatabase/fact-sheets/2014-fact-sheets-items/2014-08-04-2.html. Accessed March 20, 2017.

82. Montravers P, Perrigault PF, Timsit JF, et al. Antifungal therapy for patients with proven or suspected candida peritonitis: Amarcand2, a prospective cohort study in French intensive care units. Clin Microbiol Infect 2017;23(2):117.e1–8.

83. Timsit JF, Azoulay E, Schwebel C, et al. Empirical micafungin treatment and survival without invasive fungal infection in adults with ICU-acquired sepsis, candida colonization, and multiple organ failure: the EMPIRICUS randomized clinical trial. JAMA 2016;316(15):1555–64.

84. Leibovici L, Paul M, Nielsen AD, et al. The TREAT project: Decision support and prediction using causal probabilistic networks. Int J Antimicrob Agents 2007; 30(Supplement 1):93–102.

85. McGregor JC, Weekes E, Forrest GN, et al. Impact of a computerized clinical decision support system on reducing inappropriate antimicrobial use: a randomized controlled trial. J Am Med Inform Assoc 2006;13(4):378–84.

86. Ranji SR, Rennke S, Wachter RM. Computerised provider order entry combined with clinical decision support systems to improve medication safety: a narrative review. BMJ Qual Saf 2014;23(9):773–80.

87. White AC Jr, Atmar RL, Wilson J, et al. Effects of requiring prior authorization for selected antimicrobials: expenditures, susceptibilities, and clinical outcomes. Clin Infect Dis 1997;25(2):230–9.

88. Buising KL, Thursky KA, Robertson MB, et al. Electronic antibiotic stewardship—reduced consumption of broad-spectrum antibiotics using a computerized antimicrobial approval system in a hospital setting. J Antimicrob Chemother 2008;62(3):608–16.

89. Lewis GJ, Fang X, Gooch M, et al. Decreased resistance of *Pseudomonas aeruginosa* with restriction of ciprofloxacin in a large teaching hospital's intensive care and intermediate care units. Infect Control Hosp Epidemiol 2012;33(4): 368–73.

90. Rahal JJ, Urban C, Horn D, et al. Class restriction of cephalosporin use to control total cephalosporin resistance in nosocomial *Klebsiella*. JAMA 1998; 280(14):1233–7.

91. Tamma PD, Avdic E, Keenan JF, et al. What is the more effective antibiotic stewardship intervention: pre-prescription authorization or post-prescription review with feedback? Clin Infect Dis 2017;64(5):537–43.

92. Mehta JM, Haynes K, Wileyto EP, et al. Comparison of prior authorization and prospective audit with feedback for antimicrobial stewardship. Infect Control Hosp Epidemiol 2014;35(09):1092–9.

93. Davey P, Brown E, Charani E, et al. Interventions to improve antibiotic prescribing practices for hospital inpatients. Cochrane Database Syst Rev 2013;(4):CD003543.

94. Macy E, Contreras R. Health care use and serious infection prevalence associated with penicillin "allergy" in hospitalized patients: a cohort study. J Allergy Clin Immunol 2014;133(3):790–6.

95. MacFadden DR, LaDelfa A, Leen J, et al. Impact of reported beta-lactam allergy on inpatient outcomes: a multicenter prospective cohort study. Clin Infect Dis 2016;63(7):904–10.

96. Jeffres MN, Narayanan PP, Shuster JE, et al. Consequences of avoiding β-lactams in patients with β-lactam allergies. J Allergy Clin Immunol 2016;137(4): 1148–53.

97. Jerschow E, Lin RY, Scaperotti MM, et al. Fatal anaphylaxis in the united states 1999-2010: temporal patterns and demographic associations. J Allergy Clin Immunol 2014;134(6):1318–28.e7.

98. Albin S, Agarwal S. Prevalence and characteristics of reported penicillin allergy in an urban outpatient adult population. Allergy Asthma Proc 2014;35(6): 489–94.

99. Arroliga ME, Radojicic C, Gordon SM, et al. A prospective observational study of the effect of penicillin skin testing on antibiotic use in the intensive care unit. Infect Control Hosp Epidemiol 2003;24(5):347–50.

100. Arroliga ME, Wagner W, Bobek MB, et al. A pilot study of penicillin skin testing in patients with a history of penicillin allergy admitted to a medical ICU. Chest 2000;118(4):1106–8.

101. King EA, Challa S, Curtin P, et al. Penicillin skin testing in hospitalized patients with beta-lactam allergies: Effect on antibiotic selection and cost. Ann Allergy Asthma Immunol 2016;117(1):67–71.

102. Blumenthal KG, Shenoy ES. Editorial commentary: Fortune favors the bold: Give a beta-lactam! Clin Infect Dis 2016;63(7):911–3.

103. Elligsen M, Walker SAN, Pinto R, et al. Audit and feedback to reduce broadspectrum antibiotic use among intensive care unit patients: a controlled interrupted time series analysis. Infect Control Hosp Epidemiol 2012;33(04):354–61.

104. DiazGranados CA. Prospective audit for antimicrobial stewardship in intensive care: Impact on resistance and clinical outcomes. Am J Infect Control 2012; 40(6):526–9.

105. Fleming D, Ali KF, Matelski J, et al. When antimicrobial stewardship isn't watching: the educational impact of critical care prospective audit and feedback. Open Forum Infect Dis 2016;3(3):ofw115.

106. Elligsen M, Walker SA, Simor A, et al. Prospective audit and feedback of antimicrobial stewardship in critical care: program implementation, experience, and challenges. Can J Hosp Pharm 2012;65(1):31–6.

107. Foral PA, Anthone JM, Destache CJ, et al. Education and communication in an interprofessional antimicrobial stewardship program. J Am Osteopath Assoc 2016;116(9):588–93.

108. Goldstein EJC, Goff DA, Reeve W, et al. Approaches to modifying the behavior of clinicians who are noncompliant with antimicrobial stewardship program guidelines. Clin Infect Dis 2016;63(4):532–8.

109. Grayson ML, Macesic N, Huang GK, et al. Use of an innovative personality-mindset profiling tool to guide culture-change strategies among different health-care worker groups. PLoS One 2015;10(10):e0140509.

110. Morton JB, Curzake DJ, Morrill HJ, et al. Verbal communication with providers improves acceptance of antimicrobial stewardship interventions. Infect Control Hosp Epidemiol 2016;37(06):740–2.

111. Weiss CH, Dibardino D, Rho J, et al. A clinical trial comparing physician prompting with an unprompted automated electronic checklist to reduce empirical antibiotic utilization. Crit Care Med 2013;41(11):2563–9.

112. Weiss CH, Persell SD, Wunderink RG, et al. Empiric antibiotic, mechanical ventilation, and central venous catheter duration as potential factors mediating the effect of a checklist prompting intervention on mortality: an exploratory analysis. BMC Health Serv Res 2012;12:198.

113. Kaki R, Elligsen M, Walker S, et al. Impact of antimicrobial stewardship in critical care: a systematic review. J Antimicrob Chemother 2011;66(6):1223–30.

114. Rimawi RH, Mazer MA, Siraj DS, et al. Impact of regular collaboration between infectious diseases and critical care practitioners on antimicrobial utilization and patient outcome. Crit Care Med 2013;41(9):2099–107.

115. Curcio D, Belloni R. Strategic alliance between the infectious diseases specialist and intensive care unit physician for change in antibiotic use. J Chemother 2005;17(1):74–6.

116. Dimopoulos G, Poulakou G, Pneumatikos IA, et al. Short- vs long-duration antibiotic regimens for ventilator-associated pneumonia: a systematic review and meta-analysis. Chest 2013;144(6):1759–67.

117. Chastre J, Wolff M, Fagon JY, et al. Comparison of 8 vs 15 days of antibiotic therapy for ventilator-associated pneumonia in adults: a randomized trial. JAMA 2003;290(19):2588–98.

118. Sandberg T, Skoog G, Hermansson AB, et al. Ciprofloxacin for 7 days versus 14 days in women with acute pyelonephritis: a randomised, open-label and double-blind, placebo-controlled, non-inferiority trial. Lancet 2012;380(9840):484–90.

119. Sawyer RG, Claridge JA, Nathens AB, et al. Trial of short-course antimicrobial therapy for intraabdominal infection. N Engl J Med 2015;372(21):1996–2005.

120. Luyt CE, Brechot N, Trouillet JL, et al. Antibiotic stewardship in the intensive care unit. Crit Care 2014;18(5):480.

121. Jiang SP, Zheng X, Li X, et al. Effectiveness of pharmaceutical care in an intensive care unit from china. A pre- and post-intervention study. Saudi Med J 2012;33(7):756–62.

122. Jiang S, Zhu Z, Ma K, et al. Impact of pharmacist antimicrobial dosing adjustments in septic patients on continuous renal replacement therapy in an intensive care unit. Scand J Infect Dis 2013;45(12):891–9.

123. Whipple JK, Ausman RK, Franson T, et al. Effect of individualized pharmacokinetic dosing on patient outcome. Crit Care Med 1991;19(12):1480–5.

124. Bartal C, Danon A, Schlaeffer F, et al. Pharmacokinetic dosing of aminoglycosides: a controlled trial. Am J Med 2003;114(3):194–8.

125. Kemme DJ, Daniel CI. Aminoglycoside dosing: a randomized prospective study. South Med J 1993;86(1):46–51.

126. Welty TE, Copa AK. Impact of vancomycin therapeutic drug monitoring on patient care. Ann Pharmacother 1994;28(12):1335–9.
127. Karam CM, McKinnon PS, Neuhauser MM, et al. Outcome assessment of minimizing vancomycin monitoring and dosing adjustments. Pharmacotherapy 1999;19(3):257–66.
128. Roberts JA, Paul SK, Akova M, et al. DALI: Defining antibiotic levels in intensive care unit patients: Are current beta-lactam antibiotic doses sufficient for critically ill patients? Clin Infect Dis 2014;58(8):1072–83.
129. Kaufman SE, Donnell RW, Hickey WS. Rationale and evidence for extended infusion of piperacillin–tazobactam. Am J Health Syst Pharm 2011;68(16):1521–6.
130. Lodise TP, Lomaestro B, Drusano GL. Piperacillin-tazobactam for *Pseudomonas aeruginosa* infection: Clinical implications of an extended-infusion dosing strategy. Clin Infect Dis 2007;44(3):357–63.
131. Falagas ME, Tansarli GS, Ikawa K, et al. Clinical outcomes with extended or continuous versus short-term intravenous infusion of carbapenems and piperacillin/tazobactam: A systematic review and meta-analysis. Clin Infect Dis 2013;56(2):272–82.
132. Dulhunty JM, Roberts JA, Davis JS, et al. Continuous infusion of beta-lactam antibiotics in severe sepsis: A multicenter double-blind, randomized controlled trial. Clin Infect Dis 2013;56(2):236–44.
133. Kollef MH, Bassetti M, Francois B, et al. The intensive care medicine research agenda on multidrug-resistant bacteria, antibiotics, and stewardship. Intensive Care Med 2017. [Epub ahead of print].
134. Mertz D, Brooks A, Irfan N, et al. Antimicrobial stewardship in the intensive care setting–a review and critical appraisal of the literature. Swiss Med Wkly 2015;145:w14220.

Preventing Transmission of Multidrug-Resistant Pathogens in the Intensive Care Unit

CrossMark

Jeffrey R. Strich, MD[a], Tara N. Palmore, MD[b],*

KEYWORDS

- Intensive care unit • Infection control • Transmission • Drug resistance

KEY POINTS

- Multidrug-resistant organisms (MDRO) pose an increasing threat to critically ill patients.
- Patients, healthcare personnel, and the built environment of the intensive care unit are potential reservoirs for transmission of MDRO.
- Meticulous hand hygiene, environmental disinfection, chlorhexidine baths, and other infection control measures can interrupt spread of MDRO.
- Antimicrobial stewardship is an essential tool for improving quality of care and reducing selective pressure that promotes emergence of multidrug resistance.
- While infections with MDRO are becoming more difficult to treat with available antimicrobial drugs, intensive care unit staff can combat their spread by optimizing basic measures that are known to be effective.

INTRODUCTION

Intensive care unit (ICU) beds in the United States are increasing as a proportion of all hospital beds, reflecting increasing need for critical care, particularly among neonates and the elderly.[1] Although nosocomial infections complicate 4% of overall hospital admissions,[2] 9% to 20% of critically ill patients develop infections while in the ICU.[2–4] Nearly half of all health care–associated infections that occur in hospitals are attributable to the ICU.[2] At the same time, the proportion of nosocomial infections caused by multidrug-resistant organisms is increasing, limiting treatment options and increasing length of stay, mortality, and cost.[5] Increasing use of critical care resources and high

[a] Critical Care Medicine Department, National Institutes of Health Clinical Center, 10 Center Drive, MSC 1662, Bethesda, MD 20892-1662, USA; [b] Hospital Epidemiology Service, National Institutes of Health Clinical Center, 10 Center Drive, MSC 1899, Bethesda, MD 20892-1899, USA
* Corresponding author.
E-mail address: tpalmore@mail.nih.gov

Infect Dis Clin N Am 31 (2017) 535–550
http://dx.doi.org/10.1016/j.idc.2017.05.010
0891-5520/17/Published by Elsevier Inc.
id.theclinics.com

risk of nosocomial infection in the context of increasing antimicrobial resistance make infection prevention a leading priority in the ICU.

Guidelines from the Centers for Disease Control and Prevention (CDC) from 2006,[6] and the Society for Hospital Epidemiology of America from 2003,[7] provide infection control guidance to prevent the spread of multidrug-resistant pathogens. This article examines more recent evidence for methods of preventing the transmission of multidrug-resistant pathogens in the ICU.

Importance of Preventing Transmission of Resistant Organisms

ICU patients are highly vulnerable to nosocomial infection because of invasive devices, immune compromise caused by underlying diseases or medications, poor nutritional states, uncontrolled hyperglycemia, and sepsis, which can lead to a paradoxical immune suppression.[8] Multidrug-resistant pathogens represent a substantial proportion of nosocomial infections in the ICU, including 10% to 16% of US device-related infections.[9] Infection with multidrug-resistant organisms causes significant mortality in hospitalized patients. Approximately 23,000 persons in the United States die each year from these organisms, most of which are acquired in health care settings.[10] Nosocomial bloodstream infections with resistant gram-negative organisms can have mortality as high as 80% to 85%.[11,12]

In addition to host susceptibility, the logistics and complexity of critical care medicine put patients at risk of acquiring nosocomial organisms. Invasive procedures and indwelling devices, often essential to providing supportive care to critically ill patients, serve as portals of entry for pathogens. Lifesaving critical care treatment requires the concurrent contributions of many health care team members and the use of many patient care devices, potentially posing additive risk of transmission from personnel or fomites. Infection control precautions may not be the predominant priority in situations in which seconds matter, such as resuscitating patients suffering trauma, sepsis, cardiac arrest, and other emergencies. Antimicrobial use may select out resistant strains that are potentially transmissible from patient to patient.

Transmission of Resistant Organisms in the intensive Care Unit

Bacterial pathogens of epidemiologic concern in the ICU tend to inhabit specific sites on or in the human body, or in the hospital environment, that serve as reservoirs for transmission. The reservoirs of resistant organisms include niches in the human microbiome. The microbiota of skin, respiratory epithelium, and the gastrointestinal tract are altered within a few days in the hospital. Patients' flora can be deranged by antibiotics, chemotherapy, or acquisition of nosocomial organisms, among other sources. Patients who are colonized with resistant bacteria serve inadvertently as potential reservoirs for transmission. Colonization pressure, or the proportion of patients in a given unit who are colonized with resistant bacteria, is an independent risk factor for transmission.[13,14] Resistant organisms are generally thought to be transmitted from person to person via the hands of health care personnel, or from contaminated patient care equipment or contaminated surfaces in the health care environment. Antimicrobial stewardship, hand hygiene, and proper disinfection of equipment and hospital surfaces are thus important means of preventing spread.

Hospitals should have policies and procedures in place that outline clear infection control guidelines, along with contingency procedures for special situations. ICU staff must receive periodic training and education in infection control, which should be informed by data on infection rates, hand hygiene rates, and other relevant outcome measures. In addition, compliance with infection control procedures requires adequate staffing, infrastructure (such as handwashing sinks), and supplies (such as gloves, masks, and alcohol-based hand gel).

ANTIMICROBIAL STEWARDSHIP

Antimicrobial stewardship has an important and distinct role to play in the ICU, and has been shown to improve the treatment of critically ill patients and reduce antimicrobial resistance.[15,16] The goals of antimicrobial stewardship are to improve the quality of care and avert adverse outcomes, including antimicrobial resistance, by optimizing dosing and selection of drugs, along with reducing duration of therapy.[17] Intensivists face a challenge of balancing the need to administer broad antibiotic coverage for the immediate welfare of critically ill patients, particularly those with undifferentiated shock, with the short-term potential for drug toxicity and *Clostridium difficile* infection and the longer-term potential for generating antimicrobial resistance in individual patients and the ICU population.

The initial antimicrobial management of sepsis is critical. In patients with septic shock, delays in empiric antimicrobial administration are highly correlated with mortality.[18] The selection of appropriate initial antimicrobial therapy is also associated with a mortality benefit.[19] Empiric therapy for sepsis should consider the most likely source and pathogens, the local antibiogram, and the local epidemiology of multidrug-resistant organisms in the ward, institution, or community from which the patient arrived.

In the ICU, antimicrobial stewardship favors prospective audit and feedback by pharmacists and physicians trained in antimicrobial stewardship, reevaluating empiric therapy after 48 to 72 hours to consider deescalation if a diagnosis has been established.[20] In addition, formulary restriction of select antimicrobials and therapeutic drug monitoring are also integral to minimizing selection pressure and optimizing antimicrobial therapy in the ICU. Rapid diagnostic methods, such as matrix-assisted laser desorption ionization—time of flight (MALDI-TOF) mass spectrometry, can expedite diagnosis and thus deescalation of empiric therapy to optimal therapy.[21] In addition, guidance from serial serum concentrations of procalcitonin, a biomarker with increased levels in patients who have bacterial infections, has been shown to reduce the duration of antimicrobial therapy in ICU patients.[22] A successful antimicrobial stewardship program requires not only education of physicians, nurses, and other health care staff but also culture change, such that the program is embraced as a critical patient safety measure.

Hand Hygiene

ICU personnel who perform inadequate hand hygiene may carry multidrug-resistant organisms on their hands. Although carriage may be transient, many organisms can survive long enough to be spread to the ICU environment or directly to patients. Personnel can have longer-term carriage of bacterial pathogens in rings[23] or under long or artificial fingernails, and the recurrent role of long and artificial nails in outbreaks has led the CDC to recommend against them.[24]

Hand hygiene, prioritized as an overriding infection control goal by the CDC and the World Health Organization (WHO),[25] is one of the most challenging measures to follow consistently in the ICU. The WHO's Five Moments for Hand Hygiene is a simple, precise schema for hand hygiene opportunities, or transitions in patient care at which hand hygiene should be done in order to prevent cross-transmission.[25] Despite evidence that hand hygiene prevents nosocomial infections[26] and extensive research efforts to boost hand hygiene compliance rates in hospitals, adherence remains as low as 40% to 60%, and in some studies is lower in the ICU than in other wards.[27,28]

Investigators have attempted to understand the basis for uneven compliance in order to identify opportunities for improvement. In a recent German study, investigators measured the number of hand hygiene opportunities per ICU patient and the mean duration of hand hygiene.[29] Among an estimated 218 to 271 daily hand hygiene opportunities per patient, overall compliance was 42.6%, with an average 6.8 seconds spent on each hand hygiene episode. The investigators concluded that if hand hygiene were performed in compliance with WHO guidelines (including 20–30 seconds per hand hygiene episode), each nurse would spend an estimated 58 to 70 minutes on hand hygiene for each patient during a 12-hour shift.[29] This study shows the predicament faced by ICU personnel when patient care workload conflicts with commitment of time to meticulous hand hygiene.

Recent research studies to improve hand hygiene compliance have focused on improving monitoring of compliance and addressing behavioral and psychological barriers to consistent hand hygiene. Investigators at the University of North Carolina addressed both goals by opening compliance measurement to frontline health care personnel in a broad range of disciplines, thereby generating more robust monitoring data and improving compliance in the involved disciplines.[30] Early-generation electronic monitoring systems have had mixed results, showing that there is room for improvement in the automated systems and the study designs used to evaluate them.[31,32]

In an era in which some classes of antibiotic-resistant organisms have diminishing treatment options, hand hygiene remains the simplest and possibly the most important intervention to limit the human toll of infections caused by these organisms in the ICU. Achieving better hand hygiene compliance is a major infection control goal.

MANAGEMENT OF ANTIBIOTIC-RESISTANT ORGANISM COLONIZATION
Microbial Screening

Identification and isolation of colonized patients are standard infection control measures to reduce the risk of patient-to-patient transmission. The goal of screening patients for microbial colonization is to identify those who are carriers of antibiotic-resistant organisms and could serve as reservoirs for transmission. Such information theoretically provides an opportunity to interrupt spread through isolation precautions or decolonization. However, the efficacy of microbial surveillance as a horizontal strategy to minimize transmission of resistant pathogens is controversial. Although screening and isolation have been effective in some models and clinical settings,[33,34] widespread implementation is costly and laborious, and carries the inherent negative of placing more patients in isolation for uncertain benefit to the patient population.

In one study that shows the potential pitfalls of such an approach, investigators assessed the effect of daily surveillance cultures among ICU patients for *Staphylococcus aureus* (including methicillin-resistant *S aureus* [MRSA]), but did not report either negative or positive culture results to ICU staff, or place MRSA-colonized patients on isolation precautions.[35] Surveillance cultures and genotyping showed no cross-transmission, despite the presence of several patients colonized by methicillin-sensitive *S aureus* and MRSA, but the absence of spread was not caused by the surveillance cultures. The investigators concluded that "reporting culture results and isolating colonized patients, as suggested by some guidelines, would have falsely suggested the success of such infection control policies."[35]

The effectiveness of screening and isolation has been examined in several recent large, cluster-randomized trials. In a US cluster-randomized trial, Huskins and colleagues[36] screened patients using standard cultures for MRSA and vancomycin-resistant *Enterococcus* (VRE) within 2 days of admission, weekly thereafter, and within 2 days before or after transfer out of the ICU, with contact isolation of carriers. Control and intervention ICUs followed the same screening procedures, but control ICUs did not receive the results of their patients' screening tests. Despite more frequent identification and isolation of carriers in the intervention ICUs, there was no difference in the rate of acquisition of MRSA or VRE. Confounding the interpretation of this study, some patients' screening results may not have been available before their transfer out of the ICU, because the mean turnaround time for the screening cultures was 5.2 days.

In a large European interrupted time series trial, improved hand hygiene compliance and implementation of daily chlorhexidine baths reduced acquisition of MRSA and reduced ICU length of stay. In the next phase of the study, rapid chromogenic screening for highly resistant Enterobacteriaceae and conventional or polymerase chain reaction (PCR) screening for VRE and MRSA were implemented in intervention ICUs within 2 days of admission, twice weekly for 3 weeks, then weekly, with subsequent contact isolation of carriers. Screening, even with rapid PCR testing, and isolation did not significantly reduce acquisition of those resistant organisms in the intervention ICUs.[37] This trial is the only rigorously designed, published study that has addressed screening for resistant gram-negative pathogens.

Some hospitals have reported that ICU screening for carbapenem-resistant gram-negative bacteria as part of a larger infection control program has reduced transmission of, and clinical infections with, these organisms.[38,39] On a larger scale, Israel has achieved remarkable nationwide declines in rates of transmission of these organisms, thanks to a centralized infection control program that involves active surveillance and isolation of carriers in all health care facilities.[40] Further prospective studies are needed to better understand the benefits of screening for carbapenem-resistant bacteria in regions with low and high endemicity.

Isolation Precautions

Despite long-standing recommendations to care for patients who are known to be colonized or infected with multidrug-resistant organisms under barrier precautions,[41] there remains controversy about the benefits of isolation. As described earlier, several approaches to screening and isolating patients have shown no change in acquisition of the multidrug-resistant organisms for which they were screened,[36,37,42] which is likely to be due to a combination of colonization that screening cultures failed to detect and cross-transmission between patients.

Given the pitfalls of strategies of screening and isolation, Harris and colleagues[43] studied whether universal barrier precautions could reduce acquisition of VRE and MRSA in ICUs. In their cluster-randomized trial, personnel in intervention ICUs used gowns and gloves for all patient care, whereas control ICUs used barrier precautions only per CDC guidelines for known colonized or infected patients. Universal gowning and gloving reduced acquisition of MRSA but not VRE. Analysis of trial data showed that hand hygiene compliance improved in the intervention ICUs, and despite a lower number of health care personnel interactions with patients there was no increase in adverse events when all patients were managed under barrier precautions.[43] Implementation of universal contact isolation may be a useful intervention during an ICU-based outbreak, as suggested in several outbreak reports.[12,44,45]

Empiric Isolation

In order to be optimally effective, patient isolation should be implemented not only for confirmed transmissible infection or colonization but also for cases in which a patient is suspected of having communicable disease. For example, droplet isolation should be used when a patient has respiratory symptoms that may be consistent with influenza, airborne isolation in a negative-pressure room when a patient is being tested for pulmonary tuberculosis or chickenpox, and contact isolation when a patient has diarrhea that may be caused by an infectious pathogen. Empiric isolation is recommended until the results of diagnostic tests can confirm or counter the need for ongoing isolation. This strategy helps prevent transmission during the interval while diagnostic tests are pending.

Decolonization and Skin Antisepsis

The aim of decolonization is to eradicate carriage of potential pathogens and reduce the risk of developing invasive infections from those pathogens. Although decolonization regimens have been tested in clinical trials for several epidemiologically important pathogens, S aureus (susceptible or resistant to methicillin) is the organism for which the strongest evidence exists.[46]

Chlorhexidine gluconate baths are a widely studied strategy to reduce the microbial burden colonizing patients' skin. In addition to reducing central line–associated bloodstream infection (CLABSI) rates and MRSA in the ICU,[47] 2% chlorhexidine gluconate daily baths have been shown in some clinical trials to reduce rates of acquisition of other multidrug-resistant organisms, particularly VRE. In a study involving community hospital ICUs in North Carolina, the treatment reduced rates of all CLABSI, CLABSI caused by VRE, and total VRE infections.[48] A cluster-randomized crossover study similarly found reduced rates of CLABSI and VRE during the intervention period when chlorhexidine daily baths were used.[49] However, another such study found no reduction in CLABSI or other health care–associated infections, or occurrence of clinical cultures growing multidrug-resistant bacteria.[50]

Although the benefits of chlorhexidine baths for reducing the incidence of resistant gram-positive infections is arguable, the treatments have shown even less convincing effects on resistant gram-negative organisms in ICU patients. In a single-center, ICU-based study of 4% chlorhexidine baths, Borer and colleagues[51] reported a reduced incidence of multidrug-resistant Acinetobacter bloodstream infections. Chung and colleagues[52] reported reduction in acquisition of multidrug-resistant Acinetobacter in a single ICU with high endemicity of the organism. Rigorous, multicenter studies of the effects of chlorhexidine daily baths on multidrug-resistant gram-negative organisms are needed, involving hospitals with varying prevalence of these pathogens.

Daily baths with 2% chlorhexidine gluconate are an effective public health measure in the ICU. The antiseptic solution is applied on each patient from jaw to toes, avoiding mucous membranes and breaches in the skin, and left on to dry. The residual antimicrobial effect reduces skin colonization with epidemiologically important, antibiotic-resistant organisms, including MRSA, VRE, and carbapenemase-producing Enterobacteriaceae.[42,53,54] Because of strong, but not uniform,[50] evidence from multiple clinical trials showing reduction in CLABSI rates, chlorhexidine daily baths have become standard of care in ICUs.[55] At the present time, despite 1 study to the contrary, there are sufficiently robust data to recommend chlorhexidine daily baths as a universal, or horizontal, intervention in ICUs for prevention of bloodstream infections and reduction in gram-positive infections.[46]

Preventing transmission from the intensive care unit environment

A recent study showed that 40% of patient rooms in the hospital contained environmental contamination with multidrug-resistant organisms, most frequently VRE.[56] The viability of resistant organisms on fomites in the hospital environment is estimated from experimental studies, but is likely affected by many confounding factors (eg, organism burden and strain, temperature, moisture). Some resistant nosocomial pathogens are notoriously hardy on dry surfaces, including VRE and MRSA. Their prolonged viability presents a protracted opportunity for spread from contaminated sites. Researchers at the CDC recently found that *Acinetobacter baumannii* inoculated on steel and plastic remained cultivable at high concentrations that were undiminished throughout the 28-day study period. VRE had a 4-log reduction in concentration but remained cultivable at 28 days.[57] Organisms that prove resilient on hospital surfaces may spread to patients long after they are shed, leading to a protracted transmission cycle.

Less hardy but highly concerning pathogens such as carbapenemase-producing Enterobacteriaceae have also shown remarkable tenacity under dry conditions in experimental studies. The CDC study showed that bla_{KPC}-carrying *Klebsiella pneumoniae* was cultivable on plastic and steel for up to 5 to 6 days, and thereafter viable but noncultivable.[57]

Standard, approved hospital disinfectant cleaners are generally effective against these organisms, provided that they are applied thoroughly to contaminated surfaces and allowed to dwell for an adequate time. Patient care equipment used for patients who are known to harbor multidrug-resistant organisms should, to the greatest extent possible, be disposable to reduce the risk of cross-transmission. Equipment that is shared among patients, such as blood pressure devices, cooling blankets, and portable radiology cassettes, should be disinfected thoroughly between patients. Items like fabric privacy curtains, which are readily and widely contaminated with resistant organisms,[58] can be removed or replaced with disposable curtains.

Adjunctive methods of disinfection, such as ultraviolet light and hydrogen peroxide vapor, have been studied in experimental settings and in clinical trials.[59] Both methods reduce the burden of bacterial pathogens, including spores, in the environment. Hydrogen peroxide vapor is highly effective for eliminating pathogens that are on surfaces out of the line of sight, but takes hours and requires sealing of a patient room, including temporary closure of air supply and return. It has been used to good effect to decontaminate hospital wards undergoing outbreaks,[12] and for decontamination in the setting of high-concern pathogens.[60] Ultraviolet light is logistically easier, less time consuming, and less dependent on technical expertise to operate, but is less effective at killing organisms that are in shadows outside the path of the light.

A cluster-randomized, multicenter trial led by investigators at Duke University compared terminal cleaning with standard hospital disinfectants, enhanced cleaning with bleach-containing disinfectant, and standard or bleach cleaning in combination with ultraviolet C treatment. Despite a high rate of compliance with environmental disinfection and documented reduction in VRE and MRSA environmental contamination in bleach and ultraviolet light-treated rooms, the study results showed the complexity of linking environmental disinfection with patient outcomes. MRSA was reduced among patients who occupied rooms disinfected with ultraviolet light, VRE was reduced among those whose rooms had been treated with bleach, and *C difficile* infection was not reduced by any of the interventions.[61]

Some organisms reside in moist locations in the environment, and may inhabit biofilms from which they can potentially be transmitted to patients. Examples include waterborne bacteria such as species of *Stenotrophomonas*, *Pseudomonas*,

Aeromonas, and *Sphingomonas*, which can colonize plumbing fixtures. In multiple reported ICU outbreaks, multidrug-resistant outbreak organisms have been identified in the biofilms of sink drains, faucets, or aerators. Although circumstantial evidence may implicate the sink drain colonization in the outbreak, it is difficult to determine whether drains were truly sources of transmission or just became colonized during the course of an outbreak.

Preventing transmission from contaminated plumbing is an area of uncertainty in hospital infection control, and the subject of active research.[62] Some basic steps include ascertaining adequate levels of free chlorine in hospital water,[63] selecting sinks that have low-splash design, and avoiding placement of patient care supplies around handwashing sinks, where they could be contaminated by splash-back from the drain. In an outbreak setting in which plumbing fixtures are implicated, plumbing might require disassembly, special cleaning and disinfection procedures, or even replacement.

Preventing transmission of methicillin-resistant Staphylococcus aureus

S aureus, an important cause of severe infections in ICU patients, is carried on skin and mucous membranes in up to half of hospitalized patients.[64] MRSA causes community-acquired infections (eg, skin and soft tissue infections, endocarditis, pneumonia) that can require ICU care, and nosocomial infections (eg, wound infections, device-associated bacteremia, pneumonia) that can complicate ICU care.

Because of extensive MRSA transmission in the community, a significant proportion of patients are colonized on admission. Patients who are colonized and/or infected with MRSA can serve as reservoirs for transmission in the hospital. A long-term study showed that 22% of MRSA acquisition in a neonatal ICU could be traced to MRSA carriers in the same unit.[65] As with many other nosocomial bacteria, MRSA are thought to be spread on the hands of health care personnel, and on contaminated equipment and surfaces.

Some institutions have implemented programs of large-scale MRSA screening and isolation to reduce transmission. The Veterans Affairs hospitals began such a program in 2007, and reported sustained declines in MRSA transmission and health care–associated infections in ICUs over the subsequent 8 years. Transmission of MRSA in the ICU, defined as a newly positive screening test or clinical culture after hospital day 2, declined by 36.6%, and nosocomial MRSA infections in the ICU declined by a stunning 87%.[66] The program notably includes culture change among health care personnel around infection prevention as a major goal, in addition to tracking and quantifying preventive efforts.

Other approaches include attempts at decolonization of MRSA carriers using nasal mupirocin and chlorhexidine baths. A cluster-randomized trial by Huang and colleagues[42] showed that a strategy of screening cultures for MRSA in ICUs and isolation of carriers was less effective for reducing the incidence of MRSA than either targeted or universal decolonization with nasal mupirocin and chlorhexidine daily baths. The 2 decolonization strategies were compared in an attempt to settle controversy about whether the intervention should target those who are colonized and at high risk of infection, or should be used as a blanket public health intervention in ICUs.[46] In the study by Huang and colleagues[42] universal decolonization led to a 44% reduction in bloodstream infections caused by any pathogen and a 37% reduction in MRSA-positive clinical cultures.[42] Universal decolonization in the ICU has been shown to be a cost-effective strategy,[67] and the practice can decrease endogenous infection along with patient-to-patient transmission; however, there are concerns about development of antibiotic resistance with widespread use of chlorhexidine.[46,68]

Preventing transmission of vancomycin-resistant Enterococcus faecium

Colonization with VRE is common in the ICU, especially among patients who are immunocompromised or chronically ill, have prolonged hospital stays, and have received broad-spectrum antimicrobials. Development of VRE colonization in the ICU is associated with prolonged hospitalization and receipt of metronidazole.[69]

Although VRE bacteremia has a low attributable mortality in ICU patents, on par with that of coagulase-negative staphylococci, it does cause nosocomial infections that can be difficult to treat.[70] In VRE-colonized patients, the organisms are found primarily in the fecal flora, are shed in high numbers, and can be found on skin and throughout the patient's hospital room.[71] Because VRE can be carried on health care personnel hands and survive well on inanimate surfaces, the organisms are easily transmitted via the health care environment.

Hayden and colleagues[71] found that VRE was highly prevalent in their ICU environment, and showed that reducing environmental contamination had a marked effect on the spread of VRE in their ICU. Patients who occupy ICU rooms that previously housed patients colonized with VRE are at increased risk of acquiring VRE themselves. That risk is only partially mitigated by enhanced environmental cleaning.[72]

Preventing transmission of resistant gram-negative bacteria

Multidrug-resistant gram-negative bacteria have long posed a threat to critically ill patients. Resistant *Pseudomonas aeruginosa* and *A baumannii*, extended-spectrum β-lactamase–producing Enterobacteriaceae, and carbapenemase-producing and colistin-resistant strains of gram-negative bacteria can cause a wide range of nosocomial infections that can be difficult to treat. The most prevalent bacterial causes of nosocomial bloodstream infections have shifted from gram-positive to gram-negative organisms, with a high proportion of multidrug-resistant gram-negative strains.[73] Intensivists have a shrinking antibiotic armamentarium when patients develop device-related infections, including bacteremia and pneumonia, or other severe infections with these organisms.

Over the past 15 years, gram-negative bacteria carrying a variety of carbapenemase enzymes have emerged and disseminated around the globe, profoundly changing the epidemiology of nosocomial infections in many countries. Carbapenemase genes are often found in organisms that already harbor other significant resistance genes, such as extended-spectrum β-lactamases, and are thus extensively resistant or even pan-resistant to antibiotics.[12] Clinically significant carbapenemase genes include bla_{KPC}, bla_{OXA-48}, and $bla_{OXA-48-like}$ family, and the bla_{NDM-1}, bla_{VIM}, and bla_{IMP} metallo-β-lactamase genes. Although plasmid-borne genes for carbapenemase enzymes can be found in a broad array of gram-negative species, *K pneumoniae* and *Enterobacter* species are the most common in North America.[74] Globally, *P aeruginosa* and *A baumannii* are often multidrug resistant because of carbapenemase genes, chromosomal resistance genes (such as multidrug efflux pumps), or both. Spread of the recently discovered plasmid-borne *mcr-1* gene conferring colistin resistance may further complicate epidemiology and management of nosocomial gram-negative infections.

Like other nosocomial bacteria, resistant gram-negative organisms are likely spread on the hands of health care personnel, with contamination of the dry environment of the hospital likely playing a lesser role in nosocomial spread than is thought to occur with gram-positive bacteria. Long-term acute care hospitals serve as a deep reservoir of resistant gram-negative bacteria, in part because of poor control of transmission in those facilities, chronic illness and immunocompromised states, long-term invasive devices such as ventilators, and repeated exposure to antibiotics. Patients transferred to the ICU from these facilities are at high risk of being colonized or infected on transfer with resistant gram-negative organisms. Many hospitals target this patient population for admission surveillance with rectal or perirectal swabs to detect colonization with carbapenem-resistant or carbapenemase-producing bacteria and prevent their transmission within the ICU.

In the wake of a 2011 to 2012 outbreak of carbapenemase-producing *K pneumoniae*, our hospital conducts admission surveillance on patients of all ages, apart from those on behavioral health wards. Patients undergo carbapenemase surveillance cultures from perirectal swabs on admission, and twice weekly while in the ICU. Patients who are in the CDC's high-risk categories (those hospitalized in the United States in the previous week or outside the United States in the previous 6 months) are placed in contact isolation on admission and undergo 2 perirectal cultures to increase the sensitivity of screening. Patients who are found to be colonized with carbapenemase-producing bacteria are cohorted, or housed in a designated section of the ICU, and cared for by nurses who are assigned only to their care. An additional measure is the use of adherence monitors, staff members who are trained to observe all health care personnel and visitors who enter and exit the cohorted patient's room and ensure that all infection control precautions are followed meticulously. These measures are intended to reduce the risk of cross-transmission to other critically ill patients.[75]

Multidrug-resistant Acinetobacter baumannii

A baumannii is a nosocomial menace whose high-level resistance and worldwide dispersal have earned the bacteria the distinction of being the WHO's top antimicrobial-resistant pathogen of concern.[76] *A baumannii* is a particular problem in ICUs, where it causes device-related infections, pneumonia, bloodstream infections, and wound infections that can be extremely difficult to treat because of the paucity of effective antibiotic choices.[77] In a large international study, *Acinetobacter* species were responsible for an average of 8.8% of gram-negative ICU infections on all continents, and more than 19% in Asian ICUs.[73] More than 80% of *A baumannii* isolates are multidrug resistant,[78] with the highest rates of resistance found in residents of nursing homes.[79] Surveillance cultures for colonization can be collected from the groin, which is the most sensitive site for detection,[80] and the throat.

A baumannii develops antimicrobial resistance rapidly via chromosomal mutations and mobile genetic elements, including plasmids carrying carbapenemase genes. As noted earlier, *A baumannii* is able to withstand long periods of desiccation and can persist on ICU surfaces and equipment. The organism readily adheres to protective equipment; in one study, nearly 40% of interactions with ICU patients colonized by *A baumannii* resulted in contamination of health care personnel gloves, gowns, or both.[81] The lack of treatment options for multidrug-resistant *Acinetobacter* underscores the critical role of hand hygiene and painstaking environmental infection control in preventing spread of what is often a nearly untreatable pathogen. The authors have used the same control measures for carbapenemase-producing organisms described earlier to contain highly resistant *A baumannii* in the ICU.[44]

Candida auris

C auris is a newly emerging, global microbial threat in ICUs. *Candida* species are the most common health care–associated fungal infection and an important cause of bloodstream infections in ICU patients. Outbreaks of *C auris* have been reported in ICUs in the Americas, Europe, Africa, and Asia.[82,83] Like *A baumannii* and distinctly unlike most nosocomial *Candida* species, *C auris* tends to be multidrug resistant, spreads from colonized patients to other patients within the ICU, and contaminates surfaces with marked longevity and tenacity.[82–84] The organism has been cultured from the skin of both asymptomatic patients and health care personnel.[85] The CDC in 2016 issued a clinical alert requesting that all health care facilities report cases of *C auris*, isolate patients colonized or infected with the organism, and redouble efforts at disinfection and cleaning of their rooms.[86] This organism deserves the attention of infection control and intensive care staff, because it seems to have all the features of a fierce nosocomial pathogen.

SUMMARY

Infection control in the ICU has seen many advances, including rapid molecular screening tests for resistant organisms and chlorhexidine use in daily baths. Although these developments advance the cause of infection prevention, compliance with some of the most basic measures remains elusive. Hand hygiene, antimicrobial stewardship, and reduction in device use remain the low-technology interventions that could have a major impact on nosocomial transmission of antimicrobial-resistant organisms. Although continued research is needed on new and old ways of preventing nosocomial infections, ICU staff must persevere in improving adherence with the measures that are known to be effective.

REFERENCES

1. Halpern NA, Goldman DA, Tan KS, et al. Trends in critical care beds and use among population groups and Medicare and Medicaid beneficiaries in the United States: 2000-2010. Crit Care Med 2016;44(8):1490–9.
2. Magill SS, Edwards JR, Bamberg W, et al. Multistate point-prevalence survey of health care-associated infections. N Engl J Med 2014;370(13):1198–208.
3. Zingg W, Hopkins S, Gayet-Ageron A, et al. Health-care-associated infections in neonates, children, and adolescents: an analysis of paediatric data from the European Centre for Disease Prevention and Control point-prevalence survey. Lancet Infect Dis 2017;17(4):381–9.
4. European Centre for Disease Prevention and Control. Point prevalence survey of healthcare-associated infections and antimicrobial use in European acute care hospitals. Stockholm; 2017. Available at: http://ecdc.europa.eu/en/healthtopics/Healthcare-associated_infections/point-prevalence-survey/Pages/Point-prevalence-survey.aspx.
5. Roberts RR, Hota B, Ahmad I, et al. Hospital and societal costs of antimicrobial-resistant infections in a Chicago teaching hospital: implications for antibiotic stewardship. Clin Infect Dis 2009;49(8):1175–84.
6. Siegel JD, Rhinehart E, Jackson M, et al, and the Healthcare Infection Control Practices Advisory Committee 2006. 2007. Centers for Disease Control and Prevention. Available at: http://www.cdc.gov/ncidod/dhqp/pdf/ar/mdroGuideline2006.pdf. Accessed January 5, 2007.
7. Muto CA, Jernigan JA, Ostrowsky BE, et al. SHEA guideline for preventing nosocomial transmission of multidrug-resistant strains of *Staphylococcus aureus* and *Enterococcus*. Infect Control Hosp Epidemiol 2003;24(5):362–86.
8. Hotchkiss RS, Opal S. Immunotherapy for sepsis-a new approach against an ancient foe. N Engl J Med 2010;363(1):87–9.
9. Centers for Disease Control and Prevention. Making health care safe: protect patients from antibiotic resistance. Vital Signs; 2016. Available at: https://www.cdc.gov/vitalsigns/protect-patients/index.html. Accessed March 3, 2016.

10. Centers for Disease Control and Prevention. Antibiotic resistance threats in the United States, 2013. 2013. Available at: https://www.cdc.gov/drugresistance/threat-report-2013/pdf/ar-threats-2013-508.pdf.

11. Mathers AJ, Cox HL, Kitchel B, et al. Molecular dissection of an outbreak of carbapenem-resistant Enterobacteriaceae reveals intergenus KPC carbapenem-ase transmission through a promiscuous plasmid. MBio 2011;2(6):e00204–11.

12. Snitkin ES, Zelazny AM, Thomas PJ, et al. Tracking a hospital outbreak of carbapenem-resistant Klebsiella pneumoniae with whole-genome sequencing. Sci Transl Med 2012;4(148):148ra16.

13. Williams VR, Callery S, Vearncombe M, et al. The role of colonization pressure in nosocomial transmission of methicillin-resistant Staphylococcus aureus. Am J Infect Control 2009;37(2):106–10.

14. Masse J, Elkalioubie A, Blazejewski C, et al. Colonization pressure as a risk factor of ICU-acquired multidrug resistant bacteria: a prospective observational study. Eur J Clin Microbiol Infect Dis 2017;36(5):797–805.

15. Katsios CM, Burry L, Nelson S, et al. An antimicrobial stewardship program improves antimicrobial treatment by culture site and the quality of antimicrobial prescribing in critically ill patients. Crit Care 2012;16(6):R216.

16. Karanika S, Paudel S, Grigoras C, et al. Systematic review and meta-analysis of clinical and economic outcomes from the implementation of hospital-based antimicrobial stewardship programs. Antimicrob Agents Chemother 2016;60(8):4840–52.

17. Barlam TF, Cosgrove SE, Abbo LM, et al. Implementing an antibiotic stewardship program: guidelines by the Infectious Diseases Society of America and the Society for Healthcare Epidemiology of America. Clin Infect Dis 2016;62(10):e51–77.

18. Kumar A, Roberts D, Wood KE, et al. Duration of hypotension before initiation of effective antimicrobial therapy is the critical determinant of survival in human septic shock. Crit Care Med 2006;34(6):1589–96.

19. Kollef MH, Sherman G, Ward S, et al. Inadequate antimicrobial treatment of infections: a risk factor for hospital mortality among critically ill patients. Chest 1999;115(2):462–74.

20. Garnacho-Montero J, Gutierrez-Pizarraya A, Escoresca-Ortega A, et al. De-escalation of empirical therapy is associated with lower mortality in patients with severe sepsis and septic shock. Intensive Care Med 2014;40(1):32–40.

21. Huang AM, Newton D, Kunapuli A, et al. Impact of rapid organism identification via matrix-assisted laser desorption/ionization time-of-flight combined with antimicrobial stewardship team intervention in adult patients with bacteremia and candidemia. Clin Infect Dis 2013;57(9):1237–45.

22. de Jong E, van Oers JA, Beishuizen A, et al. Efficacy and safety of procalcitonin guidance in reducing the duration of antibiotic treatment in critically ill patients: a randomised, controlled, open-label trial. Lancet Infect Dis 2016;16(7):819–27.

23. Fagernes M, Lingaas E. Impact of finger rings on transmission of bacteria during hand contact. Infect Control Hosp Epidemiol 2009;30(5):427–32.

24. Boyce JM, Pittet D, Healthcare Infection Control Practices Advisory Committee, HICPAC/SHEA/APIC/IDSAH and Hygiene Task Force. Guideline for hand hygiene in health-care settings. Recommendations of the Healthcare Infection Control Practices Advisory Committee and the HICPAC/SHEA/APIC/IDSA Hand Hygiene Task Force. Society for Healthcare Epidemiology of America/Association for Professionals in Infection Control/Infectious Diseases Society of America. MMWR Recomm Rep 2002;51(RR-16):1–45.

25. World Health Organization. WHO guidelines on hand hygiene in health care. Geneva (Switzerland); 2009. Available at: http://www.who.int/gpsc/5may/tools/9789241597906/en/.

26. Pittet D, Hugonnet S, Harbarth S, et al. Effectiveness of a hospital-wide programme to improve compliance with hand hygiene. Infection Control Programme. Lancet 2000;356(9238):1307–12.

27. Erasmus V, Daha TJ, Brug H, et al. Systematic review of studies on compliance with hand hygiene guidelines in hospital care. Infect Control Hosp Epidemiol 2010;31(3):283–94.

28. Kowitt B, Jefferson J, Mermel LA. Factors associated with hand hygiene compliance at a tertiary care teaching hospital. Infect Control Hosp Epidemiol 2013; 34(11):1146–52.

29. Stahmeyer JT, Lutze B, von Lengerke T, et al. Hand hygiene in intensive care units: a matter of time? J Hosp Infect 2017;95(4):338–43.

30. Sickbert-Bennett EE, DiBiase LM, Schade Willis TM, et al. Reducing health care-associated infections by implementing a novel all hands on deck approach for hand hygiene compliance. Am J Infect Control 2016;44(5 Suppl):e13–6.

31. Srigley JA, Gardam M, Fernie G, et al. Hand hygiene monitoring technology: a systematic review of efficacy. J Hosp Infect 2015;89(1):51–60.

32. Ward MA, Schweizer ML, Polgreen PM, et al. Automated and electronically assisted hand hygiene monitoring systems: a systematic review. Am J Infect Control 2014;42(5):472–8.

33. Bootsma MC, Diekmann O, Bonten MJ. Controlling methicillin-resistant *Staphylococcus aureus*: quantifying the effects of interventions and rapid diagnostic testing. Proc Natl Acad Sci U S A 2006;103(14):5620–5.

34. Shadel BN, Puzniak LA, Gillespie KN, et al. Surveillance for vancomycin-resistant enterococci: type, rates, costs, and implications. Infect Control Hosp Epidemiol 2006;27(10):1068–75.

35. Nijssen S, Bonten MJ, Weinstein RA. Are active microbiological surveillance and subsequent isolation needed to prevent the spread of methicillin-resistant *Staphylococcus aureus*? Clin Infect Dis 2005;40(3):405–9.

36. Huskins WC, Huckabee CM, O'Grady NP, et al. Intervention to reduce transmission of resistant bacteria in intensive care. N Engl J Med 2011;364(15):1407–18.

37. Derde LP, Cooper BS, Goossens H, et al. Interventions to reduce colonisation and transmission of antimicrobial-resistant bacteria in intensive care units: an interrupted time series study and cluster randomised trial. Lancet Infect Dis 2014; 14(1):31–9.

38. Viale P, Tumietto F, Giannella M, et al. Impact of a hospital-wide multifaceted programme for reducing carbapenem-resistant Enterobacteriaceae infections in a large teaching hospital in northern Italy. Clin Microbiol Infect 2015;21(3):242–7.

39. Munoz-Price LS, Carling P, Cleary T, et al. Control of a two-decade endemic situation with carbapenem-resistant *Acinetobacter baumannii*: electronic dissemination of a bundle of interventions. Am J Infect Control 2014;42(5):466–71.

40. Schwaber MJ, Carmeli Y. An ongoing national intervention to contain the spread of carbapenem-resistant Enterobacteriaceae. Clin Infect Dis 2014;58(5):697–703.

41. Siegel JD, Rhinehart E, Jackson M, et al. Health care infection control practices advisory C. 2007 guideline for isolation precautions: preventing transmission of infectious agents in health care settings. Am J Infect Control 2007;35(10 Suppl 2):S65–164.

42. Huang SS, Septimus E, Kleinman K, et al. Targeted versus universal decolonization to prevent ICU infection. N Engl J Med 2013;368(24):2255–65.

43. Harris AD, Pineles L, Belton B, et al. Universal glove and gown use and acquisition of antibiotic-resistant bacteria in the ICU: a randomized trial. JAMA 2013; 310(15):1571–80.

44. Palmore TN, Michelin AV, Bordner M, et al. Use of adherence monitors as part of a team approach to control clonal spread of multidrug-resistant *Acinetobacter baumannii* in a research hospital. Infect Control Hosp Epidemiol 2011;32(12): 1166–72.

45. Klein BS, Perloff WH, Maki DG. Reduction of nosocomial infection during pediatric intensive care by protective isolation. N Engl J Med 1989;320(26):1714–21.

46. Septimus EJ, Schweizer ML. Decolonization in prevention of health care-associated infections. Clin Microbiol Rev 2016;29(2):201–22.

47. Frost SA, Alogso MC, Metcalfe L, et al. Chlorhexidine bathing and health care-associated infections among adult intensive care patients: a systematic review and meta-analysis. Crit Care 2016;20(1):379.

48. Dicks KV, Lofgren E, Lewis SS, et al. A multicenter pragmatic interrupted time series analysis of chlorhexidine gluconate bathing in community hospital intensive care units. Infect Control Hosp Epidemiol 2016;37(7):791–7.

49. Climo MW, Yokoe DS, Warren DK, et al. Effect of daily chlorhexidine bathing on hospital-acquired infection. N Engl J Med 2013;368(6):533–42.

50. Noto MJ, Domenico HJ, Byrne DW, et al. Chlorhexidine bathing and health care-associated infections: a randomized clinical trial. JAMA 2015;313(4):369–78.

51. Borer A, Gilad J, Porat N, et al. Impact of 4% chlorhexidine whole-body washing on multidrug-resistant *Acinetobacter baumannii* skin colonisation among patients in a medical intensive care unit. J Hosp Infect 2007;67(2):149–55.

52. Chung YK, Kim JS, Lee SS, et al. Effect of daily chlorhexidine bathing on acquisition of carbapenem-resistant *Acinetobacter baumannii* (CRAB) in the medical intensive care unit with CRAB endemicity. Am J Infect Control 2015;43(11): 1171–7.

53. Vernon MO, Hayden MK, Trick WE, et al. Chlorhexidine gluconate to cleanse patients in a medical intensive care unit: the effectiveness of source control to reduce the bioburden of vancomycin-resistant enterococci. Arch Intern Med 2006;166(3):306–12.

54. Lin MY, Lolans K, Blom DW, et al. The effectiveness of routine daily chlorhexidine gluconate bathing in reducing *Klebsiella pneumoniae* carbapenemase-producing Enterobacteriaceae skin burden among long-term acute care hospital patients. Infect Control Hosp Epidemiol 2014;35(4):440–2.

55. Marschall J, Mermel LA, Fakih M, et al. Strategies to prevent central line-associated bloodstream infections in acute care hospitals: 2014 update. Infect Control Hosp Epidemiol 2014;35(7):753–71.

56. Shams AM, Rose LJ, Edwards JR, et al. Assessment of the overall and multidrug-resistant organism bioburden on environmental surfaces in healthcare facilities. Infect Control Hosp Epidemiol 2016;37(12):1426–32.

57. Lyons A, Rose LJ, Noble-Wang, JA. Survival of healthcare pathogens on hospital surfaces. SHEA 2017 Spring Conference. St. Louis, March 31, 2017.

58. Ohl M, Schweizer M, Graham M, et al. Hospital privacy curtains are frequently and rapidly contaminated with potentially pathogenic bacteria. Am J Infect Control 2012;40(10):904–6.

59. Weber DJ, Rutala WA, Anderson DJ, et al. Effectiveness of ultraviolet devices and hydrogen peroxide systems for terminal room decontamination: focus on clinical trials. Am J Infect Control 2016;44(5 Suppl):e77–84.

60. Otter JA, Mepham S, Athan B, et al. Terminal decontamination of the Royal Free London's high-level isolation unit after a case of Ebola virus disease using hydrogen peroxide vapor. Am J Infect Control 2016;44(2):233–5.

61. Anderson DJ, Chen LF, Weber DJ, et al. Enhanced terminal room disinfection and acquisition and infection caused by multidrug-resistant organisms and *Clostridium difficile* (the benefits of enhanced terminal room disinfection study): a cluster-randomised, multicentre, crossover study. Lancet 2017;389(10071):805–14.

62. Kotay S, Chai W, Guilford W, et al. Spread from the sink to the patient: in situ study using green fluorescent protein (GFP)-expressing *Escherichia coli* to model bacterial dispersion from hand-washing sink-trap reservoirs. Appl Environ Microbiol 2017;83(8) [pii:e03327-16].

63. Williams MM, Armbruster CR, Arduino MJ. Plumbing of hospital premises is a reservoir for opportunistically pathogenic microorganisms: a review. Biofouling 2013;29(2):147–62.

64. Mertz D, Frei R, Periat N, et al. Exclusive staphylococcus aureus throat carriage: at-risk populations. Arch Intern Med 2009;169(2):172–8.

65. Pierce R, Lessler J, Popoola VO, et al. Meticillin-resistant *Staphylococcus aureus* (MRSA) acquisition risk in an endemic neonatal intensive care unit with an active surveillance culture and decolonization programme. J Hosp Infect 2017;95(1):91–7.

66. Evans ME, Kralovic SM, Simbartl LA, et al. Eight years of decreased methicillin-resistant *Staphylococcus aureus* health care-associated infections associated with a Veterans Affairs prevention initiative. Am J Infect Control 2017;45(1):13–6.

67. Gidengil CA, Gay C, Huang SS, et al. Cost-effectiveness of strategies to prevent methicillin-resistant *Staphylococcus aureus* transmission and infection in an intensive care unit. Infect Control Hosp Epidemiol 2015;36(1):17–27.

68. Batra R, Cooper BS, Whiteley C, et al. Efficacy and limitation of a chlorhexidine-based decolonization strategy in preventing transmission of methicillin-resistant *Staphylococcus aureus* in an intensive care unit. Clin Infect Dis 2010;50(2):210–7.

69. Mc KJ, Kunz DF, Moser SA, et al. Patient-level analysis of incident vancomycin-resistant enterococci colonization and antibiotic days of therapy. Epidemiol Infect 2016;144(8):1748–55.

70. Ong DS, Bonten MJ, Safdari K, et al. Epidemiology, management, and risk-adjusted mortality of ICU-acquired enterococcal bacteremia. Clin Infect Dis 2015;61(9):1413–20.

71. Hayden MK, Bonten MJ, Blom DW, et al. Reduction in acquisition of vancomycin-resistant enterococcus after enforcement of routine environmental cleaning measures. Clin Infect Dis 2006;42(11):1552–60.

72. Datta R, Platt R, Yokoe DS, et al. Environmental cleaning intervention and risk of acquiring multidrug-resistant organisms from prior room occupants. Arch Intern Med 2011;171(6):491–4.

73. Vincent JL, Rello J, Marshall J, et al. International study of the prevalence and outcomes of infection in intensive care units. JAMA 2009;302(21):2323–9.

74. Guh AY, Bulens SN, Mu Y, et al. Epidemiology of carbapenem-resistant enterobacteriaceae in 7 US communities, 2012-2013. JAMA 2015;314(14):1479–87.

75. Palmore TN, Henderson DK. Managing transmission of carbapenem-resistant enterobacteriaceae in healthcare settings: a view from the trenches. Clin Infect Dis 2013;57(11):1593–9.

76. World Health Organization. Global priority list of antibiotic-resistant bacteria to guide research, discovery, and development of new antibiotics. 2017. Available at: http://www.who.int/medicines/publications/global-priority-list-antibiotic-resistant-bacteria/en/.

77. Kollef MH, Niederman MS. Why is *Acinetobacter baumannii* a problem for critically ill patients? Intensive Care Med 2015;41(12):2170–2.

78. Zilberberg MD, Nathanson BH, Sulham K, et al. Multidrug resistance, inappropriate empiric therapy, and hospital mortality in *Acinetobacter baumannii* pneumonia and sepsis. Crit Care 2016;20(1):221.

79. Zilberberg MD, Kollef MH, Shorr AF. Secular trends in *Acinetobacter baumannii* resistance in respiratory and blood stream specimens in the United States, 2003 to 2012: a survey study. J Hosp Med 2016;11(1):21–6.

80. Weintrob AC, Roediger MP, Barber M, et al. Natural history of colonization with gram-negative multidrug-resistant organisms among hospitalized patients. Infect Control Hosp Epidemiol 2010;31(4):330–7.

81. Morgan DJ, Liang SY, Smith CL, et al. Frequent multidrug-resistant *Acinetobacter baumannii* contamination of gloves, gowns, and hands of healthcare workers. Infect Control Hosp Epidemiol 2010;31(7):716–21.

82. Calvo B, Melo AS, Perozo-Mena A, et al. First report of *Candida auris* in America: clinical and microbiological aspects of 18 episodes of candidemia. J Infect 2016; 73(4):369–74.

83. Lockhart SR, Etienne KA, Vallabhaneni S, et al. Simultaneous emergence of multidrug-resistant *Candida auris* on 3 continents confirmed by whole-genome sequencing and epidemiological analyses. Clin Infect Dis 2017;64(2):134–40.

84. Vallabhaneni S, Kallen A, Tsay S, et al. Investigation of the first seven reported cases of *Candida auris*, a globally emerging invasive, multidrug-resistant fungus - United States, May 2013-August 2016. MMWR Morb Mortal Wkly Rep 2016;65(44):1234–7.

85. Armstrong PA, Escandon P, Caceres DH, et al. Hospital-associated outbreaks of multidrug-resistant *Candida auris* — multiple cities, Colombia, 2016. 66th Annual EIS Conference. Atlanta, April 24, 2017.

86. Centers for Disease Control and Prevention. Clinical Alert to U.S. healthcare facilities - June 2016. Global emergence of invasive infections caused by the multidrug-resistant yeast *Candida auris* 2016. Available at: https://www.cdc.gov/fungal/diseases/candidiasis/candida-auris-alert.html.

Prevention of Central Line–Associated Bloodstream Infections

 CrossMark

Taison Bell, MD*, Naomi P. O'Grady, MD

KEYWORDS

- CLABSI • CRBSI • Central line • Central venous catheter • Blood stream infection

KEY POINTS

- The incidence of central line–associated bloodstream infection (CLABSI) has decreased with the implementation of evidence-based practice guidelines.
- Clinical factors that may reduce the risk of CLABSI include catheter choice, catheter site selection, insertion technique, and catheter maintenance.
- Newer technology, such as needleless securement devices and disinfecting caps, have been shown to be additional effective strategies to further reduce the incidence of CLABSI.

INTRODUCTION

Central venous catheters (CVCs) are often essential in the care of critically ill patients. They allow safe administration of intravenous medications that cannot be given peripherally, aid in the administration of intravenous fluid resuscitation, and help in monitoring hemodynamic parameters in the management of patients with syndromes such as septic shock, cardiogenic shock, decompensated heart failure, and pulmonary hypertension. Despite the benefits of CVCs, they also serve as potential portals for localized and systemic bloodstream infections. For this reason, considerable effort has gone into reducing the incidence of bloodstream infections from CVCs.

DEFINITIONS

There are 2 major definitions used to describe bloodstream infections related to CVCs: catheter-related bloodstream infection (CRBSI) and central line–associated

Disclosures: This work was supported by the National Instituted of Health, Clinical Center. The findings and conclusions in this report are those of the authors and do not necessarily represent the views of the National Institutes of Health, or the Department of Health and Human Services.
Critical Care Medicine Department, National Institutes of Health, 10 Center Drive, Room 2C145, Bethesda, MD 20892-1662, USA
* Corresponding author.
E-mail address: taison.bell@nih.gov

Infect Dis Clin N Am 31 (2017) 551–559
http://dx.doi.org/10.1016/j.idc.2017.05.007
0891-5520/17/Published by Elsevier Inc.

id.theclinics.com

bloodstream infection (CLABSI). CRBSI is a clinical definition based on clinical criteria related to a specific patient in whom the diagnosis is being considered. This definition is more often used for research, and in some cases of clinical care, because it requires specialized microbiological techniques to specifically identify the catheter as the source of bacteremia, and these are not available in all hospitals. In contrast, the diagnosis of CLABSI is a simplified definition based on surveillance criteria that identify bloodstream infections in patients with CVCs in whom there is no other obvious secondary source for bacteremia.[1,2] The CLABSI definition has the potential to overestimate the incidence of CRBSI, because many primary bloodstream infections do not have an obvious secondary source. However, in the years since the US Centers for Disease Control and Prevention (CDC) instituted mucosal barrier injury as a category for secondary sources of bacteremia, this overestimation has been reduced. In addition, because many states now require public reporting of hospital CLABSI rates and the Centers for Medicare and Medicaid Services instituted financial penalties for hospital reimbursements for CLABSI, there is more granularity in the reviews of bloodstream infections in some institutions, and efforts that, in years past, may not have occurred are now made to thoroughly investigate the possibility of secondary sources. These public policy changes and financial incentives to produce low CLABSI rates have raised concerns that partially subjective surveillance definitions (eg, the National Healthcare Safety Network) applied inconsistently could be exploited or be prone to subconscious cognitive bias to reduce infection rates.[3] Because CLABSI is the more commonly used definition for quality initiatives, it is the focus of this article. However, it is important to understand the differences between the two definitions (**Table 1**).

CLABSIs are an important cause of morbidity and mortality in the intensive care unit, and lead to increased costs to the health care system. Although there was a 46% reduction in CLABSI rates in the United States between 2008 and 2013, an estimated 30,100 CLABSIs still occur in intensive care units and acute care wards each year.[4] Other studies have estimated that CLABSIs account for between 84,000 and 204,000 infections per year, resulting in up to 25,000 preventable deaths at a cost of up to $21 billion per year.[5] There are several measures that can be taken to decrease the incidence of CLABSI, and the introduction of the first widely adopted set of guidelines for the prevention of CLABSI in 2002 led to a substantial reduction in the incidence of CLABSI.[6] Between 2001 and 2009 the incidence of CLABSI declined by 58%, with a reduction in *Staphylococcus aureus* infections of 73%. The

Table 1	
Comparison of catheter-related bloodstream infection and central line–associated bloodstream infection	
CRBSI	Clinical signs of sepsis and positive peripheral blood culture in absence of an obvious source other than CVC with 1 of the following: • Positive semiquantitative (>15 CFU) or quantitative (>10^3 CFU) culture from a catheter segment with the same organisms isolated peripherally • Simultaneous quantitative blood cultures with a ratio of ≥3:1 (CVC vs peripheral) • Time to culture positivity difference no more than 2 h between CVC cultures and peripheral cultures
CLABSI	Primary bloodstream infection in a patient who had a central line within the 48-h period before development • Infection must not be related to an alternative cause

Abbreviation: CFU, colony-forming units.

updated guideline released in 2011,[1] along with newer studies, highlights new strategies to reduce the cost and burden of CLABSI even further.

CLOSED INTENSIVE CARE UNIT VERSUS OPEN INTENSIVE CARE UNIT

Intensive care is frequently practiced in a multidisciplinary fashion, in which the primary treatment team is tasked with providing care for patients with the input from specialty providers, pharmacists, therapists, nutritionists, and other health care professionals. Such an environment can lead to differing opinions on the approach to care and methods to implement plans of care. In an effort to centralize critical decision making for critically ill patients and standardize care, many intensive care units have implemented a closed-unit model in which the intensive care unit team assumes primary responsibility for the patients to implement diagnostic and treatment decisions. The benefits of this model include streamlining treatment decisions and an enhanced ability to implement treatment protocols. This approach may also lead to better clinical outcomes for hospital-acquired conditions. A single-center study showed that implementing a closed-unit model led to a 52% reduction in ventilator-associated pneumonia (confidence interval [CI] = 49.1%–54.9%) and a 25% reduction in CLABSI (CI = 22.5%–27.5%), although the latter finding was nonsignificant.[7]

Site Selection for Catheterization

There are 3 commonly used sites for central venous catheterization: the internal jugular vein, the subclavian vein, and the femoral vein. All are associated with infectious, thrombotic, and mechanical complications, with each risk differing according to the site of insertion.[8] The subclavian site is the preferred site for the sole purposes of reducing CLABSI.[9] However, there are many other practical considerations when determining the site of catheter placement. Patients may not be suitable candidates for subclavian access if they have coagulopathies or anatomic considerations such as lymphadenopathy distorting normal anatomic features. In acute situations in which vascular access needs to be rapidly obtained, femoral catheterization may be preferred to avoid the risk of pneumothorax with either subclavian or internal jugular catheterization. In addition, for patients with end-stage renal disease or those at risk for its development, subclavian catheterization should be avoided given the risk of subsequent subclavian stenosis complicating long-term arteriovenous fistula access.[1]

Femoral catheters should be avoided, when possible, because of their higher rates of infectious and thrombotic complications compared with the internal jugular and subclavian sites.[1,9,10] Femoral catheters are also associated with a higher rate of deep venous thrombosis compared with subclavian and internal jugular access.[9,11] Although there may be good reasons to select the femoral site for insertion of a CVC in the acute setting, it may be prudent to select an alternative site if the catheter is anticipated to stay in place for more than 2 days.

Do all Catheter Placements Require Ultrasonography Guidance?

The use of real-time two-dimensional ultrasonography for the placement of CVCs substantially decreased mechanical complications and reduced the number of attempts required for successful cannulation and failed attempts at cannulation compared with the standard landmark placement.[12,13] Patients who have catheters placed after several failed attempts are more likely to develop complications related to their catheters than patients whose initial attempt was successful. For this reason, all efforts should be made to ensure successful cannulation and bedside ultrasonography should be used.

What Kind of Venous Catheter Should Be Used?

The type of venous catheter used can have an influence on the likelihood of bacterial colonization and subsequent infection. Two major decisions for the type of catheter to use are single-lumen versus multilumen catheters and the use of catheters impregnated with antibiotics or antiseptics.

Single-lumen versus multilumen catheters

Limited data exist regarding the risk of CLABSI with singe-lumen versus multilumen catheters. Although multilumen catheters are convenient for patients requiring multiple infusions or blood draws for laboratory tests, they also provide additional potential pathways for infection. Multiple studies have shown increased infections in multilumen catheters compared with single-lumen catheters in varied patient populations, including the critically ill and patients with cancer[14–16]; however, a meta-analysis did not detect a significant difference when excluding many studies assessed as low quality.[17] On balance, guidelines recommend using a catheter "with the minimum number of ports or lumens essential for the management of the patient."[1] This approach is reasonable, rather than abandoning the convenience of multilumen catheters.

Antibiotic-impregnated and antiinfective-impregnated catheters

Catheters impregnated with antiseptics (chlorhexidine/silver sulfadiazine) or antibiotics (minocycline/rifampin) have been shown to reduce the risk of CLABSI and potentially decrease hospital costs associated with CLABSI despite the additional cost of acquiring the more expensive catheters.[18–20] A recent meta-analysis showed a 2% absolute risk reduction and relative risk of 0.62.[21,22] The benefits of using impregnated catheters vary according to clinical setting, with the most significant benefits being realized in settings that have a higher risk for CLABSI (eg, ICU) than in settings in which the risk for CLABSI is low (eg, general ward). For this reason, and in combination with the additional cost that these catheters add, widespread use across all clinical settings has not been broadly recommended. However, in targeted settings such as the intensive care unit and in areas in which CLABSI rates remain higher than institutional goals, antibiotic-impregnated or antiseptic-impregnated catheters are recommended for routine use.[1]

Catheter removal

The risk of CVC colonization increases with catheter duration, and catheter colonization is the precursor to CLABSI. Thus, one of the most effective ways to reduce CLABSIs is to remove CVCs as soon as they are no longer necessary for the care of the patient. Observational studies suggest that a systemic approach to addressing the need for continued catheter use on a daily basis is highly effective.[23,24] Such approaches include incorporation on a daily goals sheet and nurse-driven protocols. Catheter removal is also strongly advised if there is any suspicion of bloodstream infection, such as unexplained fever and signs of sepsis. Scheduled catheter replacement or exchange has been studied as a potential strategy to prevent CLABSIs. However, a randomized trial investigated a strategy of using scheduled catheter exchange over a guidewire or replacement at a new site after 3 days versus exchange or replacement when clinically indicated and found no difference in the rate of CRBSI.[25] This study was later followed by a systematic review of scheduled replacement strategies compared with clinically indicated removal of CVCs and found no difference in CLABSI rates, although mechanical complications were higher in the groups of patients with scheduled catheter replacements.[26] To date, there are no data published in support of a scheduled replacement strategy on any schedule as an effective means for the prevention of CLABSI.

Guidewire exchange

Catheter replacement over a guidewire is an accepted strategy for replacing malfunctioning catheters or replacing specialty catheters (such as a pulmonary-arterial catheter or a sheath introducer) with a standard CVC. However, in the setting of CLABSI, replacement with a new venous puncture site is preferred to exchange over a guidewire. In the systematic review of catheter replacements, catheters exchanged over a guidewire had higher rates of colonization, exit site infection, and catheter-related bacteremia than those placed at a new site.[26] There are small nonrandomized studies suggesting that, in difficult circumstances in which obtaining access is difficult or may lead to further long-term complications (such as patients on dialysis), exchange over a guidewire may be considered.[27,28]

Insertion Technique

A sterile insertion technique is crucial to maintaining low rates of CLABSI. In a large multicenter cohort study, the rate of CRBSI was followed over the course of implementation of a 5-point evidence-based strategy developed by the CDC.[23] This strategy included the measures listed in **Box 1** accompanied by an aggressive education campaign targeted to clinicians and a third-party compliance observer.

By 3 months from the beginning of the intervention, the median rate of CRBSI had decreased from 2.7 infections per 1000 catheter days to 0 ($P \leq .002$). The regression model showed a significant decrease in infection rates from baseline, with incidence-rate ratios continuously decreasing from 0.62 (95% CI, 0.47–0.81) at 0 to 3 months after implementation of the intervention to 0.34 (95% CI, 0.23–0.50) at 16 to 18 months. Overall, a sustained reduction of 66% was observed, emphasizing the importance of these basic measures in preventing CRBSI.

Catheter Dressing and Maintenance

Chlorhexidine-impregnated dressings

Two types of chlorhexidine gluconate–impregnated dressings are widely available: the Biopatch (http://www.ethicon.com/healthcare-professionals/infection-prevention/biopatch-protective-disk-chg) and the Tegaderm chlorhexidine gluconate intravenous securement dressing (http://www.3m.com/3M/en_US/company-us/all-3m-products/~/3M-Tegaderm-CHG-Chlorhexidine-Gluconate-I-V-Securement-Dressing?N=5002385+3293321978&rt=rud). Both are considered to be members of the same product class because they both have chlorhexidine as the active agent, both have the same anatomic site of action (skin around catheter insertion site), both have local

---

Box 1
Evidence-based strategies to reduce central line–associated bloodstream infection

1. Handwashing with soap and water
2. Sterile insertion with full barrier precautions (cap, mask, sterile gown, sterile gloves, and full sterile drape)
3. Use of 2% chlorhexidine solution with proper air drying before insertion
4. Avoiding femoral site for catheterization
5. Prompt removal of unnecessary catheters

elution of chlorhexidine directly to the catheter insertion site and surrounding skin, and both have a similar time span of delivery (eg, while dressing is present).[29] Both have been shown to reduce catheter colonization and catheter-related infections.[30-33] A Cochrane Review found moderate-quality evidence showing that chlorhexidine-impregnated dressings reduce the frequency of catheter-related blood stream infection per 1000 patient days compared with standard polyurethane dressings (relative risk [RR], 0.51; 95% CI, 0.33–0.78) and reduce catheter tip colonization compared with standard dressings (RR, 0.58; 95% CI, 0.47–0.73).[34]

Needleless securement devices

During the course of their use, CVCs commonly encounter shear forces capable of shifting catheter position or dislodging the device. Examples range from gentle forces, such as gentle tugging from manipulation, to stronger forces like accidental pulls/entanglements or pulls from agitated or delirious patients. For securement, CVCs are commonly sutured to the surrounding skin to prevent accidental dislodging. Although a secure way to ensure catheters remain in place, it does increase the potential for localized skin infections and can be uncomfortable for patients. Sutureless securement devices (SSDs) are systems that can achieve this goal without violating the skin. SSDs secure catheters to the skin using a strong adhesive and often use the catheter hub suture wings as a key contact area.[35] Examples include the Bard StatLock CV Plus Stabilization Device (http://www.bardaccess.com/products/stabilization/other-universal-plus) and the 3M PICC/CVC needleless securement device (http://www.3m.com/3M/en_US/company-us/all-3m-products/~/All-3M-Products/Health-Care/Medical/Securement-Immobilization-Dressing-Securement/Securement-Devices/?N=5002385+8707795+8707798+8710892+8711017+8711097+3294857497&rt=r3).

A growing body of literature has described how these devices can be used as safe and effective alternatives to suturing CVCs and other vascular access catheters, reducing catheter dislodgement, CLABSI, and occupational needlestick injury.[36-38] Given the benefits of using SSDs in reducing CLABSI, they are recommended by guidelines for the securement of CVCs.[1]

Disinfection caps

Catheter manipulation for drug administration presents an opportunity for contamination, and preventive measures should be taken to prevent the potential transmission of pathogenic organisms. When access ports are manipulated, they should be scrubbed with an antiseptic solution, such as chlorhexidine, povidone iodine, an iodophor, or 70% alcohol.[1] The optimum duration of scrubbing is not known. However, a study comparing scrub times of 3, 10, and 15 seconds with 70% alcohol on catheters contaminated with a solution containing S aureus, Staphylococcus spp, Escherichia coli, and Pseudomonas aeruginosa showed a reduction of nearly 20-fold in colony-forming units (CFU) per milliliter between the 3-second time and the 15-second time.[39] This difference did not reach statistical significance ($P = .09$), although the study was likely underpowered. The difference in effectiveness between scrub times introduces human factors into successful decontamination efforts. In contrast, passive hub decontamination relies on hub and port covers that maintain contact between catheter hubs and disinfecting solution (http://www.3m.com/3M/en_US/company-us/all-3m-products/~/All-3M-Products/Health-Care/Medical/Curos/?N=5002385+8707795+8707798+8711017+8717585+3294857497&rt=r3).

Caps do not require scrubbing before infusions or draws once they are removed. Several disinfection cap products are available and have been shown to be effective in reducing hub colonization and CLABSI. In a retrospective study investigating the introduction of disinfection caps, CLABSI rates decreased from 1.682 per 1000 catheter days to 0.6461 per 1000 catheter days after implementing disinfection caps, achieving statistical significance.[40] In an observational study in an oncology unit, a total of 3005 catheter days and 1 CLABSI (0.3 infections per 1000 catheter days) were documented during an intervention period in which alcohol-impregnated port protectors were introduced, compared with 6851 catheter days and 16 CLABSIs (2.3 infections per 1000 catheter days) during the control period (RR, 0.14; 95% CI, 0.02–1.07; $P = .03$).[41] As an effective antiseptic method that does not rely on active human intervention, disinfection caps are an attractive way to complement a comprehensive CLABSI reduction strategy.

SUMMARY

Preventing CLABSIs in the ICU usually requires multiple strategies. Insertion strategies including education and training of those who insert catheters, use of chlorhexidine for skin antisepsis, and use of maximal sterile barrier precautions have a long record of preventing CLABSI. Novel technologies, such as antibiotic-impregnated or antiseptic-impregnated catheters, SSDs, and disinfection caps, should be added to the armamentarium of tools to further reduce CLABSI rates.

REFERENCES

1. O'Grady NP, Alexander M, Burns LA, et al. Guidelines for the prevention of intravascular catheter-related infections. Clin Infect Dis 2011;52(9):e162–93.
2. Available at: https://www.cdc.gov/nhsn/acute-care-hospital/clabsi/index.html. Accessed March 23, 2017.
3. Mayer J, Greene T, Howell J, et al. Agreement in classifying bloodstream infections among multiple reviewers conducting surveillance. Clin Infect Dis 2012; 55(3):364–70.
4. CDC National and State Healthcare Progress Report. 2014. Available at: https://www.cdc.gov/HAI/pdfs/progress-report/hai-progress-report.pdf. Accessed April 3, 2017.
5. Umscheid CA, Mitchell MD, Doshi JA, et al. Estimating the proportion of healthcare-associated infections that are reasonably preventable and the related mortality and costs. Infect Control Hosp Epidemiol 2011;32(2):101–14.
6. O'Grady NP, Alexander M, Dellinger EP, et al. Guidelines for the prevention of intravascular catheter-related infections. Centers for Disease Control and Prevention. MMWR Recomm Rep 2002;51(RR-10):1–29.
7. El-Kersh K, Guardiola J, Cavallazzi R, et al. Open and closed models of intensive care unit have different influences on infectious complications in a tertiary care center: a retrospective data analysis. Am J Infect Control 2016;44(12):1744–6.
8. Parienti JJ, du Cheyron D, Timsit JF, et al. Meta-analysis of subclavian insertion and nontunneled central venous catheter-associated infection risk reduction in critically ill adults. Crit Care Med 2012;40(5):1627–34.
9. Parienti JJ, Mongardon N, Mégarbane B, et al. Intravascular complications of central venous catheterization by insertion site. N Engl J Med 2015;373(13): 1220–9.
10. Parienti JJ, Thirion M, Mégarbane B, et al. Femoral vs jugular venous catheterization and risk of nosocomial events in adults requiring acute renal replacement therapy: a randomized controlled trial. JAMA 2008;299(20):2413–22.

11. Merrer J, De Jonghe B, Golliot F, et al. Complications of femoral and subclavian venous catheterization in critically ill patients: a randomized controlled trial. JAMA 2001;286(6):700–7.

12. Rabindranath KS, Kumar E, Shail R, et al. Use of real-time ultrasound guidance for the placement of hemodialysis catheters: a systematic review and meta-analysis of randomized controlled trials. Am J Kidney Dis 2011;58(6):964–70.

13. Brass P, Hellmich M, Kolodziej L, et al. Ultrasound guidance versus anatomical landmarks for subclavian or femoral vein catheterization. Cochrane Database Syst Rev 2015;(1):CD011447.

14. Early TF, Gregory RT, Wheeler JR, et al. Increased infection rate in double-lumen versus single-lumen Hickman catheters in cancer patients. South Med J 1990; 83(1):34–6.

15. Yeung C, May J, Hughes R. Infection rate for single lumen v triple lumen subclavian catheters. Infect Control Hosp Epidemiol 1988;9(4):154–8.

16. Templeton A, Schlegel M, Fleisch F, et al. Multilumen central venous catheters increase risk for catheter-related bloodstream infection: prospective surveillance study. Infection 2008;36(4):322–7.

17. Dezfulian C, Lavelle J, Nallamothu BK, et al. Rates of infection for single-lumen versus multilumen central venous catheters: a meta-analysis. Crit Care Med 2003;31(9):2385–90.

18. Harron K, Mok Q, Hughes D, et al. Generalisability and cost-impact of antibiotic-impregnated central venous catheters for reducing risk of bloodstream infection in paediatric intensive care units in England. PLoS One 2016;11(3):e0151348.

19. Gilbert RE, Mok Q, Dwan K, et al. Impregnated central venous catheters for prevention of bloodstream infection in children (the CATCH trial): a randomised controlled trial. Lancet 2016;387(10029):1732–42.

20. Veenstra DL, Saint S, Sullivan SD. Cost-effectiveness of antiseptic-impregnated central venous catheters for the prevention of catheter-related bloodstream infection. JAMA 1999;282(6):554–60.

21. Brun-Buisson C, Doyon F, Sollet JP, et al. Prevention of intravascular catheter-related infection with newer chlorhexidine-silver sulfadiazine-coated catheters: a randomized controlled trial. Intensive Care Med 2004;30(5):837–43.

22. Lai NM, Chaiyakunapruk N, Lai NA, et al. Catheter impregnation, coating or bonding for reducing central venous catheter-related infections in adults. Cochrane Database Syst Rev 2016;(3):CD007878.

23. Pronovost P, Needham D, Berenholtz S, et al. An intervention to decrease catheter-related bloodstream infections in the ICU. N Engl J Med 2006;355(26): 2725–32.

24. Berenholtz SM, Pronovost PJ, Lipsett PA, et al. Eliminating catheter-related bloodstream infections in the intensive care unit. Crit Care Med 2004;32(10):2014–20.

25. Cobb DK, High KP, Sawyer RG, et al. A controlled trial of scheduled replacement of central venous and pulmonary-artery catheters. N Engl J Med 1992;327(15): 1062–8.

26. Cook D, Randolph A, Kernerman P, et al. Central venous catheter replacement strategies: a systematic review of the literature. Crit Care Med 1997;25(8): 1417–24.

27. Chaftari AM, El Zakhem A, Jamal MA, et al. The use of minocycline-rifampin coated central venous catheters for exchange of catheters in the setting of staphylococcus aureus central line associated bloodstream infections. BMC Infect Dis 2014;14:518.

28. Hou SM, Chou PC, Huang CH, et al. Is guidewire exchange a better approach for subclavian vein re-catheterization for chronic hemodialysis patients? Thromb Res 2006;118(4):439–45.
29. U.S. Department of Health and Human Services Centers for Disease Control and Prevention HIPAC Meeting November 2015. Available at: http://www.cdc.gov/HICPAC/presentations.html. Accessed March 21, 2017.
30. Arvaniti K, Lathyris D, Clouva-Molyvdas P, et al. Comparison of Oligon catheters and chlorhexidine-impregnated sponges with standard multilumen central venous catheters for prevention of associated colonization and infections in intensive care unit patients: a multicenter, randomized, controlled study. Crit Care Med 2012;40(2):420–9.
31. Ruschulte H, Franke M, Gastmeier P, et al. Prevention of central venous catheter related infections with chlorhexidine gluconate impregnated wound dressings: a randomized controlled trial. Ann Hematol 2009;88(3):267–72.
32. Timsit JF, Mimoz O, Mourvillier B, et al. Randomized controlled trial of chlorhexidine dressing and highly adhesive dressing for preventing catheter-related infections in critically ill adults. Am J Respir Crit Care Med 2012;186(12):1272–8.
33. Timsit JF, Schwebel C, Bouadma L, et al. Chlorhexidine-impregnated sponges and less frequent dressing changes for prevention of catheter-related infections in critically ill adults: a randomized controlled trial. JAMA 2009;301(12):1231–41.
34. Ullman AJ, Cooke ML, Mitchell M, et al. Dressings and securement devices for central venous catheters (CVC). Cochrane Database Syst Rev 2015;(9):CD010367.
35. Krenik KM, Smith GE, Bernatchez SF. Catheter securement systems for peripherally inserted and nontunneled central vascular access devices: clinical evaluation of a novel sutureless device. J Infus Nurs 2016;39(4):210–7.
36. Stephenson C. The advantages of a precision-engineered securement device for fixation of arterial pressure-monitoring catheters. J Assoc Vasc Access 2005; 10(3):130–2.
37. Frey AM, Schears GJ. Why are we stuck on tape and suture? A review of catheter securement devices. J Infus Nurs 2006;29(1):34–8.
38. Yamamoto AJ, Solomon JA, Soulen MC, et al. Sutureless securement device reduces complications of peripherally inserted central venous catheters. J Vasc Interv Radiol 2002;13(1):77–81.
39. Simmons S, Bryson C, Porter S. "Scrub the hub": cleaning duration and reduction in bacterial load on central venous catheters. Crit Care Nurs Q 2011;34(1):31–5.
40. Schears, G. "Cap the connector: save the patient," in Proceedings of the AVA Annual Scientific Meeting. 2011.
41. Sweet MA, Cumpston A, Briggs F, et al. Impact of alcohol-impregnated port protectors and needleless neutral pressure connectors on central line-associated bloodstream infections and contamination of blood cultures in an inpatient oncology unit. Am J Infect Control 2012;40(10):931–4.

High-Containment Pathogen Preparation in the Intensive Care Unit

 CrossMark

Brian T. Garibaldi, MD[a], Daniel S. Chertow, MD, MPH[b],*

KEYWORDS

- Preparedness • Supportive critical care • High-containment pathogens
- Biocontainment unit

KEY POINTS

- Providing state-of-the-art critical care to patients with highly infectious diseases presents unique challenges to health care providers and hospitals.
- Specialized biocontainment units or modification of existing care environments are needed to facilitate the delivery of safe and effective high-containment care.
- Multidisciplinary teams, protocol development, appropriate staffing, and training optimize the likelihood of a successful clinical outcome, including prevention of health care worker infections.
- Coordination at the local, state, regional, and national level is required to care for patients infected with high-containment pathogens.

INTRODUCTION

The recent Ebola virus disease (EVD) outbreak in West Africa in 2014 to 2016 highlighted the capabilities of dedicated biocontainment units (BCUs) at the National Institutes of Health (NIH), Emory University, and the Nebraska Medical Center to provide care for patients with highly infectious diseases.[1–3] In order to increase national capacity, the Centers for Disease Control and Prevention (CDC) called for the creation

Disclosure Statement: None of the authors are aware of any affiliations, memberships, funding, or financial holdings that might be perceived as affecting the objectivity of this review. The Intramural Research Programs of National Institutes of Health (Clinical Center, Critical Care Medicine Department) supported this work. The content of this publication does not necessarily reflect the views or policies of the US Department of Health and Human Services; mention of trade names, commercial products, or organizations does not imply endorsement by the US government.

[a] Division of Pulmonary and Critical Care, Johns Hopkins University School of Medicine, 1830 East Monument Street, 5th Floor, Baltimore, MD 21205, USA; [b] Critical Care Medicine Department, Clinical Center, National Institutes of Health, 10 Center Drive, Room 2C-145, Bethesda, MD 20892-1662, USA
* Corresponding author.
E-mail address: chertowd@cc.nih.gov

Infect Dis Clin N Am 31 (2017) 561–576
http://dx.doi.org/10.1016/j.idc.2017.05.008
0891-5520/17/Published by Elsevier Inc.

id.theclinics.com

of a tiered network of US hospitals, including frontline hospitals, assessment hospitals, and Ebola Treatment Centers (ETCs).[4] The Office of the Assistant Secretary for Preparedness and Response (ASPR) also funded the creation of 10 Regional Ebola and Special Pathogen Treatment Centers (RESPTCs).[5]

There are no definitive guidelines outlining the optimal environment of care for patients with highly infectious diseases.[5] Several of the RESPTCs and some of the ETCs built new stand-alone BCUs.[6] Other hospitals, such as Bellevue Health Center in New York City, transitioned existing intensive care unit (ICU) or other patient-care space into high-containment areas to be used on an as-needed basis.[7] Regardless of the chosen solution, there are several core principles that underlie the creation of containment areas that can provide care for patients with highly infectious diseases[3,8] (**Box 1**). In this article, the authors review the key aspects of high-containment care and provide a framework for successful critical care in this environment.

THE ENVIRONMENT

The physical structure of the care space is critical to ensuring health care worker, staff, and patient safety in the context of highly infectious diseases. The European Network of Infectious Diseases as well as a group from US centers with experience in highly infectious diseases have published consensus guidelines on the design and operation of BCUs.[3,8] Lessons learned from the 2014 to 2016 EVD outbreak have further informed design considerations.[6]

Location of the Unit

The ideal containment area should be located away from other clinical areas with secured entry and exit points. This location will limit unnecessary traffic through the space. There should also be clearly identifiable transport routes into and out of the unit to allow entry of new patients and to evacuate patients and staff in the event of an emergency.[3]

Layout of the Care Space

The layout of the unit needs to support infection control practices, such as the donning and doffing of personal protective equipment (PPE) as well as the prevention of cross-contamination of clean areas. At a minimum, each patient room should have an

---

Box 1
Common features of biocontainment units

- Secure entry and exit points
- Onsite laboratory
- Advanced air-handling system for airborne and droplet transmission
- Highly trained nurse and clinician provider team
- Critical care capabilities
- Onsite portable radiology and ultrasound
- Advanced telecommunication capabilities
- Pass-through autoclaves for waste management
- Dedicated donning and doffing areas
- Unidirectional flow of staff through patient care areas where possible

anteroom for donning and doffing. Some facilities include an anteroom for donning and then a separate exit-room for doffing.[6] Although an exit-room is not necessary for an airborne pathogen, this design allows for unidirectional flow of patients, staff, and materials through the care space to limit the possibility of cross-contamination, particularly in the context of contact-transmitted pathogens, such as Ebola virus (EBOV) or other viral hemorrhagic fevers. This principle of unidirectional flow is a cornerstone of Ebola Treatment Centers in Africa.[9] Each unit should have an exit space where staff can shower after their care shift and change into clean clothing before exiting the unit. The unit should be equipped to provide critical care services and, depending on the local need, should anticipate caring for additional patient populations, including children and pregnant women.[6]

In addition to the care space, there should also be a staff break area for personnel to gather before and after their shift. This space needs to be separate from the rest of the unit and ideally should be on a separate air-handling system to ensure safety.

Fig. 1 shows the layout of the Johns Hopkins BCU, which was built in response to the 2014 to 2016 EVD outbreak.

Air Handling

In order to support the care of patients with diseases transmitted by droplet and airborne routes, the containment space should have an air-handling system that provides a negative pressure environment for contaminated areas. Such a system also protects health care workers and other patients in situations whereby infectious particles might be aerosolized (eg, coughing, sneezing, procedures, such as endotracheal intubation, and so forth).[10] There are no existing regulations for air-handling

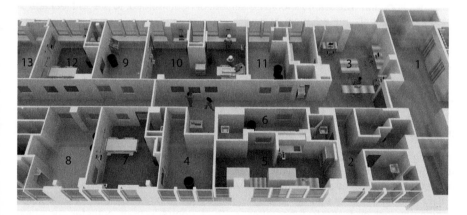

Fig. 1. General layout of the Johns Hopkins BCU. Patient rooms and the laboratory have dedicated space for donning and doffing PPE. This space allows unidirectional flow to reduce the risk of cross-contamination. Green indicates clean space, red indicates contaminated space, and yellow indicates doffing rooms. (1) Off-unit area with dedicated elevators, locker room, changing area, and lounge for staff; (2) clean entry and exit space for staff; (3) nurse station; (4) shared donning room for laboratory and patient room 3; (5) laboratory; (6) doffing room for laboratory; (7) patient room 3; (8) doffing room for patient room 3; (9) shared donning room for patient rooms 1 and 2; (10) patient room 1 with 2 ICU headwalls; (11) doffing room for patient room 1; (12) patient room 2; (13) doffing room for patient room 2. (*Reprinted from* Garibaldi BT, Kelen GD, Brower RG, et al. The creation of a biocontainment unit at a tertiary care hospital. The Johns Hopkins medicine experience. Ann Am Thorac Soc 2016;13(5):603; with permission from American Thoracic Society.)

systems in an entire containment unit. Guidelines for airborne infection isolation (AII) rooms from the CDC, American Society of Heating, Refrigerating, and Air-Conditioning Engineers, American National Standards Institute, and American Society for Healthcare Engineering can inform the design of the air-handling system for an entire unit.[6,11]

For example, the entire Johns Hopkins BCU is negative pressure relative to the rest of the hospital. Each contaminated area is designed to have a pressure differential of at least −0.02-in water gauge to adjacent areas (twice the requirement for an AII). This design ensures that air does not travel from a contaminated to a clean space. All intake air is filtered using a minimum efficiency reporting value 16 filter that captures 99% of 1.0 μm particles; no air is recirculated. The anteroom air is changed at least 10 times per hour, whereas the patient room air is changed 12 to 15 times per hour, in accordance with AII guidelines. The air intake is on the ceiling, whereas the exhaust ports are on the wall close to the floor. This location creates laminar flow, away from a health care worker's face. The negative pressure for the unit is maintained by 2 rooftop fans, each equipped with high-efficiency particulate air (HEPA) filters that capture 99.99% of particles with a size of 0.3 μm. Each fan can maintain the negative pressure for the entire unit in the case of a single fan failure or the need for maintenance.[6] Such redundancies improve the safety of the care space but may not be possible in all environments.

Decontamination of the Environment

Decontamination of the environment is an important consideration when designing an isolation unit. Floors and walls must be constructed of materials that can resist breakdown from hospital disinfectants, such as bleach and quaternary ammonium. Where possible, floor and wall seams should be sealed, or heat-welded, to prevent leakage of infectious materials into adjacent areas.[3,6]

The use of either UV light or vaporized hydrogen peroxide to decontaminant the health care environment after patients are discharged may require additional design considerations, such as UV reflective paint or special exhaust covers for the air-handling system.[12,13]

Equipment

In addition to the standard medical equipment required to care for critically ill patients, there are several equipment issues that are unique to the containment environment.

Imaging and other diagnostic technology Because patients are often not able to be transported outside of the containment environment for diagnostic testing or invasive procedures, it is necessary to provide advanced imaging and procedural capabilities onsite.[8] Portable ultrasound devices allow for chest, abdomen, cardiac, and obstetric imaging as well as facilitate procedures, such as central venous catheter and chest tube insertion. Other point-of-care devices, such as digital stethoscopes, can overcome some of the limitations of PPE and enhance the diagnostic yield of the physical examination.[6] Portable digital x-ray devices also allow for chest and abdominal imaging, although the need to process the plate and decontaminate the equipment presents additional logistical problems.[14]

Communication Communication is critical in a BCU environment, both for staff and for patients and their families. It can be difficult for providers to hear one another while wearing powered air purifying respirators (PAPRs), and visibility and facial recognition may be constrained by visors or PAPR hoods. Visitors are usually not allowed in the unit, which can contribute to a sense of isolation. There are several potential solutions, ranging from less expensive choices (eg, smartphones and tablets) to advanced telecommunications systems that could include PAPR-integrated microphones and headsets. The goal of these devices is to allow patients and staff to effectively communicate with each other in the unit but also with individuals outside of the containment environment. This communication can facilitate consultation by health care providers and other ancillary services that do not need to enter into the contaminated space as well as allow patients to spend time with family and friends in a more intimate environment.

Reusing equipment and supplies In addition to the equipment mentioned earlier, there is a need to develop policies and procedures surrounding the reuse of specific critical care devices, such as mechanical ventilators and continuous renal replacement therapy machines. The CDC has published interim guidance on the decontamination of dialysis machines, but individual manufacturers may need to provide specific instructions on how best to clean a device after use.[15] If there is any doubt as to the ability to safely decontaminate a device, the device should be discarded or, at the very least, kept out of clinical circulation until an effective decontamination strategy is developed.

Waste management

The safe handling of highly infectious waste is one of the most challenging issues in a containment environment.[16–19] Category A infectious substances, defined as substances that can cause life-threatening or permanent injury on exposure to humans, have strict federal regulations surrounding their packaging, transport, and disposal.[20] Only a handful of civilian facilities process category A substances, and the cost of transport and disposal is substantial.[21] The potential high volume of waste, both in the form of patient secretions and disposable products, such as PPE, present additional challenges.[18,19,21,22] The CDC and ASPR recommend that facilities planning to care for patients with EVD consider installing steam sterilizers, or autoclaves, to sterilize waste before transport out of the containment facility.[17] It is critical that facilities using onsite autoclaves validate their protocols using simulated patient waste and biological indicators to ensure successful sterilization.[21] In a recent survey of 43 ETCs, 10 had onsite autoclave capabilities. The remaining centers had alternative plans that included packaging waste according to Department of Transportation's guidelines and transporting it to a certified processing facility. Onsite incineration is also a possibility but not currently planned by any ETC.[23]

In addition to waste that is packaged for transport, facilities must have a plan to dispose of liquid waste from patient secretions (eg, urine, feces, vomit, and so forth) and procedures, such as dialysis. Specific protocols will vary depending on municipal regulations and water treatment facilities, but most call for the addition of a disinfectant for a designated period of time before allowing waste water to enter the sewage system.[17–19]

Transportation

Transportation is a critical issue in the care of patients with highly infectious diseases. Guidelines and recommendations for the aeromedical transport of patients exist but are beyond the scope of this current review.[24–26] Although some facilities have their own dedicated ground transport units,[6,27–29] every facility with biocontainment capabilities should be prepared to accept the handoff of patients from a ground transport team.

Ground transportation requires careful coordination of local and state agencies, including law enforcement, public health, and emergency medical services.[22] There is no clear consensus on how best to prepare an ambulance for transport. Many

US centers recommend wrapping the ambulance in impermeable material, such as plastic, to aid in ambulance decontamination,[28,29] although this practice is not universally followed. Although some countries in Europe have invested in specially designed ambulances with HEPA filtration,[8] it is likely sufficient to separate the driver's compartment from the care bay to limit the potential for exposure to aerosolized or airborne pathogens.[29] Ambulance staff should be properly trained in the use of appropriate PPE.[30] Patients can be placed in PPE to prevent excessive spillage of contaminated bodily fluids.[28,29] A transport isolation system can also be used, although this might limit access to patients if the need for interventions during transport arises.[8]

On arrival to the biocontainment facility, a facility-specific transport team can take over the care of patients, while the ambulance team prepares to decontaminate their equipment in a dedicated and secure area.[27–29] Once inside the facility, there should be a clearly delineated path from the point of entry to the BCU. This path should be easily securable and ideally would not pass through other clinical areas.[8]

CLINICAL CARE

State-of-the-art critical care can be provided to patients with highly infectious diseases while maintaining staff safety and preventing nosocomial transmission.[7] Success in this setting is defined both by achieving the desired clinical outcome of patient survival with limited morbidity and by preventing secondary infections among hospital staff and patients.[31] Critical care planning for high-containment pathogens benefits from a detailed understanding of disease natural history including routes of pathogen transmission, infectious period, and expected time course of organ dysfunction.[32–35] Although some of these data are incomplete for emerging or reemerging pathogens, available information can be used to guide likely resources (staff, space, equipment, supplies) needed to facilitate the desired clinical outcome while maintaining staff safety. A prior knowledge of disease natural history will also assist in predicting the supportive care procedures and interventions that may be required during illness, so that risks associated with these interventions may be mitigated through planning and practice.[35,36]

Experiences from the care of patients infected with severe acute respiratory syndrome coronavirus (SARS-CoV), middle east respiratory syndrome coronavirus (MERS-CoV), and EBOV emphasize the need for multidisciplinary coordination before, during, and after the care of these patients.[37,38] **Fig. 2** summarizes some of the essential planning and intervention elements required during this care continuum. In this section, the authors summarize recommendations for effective multidisciplinary team building, staffing, use of PPE, development of clinical protocols, clinical laboratory testing, and training to facilitate the delivery of safe and effective critical care in high-containment environments.

Multidisciplinary Teams

Developing and maintaining multidisciplinary teams is an essential first step to plan for and deliver care to patients infected with high-containment pathogens.[31] Intensive care teams include critical care physicians, nurses, therapists, consulting providers, pharmacists, dieticians, technicians, ethicists, and administrative staff.[39,40] Additional close partnerships with hospital administrators, facilities engineers, infection control specialists, waste management experts, laboratory and radiology staff, and others are also required.[6]

Beyond internal stakeholders, external stakeholders should be identified and engaged. External stakeholders might include local, state, and federal public health

Prior to Care

Establish multidisciplinary team
- Engage stakeholders
- Establish communication plan

Prepare the physical environment
- Design and or modify facility
- Stage equipment and supplies

Develop a staffing plan
- Recruit staff
- Establish sustainable schedule
- Initiate occupational health plan

Develop clinical protocols
- Identify best practices in other facilities
- Vet procedures among stakeholders
- Establish laboratory testing capacity

Implement training
- Practice donning and doffing PPE
- Practice procedures in full PPE
- Establish proficiency standards

During Care

Maintain internal/external communication
- Conduct frequent team meetings
- Designate public information officer

Implement staffing and care plans
- Use observers to assure proper PPE use
- Follow clinical protocols
- Troubleshoot unexpected challenges

Facilitate staff well-being
- Monitor for fatigue
- Promote morale and recognition
- Actively monitor for illness

Maintain equipment and consumables
- Monitor and resupply stocks
- Allow only essential equipment in BCU
- Avoid cross-contamination

Manage waste and the environment
- Autoclaved waste when possible
- Disinfect liquid waste
- Decontaminate work space often

Following Care

Establish lessons learned
- Debrief stakeholders
- Identify system's strengths
- Identify areas for improvement

Decontaminate environment/equipment
- Following CDC and manufacturer's guidance
- Repair, maintain, modify physical space

Update protocols and training
- Review and refine protocols
- Perform refresher training (PPE, skills)

Support workforce
- Monitor for illness
- Provide mental health services
- Establish formal recognition

Fig. 2. Timeline of activities caring for patients infected with high-containment pathogens.

officials; local community members and government representatives; medical waste management providers; and emergency medical transportation providers, among others.[41,42] These stakeholders should be engaged by a designated spokesperson with a clear communication plan and well-defined objectives to facilitate exchange of ideas and expertise, maintain transparency, and provide a platform to troubleshoot operational challenges as they arise. Establishing points of contact and a collaborative approach will allow for standardization of protocols and common training and drilling in advance of patient care.

Staffing

Staffing of BCUs must take into account the need for first-line and backup personnel, the role of consultants, volunteer versus mandatory staff participation, and impact on patient care units elsewhere in the hospital. Staff members likely to provide direct patient care include critical care and infectious diseases physicians, medical and intensive care nurses, respiratory therapists, and radiology technicians.[39] Clinical consultants, including nephrologists, neurologists, ophthalmologists, surgeons, and other subspecialists, may also be called on to provide direct patient care.[43,44] Support staff that are likely to be involved include infection control observers and dedicated laboratory, housekeeping, and administrative staff. The ability of care teams to deliver specialized obstetric, pediatric, or complicated surgical care would need to be defined in advance with appropriate facilities, staffing, and care protocols in place.[45,46]

Staffing models should take into account excess physical demand placed on health care workers related to prolonged use of PPE[39,47] and excess emotional demand associated with caring for critically ill patients who may be highly infectious.[48] During the 2014 to 2016 EVD outbreak, health care workers were on occasion stigmatized in the workplace and in their communities, exacerbating emotional strain.[39,49] Backup providers should be identified and formalized backup schedules established when possible to provide redundancy if first-line providers become unavailable.

The decision to request volunteer or required staff participation must allow adequate time for staff recruitment, education, and training as staffing levels needed to care for patients infected with high-containment pathogens exceed those of routine care.[31] A single critically ill patient infected with EBOV cared for at NIH required 4 nurses (2 ICU nurses and 2 medical floor nurses) per 8-hour shift and 2 physicians (1 ICU and 1 infectious diseases physician) per 12-hout shift to participate in direct patient care. Multiple additional support staff per shift was needed.[43] The decision to cohort staff to the care of patients on BCUs will also increase staffing demands on other clinical care units.

Personal Protective Equipment

The US Department of Labor Occupational Safety and Health Administration regulates the availability and use of PPE to assure proper fit and function among health care workers (29 CFR 1910.132 and 29 CFR 1910.134). Recommendations for the use of PPE are pathogen dependent with detailed guidance for US health care facilities provided by the CDC.[50] Specific guidance on the use of PPE for EVD is available.[51] Standard universal precautions mandate hand hygiene on entering and exiting patient rooms; contact precautions recommend use of gloves and gowns; droplet precautions require use of a surgical mask; and airborne precautions require the use of a respirator, such as an N-95 mask or PAPR. Under routine circumstances, compliance with these precautions is less than 100%, and so added emphasis and oversight is needed in the care of patients with highly infectious diseases.

Although some pathogens are thought to primarily spread via large respiratory droplets (eg, influenza virus, MERS-CoV), added precautions, including use of a respirator and eye protection, are needed during aerosol-generating procedures. Procedures associated with increased risk of health care worker exposure include endotracheal intubation and noninvasive positive pressure mechanical ventilation.[52] Other procedures, including bronchoscopy and high-flow oxygen delivery, may also increase risk.[53] External surfaces of PPE and the environment may become contaminated, emphasizing the need for caution in removing PPE and the need for frequent environmental decontamination.[54,55]

The low infectious dose of EBOV[56] and prior examples of inadvertent health care worker exposures contributed to the CDC's recommendation that PPE cover all exposed skin and mucous membranes and that trained observers facilitate donning and doffing PPE.[37] EBOV has been shown to survive on inanimate surfaces for days to weeks at temperature and humidity observed in hospital settings, further emphasizing the need for caution in removing PPE and frequent environmental decontamination.[55] Detailed recommendations for environmental decontamination in the care of patients infected with EBOV are available.[57] Educational videos and training materials on the use of PPE from facilities with experience in the care of EBOV-infected patients are also available online.[58–60]

Hospitals should take into account the type and amount of PPE required to maintain on hand for training, drills, and actual patient care and how often these supplies need to be replaced or replenished. Shortages of PPE may occur during outbreak situations or during periods of perceived increased risk. Local health officials may guide PPE availability when supplies are limited, with preference given to facilities designated as specialized treatment centers.

Clinical Protocols

Development of written protocols facilitates identification of care processes that might place health care workers at increased risk of exposure. These processes can then be modified to mitigate risks.[40] Outlining individual steps of otherwise routine procedures allows clinical stakeholders to closely review and vet processes, standardizes expectation among staff, and provides a template for staff training and proficiency testing.

Although few data exist to mandate specific clinical protocols in the care of patients in BCUs, practical suggestions may be derived from best practice among organizations with experience caring for patients with EVD. Practice modifications should take into account risks associated with invasive procedures (blood-borne exposures), aerosol-generating procedures (small or large droplet exposures), and procedures that result in significant environmental contamination (indirect fomite exposures).

Although safe sharp practices are routinely recommended in all care settings (eg, use of smart sharp devices, avoiding recapping needles), additional considerations might further reduce the risk of needle sticks in the care of patients in BCUs. For example, procedures for placement of central venous catheters in EBOV-infected patients may require that all catheters be placed under ultrasound guidance and that only one sharp be placed on the sterile procedural field at a time.

Aerosol-generating procedures in patients with acute respiratory infections have been associated with increased risk of secondary health care worker infection.[52] Therefore, consideration should be given to modifying routine respiratory care practices, such as limiting the use of noninvasive positive pressure ventilation and avoiding discontinuity of the respiratory circuit during invasive positive-pressure ventilation. Additional research is needed in this area to better guide practice.

Box 2 provides a list of procedures that might benefit from the development of detailed standardized protocols.

Laboratory Testing

Accurate and timely laboratory testing is essential for effective management of patients in BCUs. Common point-of-care tests might include comprehensive chemistry panels, arterial blood gas analyses, complete blood counts with differential, coagulation studies, blood cultures, and microscopy (eg, thick and thin blood smear).[61] A recent survey of the 55 hospitals in the United States designated as ETCs revealed that 87% of responding hospitals planned to provide point-of-care testing within the isolated patient room and 91% had biosafety level 3 laboratory support through their clinical laboratory or jurisdictional public health laboratory.[62]

Adequate planning and preparation is required to successfully implement laboratory testing in BCUs. This planning must take into account the timing and availability of specific tests and protocols for handling, transporting, and evaluating specimens.[63] The CDC provides guidance for the management of clinical specimens when there is a concern for EVD.[64]

Training

Training is required to assure staff familiarity and proficiency in use of PPE, clinical protocols, and waste and environmental management. When caring for patients with EVD, the use of trained observers is recommended to assure proper donning and doffing of PPE. Although high-quality studies are limited, stepwise and orchestrated removal of PPE seems to significantly reduce the risk of self-contamination.[65] Training may be implemented via online learning, video presentations, in-person didactics, and experiential hands-on sessions. Multiple existing training materials are publically available, including clear and concise videos for the safe donning and doffing of PPE as noted earlier.

It is prudent for staff to practice routine ICU procedures (eg, central venous catheter placement, endotracheal intubation) in simulated care scenarios while wearing full PPE, as PPE may alter manual dexterity as well as tactile, auditory, and visual cues.[66] Training should familiarize staff with limitations imposed by PPE and provide an opportunity to assess and improve procedural proficiency while prioritizing safety.[67] Multidisciplinary training for complex tasks, such as delivering advanced cardiac life support in a code blue scenario or extraction of an impaired health care worker, facilitates team building and effective communication and provides a common venue to clearly define processes and parameters of care.

All designated team members should undergo initial training. Given that care of patients infected with high-containment pathogens is likely to be a rare event, recurrent training to maintain baseline proficiency is also prudent and rational. Ideal frequency of

---

Box 2
Standardized protocols for a high-containment environment

- Invasive procedures (eg, central line placement)
- Advanced respiratory care (eg, endotracheal intubation, invasive mechanical ventilation)
- Renal replacement therapy
- Advanced cardiac life support (ie, code blue response)
- Extraction of an impaired health care worker
- Health care worker infectious exposure (ie, occupational medicine plan)

repeat training has not been established and requires objective, prospective evaluation. While just-in-time training should not be relied on as a primary approach, it does offer the opportunity to rapidly refresh competencies of previously trained providers or to establish baseline competencies of newly recognized providers.

DISCUSSION

During the 2014 to 2016 EVD outbreak, 40% mortality was observed among more than 28,000 Ebola cases in West Africa.[68] Twenty-seven patients were treated in Europe and the United States. Most of these patients (82%) survived, largely because they received high-quality, supportive critical care.[7] Planning and delivering care to these patients was labor and resource intensive and took place in a few specialized centers. The cost to establish an Ebola treatment center in the United States has been estimated to be $1,200,000, whereas the cost to care for a single patient in this setting may be as high as $30,000 per day.[69,70] Secondary transmission of EBOV to health care workers in a community hospital in Texas served as a stark reminder of the risks associated with caring for patients with EVD and the need for adequate resources, planning, and training to mitigate risk.[71]

Although EVD is the most recent example of a highly infectious disease necessitating ICU care, SARS-CoV and MERS-CoV serve as other important examples. The 2003 to 2004 SARS-CoV epidemic resulted in more than 8000 infections and 700 deaths worldwide. In Toronto, Canada, 375 probable and suspected cases of SARS-CoV occurred, with 72% related to a health care exposure.[72,73] Similarly, MERS-CoV has resulted in large nosocomial outbreaks in Saudi Arabia and Korea. During an August-September 2015 nosocomial outbreak of MERS-CoV in Saudi Arabia, 63 patients, including 8 health care workers, were admitted to 3 MERS-CoV-designated ICUs. Hospital mortality among these patients was 63%.[35]

Given existing and emerging serious infectious disease threats, including the ever-looming threat of a severe influenza pandemic, it seems prudent to continue to build capacity to provide high-quality ICU level care for affected patients under safe conditions. An important step forward in this process was the establishment of the National Ebola Training and Education Center (NETEC) through the ASPR and CDC.[74] This collaboration provides funding to Emory University, University of Nebraska, and Bellevue Hospital Center, all centers with a successful track record of caring for patients with EVD, to train and prepare other US health care facilities for emerging threats. NETEC will work with the other federally funded RESPTCS as well as the NIH Special Clinical Studies Unit, to advance the clinical science behind high-containment care and to ensure the safety of patients, health care workers, and their surrounding communities.

Hospitals must take stock of existing capacity to care for patients with highly infectious diseases. Although not all facilities will be called on to provide ICU-level care, all hospitals must have protocols, plans, and training in place to identify, isolate, and provide short-term care for patients infected with high-containment pathogens. Hospitals designated to provide definitive ICU care must maintain staff and facility readiness through ongoing training and pursuit of best practices. Improved coordination and communication among existing centers as well as with local, state, and federal health officials will further the goal of establishing a sustainable infrastructure to address the persistent threat of severe infectious disease outbreaks.

ACKNOWLEDGMENTS

The authors would like to thank their colleagues at the National Ebola Treatment and Education Center, as well as the staff of all the units that are preparing to provide care for patients with highly infectious diseases, for their ongoing contributions to high-containment care.

REFERENCES

1. Connor MJ Jr, Kraft C, Mehta AK, et al. Successful delivery of RRT in Ebola virus disease. J Am Soc Nephrol 2015;26:31–7.
2. Johnson DW, Sullivan JN, Piquette CA, et al. Lessons learned: critical care management of patients with Ebola in the United States. Crit Care Med 2015;43:1157–64.
3. Smith PW, Anderson AO, Christopher GW, et al. Designing a biocontainment unit to care for patients with serious communicable diseases: a consensus statement. Biosecur Bioterror 2006;4:351–65.
4. Interim guidance for preparing Ebola treatment centers. Available at: http://www.cdc.gov/vhf/ebola/healthcare-us/preparing/treatment-centers.html. Accessed February 2, 2017.
5. HHS selects nine regional Ebola and other special pathogen treatment centers. Available at: http://www.hhs.gov/about/news/2015/06/12/hhs-selects-nine-regional-ebola-and-other-special-pathogen-treatment-centers.html. Accessed February 2, 2017.
6. Garibaldi BT, Kelen GD, Brower RG, et al. The creation of a biocontainment unit at a Tertiary Care Hospital. The Johns Hopkins Medicine Experience. Ann Am Thorac Soc 2016;13:600–8.
7. Uyeki TM, Mehta AK, Davey RT Jr, et al, Working Group of the U.S.–European Clinical Network on Clinical Management of Ebola Virus Disease Patients in the U.S. and Europe. Clinical Management of Ebola Virus Disease in the United States and Europe. N Engl J Med 2016;374:636–46.
8. Bannister B, Puro V, Fusco FM, et al. Framework for the design and operation of high-level isolation units: consensus of the European Network of Infectious Diseases. Lancet Infect Dis 2009;9:45–56.
9. Manual for the care and management of patients in Ebola care units/community care centres: interim emergency guidance. Available at: http://www.who.int/csr/resources/publications/ebola/patient-care-CCUs/en/. Accessed February 2, 2017.
10. Kortepeter MG, Kwon EH, Hewlett AL, et al. Containment care units for managing patients with highly hazardous infectious diseases: a concept whose time has come. J Infect Dis 2016;214:S137–41.
11. ASHRAE position document on airborne infectious diseases. Available at: https://www.ashrae.org/about-ashrae/position-documents. Accessed February 2, 2017.
12. Boyce JM, Havill NL, Moore BA. Terminal decontamination of patient rooms using an automated mobile UV light unit. Infect Control Hosp Epidemiol 2011;32:737–42.
13. Weber DJ, Rutala WA, Anderson DJ, et al. Effectiveness of ultraviolet devices and hydrogen peroxide systems for terminal room decontamination: focus on clinical trials. Am J Infect Control 2016;44:e77–84.
14. Mollura DJ, Palmore TN, Folio LR, et al. Radiology preparedness in Ebola virus disease: guidelines and challenges for disinfection of medical imaging equipment for the protection of staff and patients. Radiology 2015;275:538–44.
15. Recommendations for safely performing acute hemodialysis in Patients with Ebola virus disease (EVD) in U.S. hospitals. Available at: https://www.cdc.gov/vhf/ebola/healthcare-us/hospitals/acute-hemodialysis.html. Accessed February 2, 2017.

16. Safe handling, treatment, transport and disposal of Ebola-contaminated waste. Available at: https://www.osha.gov/Publications/OSHA_FS-3766.pdf. Accessed February 2, 2017.

17. Ebola-associated waste management. Available at: http://www.cdc.gov/vhf/ebola/healthcare-us/cleaning/waste-management.html. Accessed February 2, 2017.

18. Lowe JJ, Gibbs SG, Schwedhelm SS, et al. Nebraska Biocontainment Unit perspective on disposal of Ebola medical waste. Am J Infect Control 2014;42:1256–7.

19. Lowe JJ, Olinger PL, Gibbs SG, et al. Environmental infection control considerations for Ebola. Am J Infect Control 2015;43:747–9.

20. Transporting infectious substances safely. US Department of Transportation. Pipeline and Hazardous Materials Safety Administration. Available at: http://www.phmsa.dot.gov/staticfiles/PHMSA/DownloadableFiles/Files/Transporting_Infectious_Substances_brochure.pdf. Accessed February 2, 2017.

21. Garibaldi BT, Reimers M, Ernst N, et al. Validation of autoclave protocols for successful decontamination of category a medical waste generated from care of patients with serious communicable diseases. J Clin Microbiol 2017;55:545–51.

22. Hewlett AL, Varkey JB, Smith PW, et al. Ebola virus disease: preparedness and infection control lessons learned from two biocontainment units. Curr Opin Infect Dis 2015;28:343–8.

23. Herstein JJ, Biddinger PD, Kraft CS, et al. Current capabilities and capacity of Ebola treatment centers in the United States. Infect Control Hosp Epidemiol 2016;37:313–8.

24. Guidance on air medical transport (AMT) for patients with Ebola virus disease (EVD). Available at: https://www.cdc.gov/vhf/ebola/healthcare-us/emergency-services/air-medical-transport.html. Accessed February 2, 2017.

25. Christopher GW, Eitzen EM Jr. Air evacuation under high-level biosafety containment: the aeromedical isolation team. Emerg Infect Dis 1999;5:241–6.

26. Withers MR, Christopher GW. Aeromedical evacuation of biological warfare casualties: a treatise on infectious diseases on aircraft. Mil Med 2000;165:1–21.

27. Isakov A, Jamison A, Miles W, et al. Safe management of patients with serious communicable diseases: recent experience with Ebola virus. Ann Intern Med 2014;161:829–30.

28. Isakov A, Miles W, Gibbs S, et al. Transport and management of patients with confirmed or suspected Ebola virus disease. Ann Emerg Med 2015;66:297–305.

29. Lowe JJ, Jelden KC, Schenarts PJ, et al. Considerations for safe EMS transport of patients infected with Ebola virus. Prehosp Emerg Care 2015;19:179–83.

30. Interim guidance for emergency medical services (EMS) systems and 9-1-1 public safety answering points (PSAPs) for management of patients under investigation (PUIs) for Ebola virus disease (EVD) in the United States. Available at: https://www.cdc.gov/vhf/ebola/healthcare-us/emergency-services/ems-systems.html. Accessed February 2, 2017.

31. Decker BK, Sevransky JE, Barrett K, et al. Preparing for critical care services to patients with Ebola. Ann Intern Med 2014;161:831–2.

32. de Wit E, van Doremalen N, Falzarano D, et al. SARS and MERS: recent insights into emerging coronaviruses. Nat Rev Microbiol 2016;14:523–34.

33. Yildirmak T, Tulek N, Bulut C. Crimean-Congo haemorrhagic fever: transmission to visitors and healthcare workers. Infection 2016;44:687–9.

34. Baseler L, Chertow DS, Johnson KM, et al. The pathogenesis of Ebola virus disease. Annu Rev Pathol 2016;12:387–418.

35. Al-Dorzi HM, Aldawood AS, Khan R, et al. The critical care response to a hospital outbreak of Middle East respiratory syndrome coronavirus (MERS-CoV) infection: an observational study. Ann Intensive Care 2016;6:101.

36. Sampathkumar P, Temesgen Z, Smith TF, et al. SARS: epidemiology, clinical presentation, management, and infection control measures. Mayo Clin Proc 2003;78: 882–90.

37. Cummings KJ, Choi MJ, Esswein EJ, et al. Addressing infection prevention and control in the first U.S. community hospital to care for patients with Ebola virus disease: context for national recommendations and future strategies. Ann Intern Med 2016;165:41–9.

38. Booth CM, Stewart TE. Severe acute respiratory syndrome and critical care medicine: the Toronto experience. Crit Care Med 2005;33:S53–60.

39. Johnson SS, Barranta N, Chertow D. Ebola at the National Institutes of Health: perspectives from critical care nurses. AACN Adv Crit Care 2015;26:262–7.

40. Torabi-Parizi P, Davey RT Jr, Suffredini AF, et al. Ethical and practical considerations in providing critical care to patients with Ebola virus disease. Chest 2015;147:1460–6.

41. Kabore HJ, Desamu-Thorpe R, Jean-Charles L, et al. Monitoring of persons with risk for exposure to Ebola virus - United States, November 3, 2014-December 27, 2015. MMWR Morb Mortal Wkly Rep 2016;65:1401–4.

42. Zucker HA, Whalen D, Raske KE. Lessons from New York State's preparedness efforts for Ebola. Disaster Med Public Health Prep 2016;10:1–6.

43. Chertow DS, Nath A, Suffredini AF, et al. Severe meningoencephalitis in a case of Ebola virus disease: a case report. Ann Intern Med 2016;165:301–4.

44. Sueblinvong V, Johnson DW, Weinstein GL, et al. Critical care for multiple organ failure secondary to Ebola virus disease in the United States. Crit Care Med 2015; 43:2066–75.

45. DeBiasi RL, Song X, Cato K, et al, CNHS Ebola Response Task Force. Preparedness, evaluation, and care of pediatric patients under investigation for Ebola virus disease: experience from a pediatric designated care facility. J Pediatr Infect Dis Soc 2016;5:68–75.

46. Kamali A, Jamieson DJ, Kpaduwa J, et al. Pregnancy, labor, and delivery after Ebola virus disease and implications for infection control in obstetric services, United States. Emerg Infect Dis 2016;22:1156–61.

47. Chertow DS, Kleine C, Edwards JK, et al. Ebola virus disease in West Africa - clinical manifestations and management. N Engl J Med 2014;371:2054–7.

48. Gershon R, Dernehl LA, Nwankwo E, et al. Experiences and psychosocial impact of West Africa Ebola deployment on US health care volunteers. PLoS Curr 2016;8: 1–29.

49. Lewis JD, Enfield KB, Perl TM, et al. Preparedness planning and care of patients under investigation for or with Ebola virus disease: a survey of physicians in North America. Am J Infect Control 2017;45:65–8.

50. 2007 guideline for isolation precautions: preventing transmission of infectious agents in healthcare settings. Available at: https://www.cdc.gov/hai/pdfs/ isolation2007.pdf. Accessed February 2, 2017.

51. Infection prevention and control recommendations for hospitalized patients under investigation (PUIs) for Ebola virus disease (EVD) in U.S. hospitals. Available at: https://www.cdc.gov/vhf/ebola/healthcare-us/hospitals/infection-control.html. Accessed February 2, 2017.

52. Tran K, Cimon K, Severn M, et al. Aerosol generating procedures and risk of transmission of acute respiratory infections to healthcare workers: a systematic review. PLoS One 2012;7:e35797.

53. Thompson KA, Pappachan JV, Bennett AM, et al, EASE Study Consortium. Influenza aerosols in UK hospitals during the H1N1 (2009) pandemic–the risk of aerosol generation during medical procedures. PLoS One 2013;8:e56278.

54. Kim SH, Chang SY, Sung M, et al. Extensive viable Middle East respiratory syndrome (MERS) coronavirus contamination in air and surrounding environment in MERS isolation wards. Clin Infect Dis 2016;63:363–9.

55. Fischer R, Judson S, Miazgowicz K, et al. Ebola virus stability on surfaces and in fluids in simulated outbreak environments. Emerg Infect Dis 2015;21:1243–6.

56. Franz DR, Jahrling PB, Friedlander AM, et al. Clinical recognition and management of patients exposed to biological warfare agents. JAMA 1997;278:399–411.

57. Interim guidance for environmental infection control in hospitals for Ebola virus. Available at: https://www.cdc.gov/vhf/ebola/healthcare-us/cleaning/hospitals.html. Accessed February 2, 2017.

58. Personal protective equipment (PPE) training. Available at: https://www.cdc.gov/vhf/ebola/healthcare-us/ppe/training.html. Accessed February 2, 2017.

59. Ebola courses for the general public & clinicians. Available at: http://www.nebraskamed.com/biocontainment-unit/ebola. Accessed February 2, 2017.

60. Ebola preparedness protocols. Available at: http://www.emoryhealthcare.org/ebola-protocol. Accessed February 2, 2017.

61. Hill CE, Burd EM, Kraft CS, et al. Laboratory test support for Ebola patients within a high-containment facility. Lab Med 2014;45:e109–11.

62. Jelden KC, Iwen PC, Herstein JJ, et al. U.S. Ebola treatment center clinical laboratory support. J Clin Microbiol 2016;54:1031–5.

63. Iwen PC, Garrett JL, Gibbs SG, et al. An integrated approach to laboratory testing for patients with Ebola virus disease. Lab Med 2014;45:e146–51.

64. Guidance for U.S. laboratories for managing and testing routine clinical specimens when there is a concern about Ebola virus disease. Available at: https://www.cdc.gov/vhf/ebola/healthcare-us/laboratories/safe-specimen-management.html. Accessed February 2, 2017.

65. Verbeek JH, Ijaz S, Mischke C, et al. Personal protective equipment for preventing highly infectious diseases due to exposure to contaminated body fluids in healthcare staff. Cochrane Database Syst Rev 2016;(4):CD011621.

66. Grillet G, Marjanovic N, Diverrez JM, et al. Intensive care medical procedures are more complicated, more stressful, and less comfortable with Ebola personal protective equipment: a simulation study. J Infect 2015;71:703–6.

67. Wiechmann W, Toohey S, Majestic C, et al. Intubating Ebola patients: technical limitations of extensive personal protective equipment. West J Emerg Med 2015;16:965.

68. World Health Organization. Situation report. Ebola virus disease 10 June 2016. Available at: Interim guidance for environmental infection control in hospitals for Ebola virus. Available at: https://www.cdc.gov/vhf/ebola/healthcare-us/cleaning/hospitals.html. Accessed May 1, 2017.

69. Herstein JJ, Biddinger PD, Kraft CS, et al. Initial costs of Ebola treatment centers in the United States. Emerg Infect Dis 2016;22:350–2.

70. Sun LH. Cost to treat Ebola in the U.S.: $1.16 million for 2 patients. Available at: https://www.washingtonpost.com/news/post-nation/wp/2014/11/18/cost-to-treat-ebola-in-the-u-s-1-16-million-for-2-patients/?utm_term=.894ccd9d6105. Accessed May 1, 2017.

71. Wallis L. First U.S. nurse to contract Ebola sues Texas health resources. Am J Nurs 2015;115:16.
72. Skowronski DM, Petric M, Daly P, et al. Coordinated response to SARS, Vancouver, Canada. Emerg Infect Dis 2006;12:155–8.
73. McDonald LC, Simor AE, Su IJ, et al. SARS in healthcare facilities, Toronto and Taiwan. Emerg Infect Dis 2004;10:777–81.
74. National Ebola Training and Education Center (NETEC). Available at: http://netec.org/. Accessed February 2, 2017.

Inhaled Antibiotics for Ventilator-Associated Infections

Lucy B. Palmer, MD

KEYWORDS

- Inhaled antibiotics • Ventilator-associated pneumonia
- Ventilator-associated tracheobronchitis • Multidrug-resistant bacteria

KEY POINTS

- Inhaled antibiotics provide high concentrations of antibiotics with fewer systemic effects than intravenous therapy.
- Devices that are well characterized ensure delivery to the right location with the right concentration.
- Multisite studies are needed to better assess the indications and efficacy of inhaled antibiotics and to determine whether their use can lessen the amount or duration of systemic antibiotic use.
- Early data suggest that inhaled antibiotics decrease rather than increase resistance compared with systemic antibiotics, and this is an important area of future investigation.

INTRODUCTION

Ventilator-associated pneumonia (VAP) remains the leading cause of death related to nosocomial infection in critically ill patients.[1–3] Equally important, it accounts for more than 50% of the antibiotic use in the intensive care unit (ICU).[4,5]

There is much discussion about the current incidence of VAP, with a range from 10% to 27%.[2,4,6] The morbidity and mortality related to respiratory infections remain significant and may vary with the causative organism.[5,7–10] In a 2009 review of clinical outcomes of health care–related infection in European ICUs, 4457 patients were identified with VAP caused by *Pseudomonas aeruginosa*, *Acinetobacter baumannii*, *Escherichia coli*, or *Staphylococcus aureus*.[5] The excess risk of death from VAP

Disclosure: Dr L.B. Palmer and her associate Dr G.C. Smaldone have a patent with the Research Foundation of SUNY Stony Brook for the use of endobronchial antibiotics, which is licensed to Nektar Therapeutics (Grant # W8BNMSWD). A primary investigator–driven study of inhaled antibiotics was funded by Nektar Therapeutics.
Pulmonary, Critical Care and Sleep Division, SUNY at Stony Brook, HSC T17-040, Stony Brook, NY 11794-8172, USA
E-mail address: lucy.b.palmer@stonybrook.edu

(hazard ratio) was 1.7 (95% confidence interval [CI], 1.4–1.9) for drug-sensitive *S aureus* and 3.5 (95% CI, 2.9–4.2) for ceftazidime-resistant *Pseudomonas*. Now that multidrug-resistant (MDR) pathogens in ICU patients are outpacing Pharma's motivation to create new systemic antibiotics, there is an urgent call for new therapies.[11,12] Some regions of the world now have gram-negative pathogens that are extensively drug resistant (XDR); that is, resistant to all antibiotics, including colistin.[13]

ICU physicians in regions of the world with endemic MDR or XDR gram-negatives are responding to the lack of effective systemic antibiotics by adding inhaled antibiotics empirically to their VAP treatment regimens.[14–25] Empiric therapy with off-the-shelf nebulizers and off-label use of antibiotics is their only choice because, 45 years after the initial instillation of antibiotics into an endotracheal tube or a tracheostomy, there are no commercially available US Food and Drug Administration (FDA)–approved inhaled drugs on the market for ventilated patients. The 2016 American Thoracic Society (ATS) guidelines state that, "For patients with VAP due to gram-negative bacilli that are susceptible to only aminoglycosides or polymyxins (colistin or polymyxin B), we suggest both inhaled and systemic antibiotics, rather than systemic antibiotics alone (weak recommendation)."[3]

This article reviews the literature, with an emphasis on the most recent data concerning:

- Rationale and indications for treatment
- Clinical outcomes
- Microbial effects of inhaled antibiotics.

BACKGROUND

The earliest studies of inhaled antibiotic therapy were driven by the same clinical problem that exists now: the emergence of resistance to the currently available antibiotics. Resistant gram-negative organisms, in particular *Pseudomonas* species, were causing respiratory infections in intubated patients and clinical response to intravenous (IV) therapy was poor.[26–29] At that time, aminoglycosides given intravenously were the primary treatment of gram-negative organisms and treatment failure occurred in up to 60% of patients. These poor outcomes were thought primarily to be caused by poor penetration of the aminoglycosides into the lung so methods of increasing the concentration via direct delivery were investigated.

Early investigations used endotracheal instillation of the antibiotic.[28,29,31] The peripheral parenchymal distribution of this method is unknown but concentrations of the aminoglycoside in bronchial secretions were shown to be 1000-fold higher than serum concentrations of patients receiving IV therapy, and bactericidal activity was more than 30-fold greater than that in serum.[28] These investigators showed clinical benefit from instillation of aminoglycosides for the treatment of bronchial infections in intubated patients (now called ventilator-associated tracheobronchitis [VAT]), as well as in bronchopneumonia.[26,27] At that time, the investigators wrote, "endotracheal administration might thus represent the ideal adjunct to systemic antimicrobial therapy for bronchopneumonina."[26] However, these early studies of the 1970s did not lead to multisite clinical randomized trials of inhaled antimicrobials for treatment of respiratory infection in mechanically ventilated patients. Instead, almost all aerosol treatment of VAT or VAP in patients without cystic fibrosis is used off label with no well-validated dosing or defined devices for most studies (**Box 1**). **Table 1** shows the common side effects related to their use.

There is 1 phase 3 randomized controlled trial (RCT) in ventilated patients for VAP that is currently enrolling patients. This delay of research and development in

---

Box 1
Inhaled antibiotics used in mechanically ventilated patients for respiratory infection: off-label use and Food and Drug Administration approved

Amikacin

Amikacin proprietary preparation[a]

Amikacin/fosfomycin proprietary preparation[b]

Colistin

Colistin methanesulfonate[c]

Ceftazidime

Gentamicin

Tobramycin

Tobramycin proprietary preparation[d]

Sisomicin

Vancomycin

[a] Phase 3 enrolling patients. Delivered by Bayer Healthcare with proprietary pulmonary drug delivery system.
[b] Phase 1 completed. Delivered with Pari investigational eFlow inline nebulizer.
[c] Prodrug of colistin polymyxin E.
[d] FDA approved for spontaneous breathing patients with cystic fibrosis known to be colonized with *P aeruginosa*.
From Palmer LB. Ventilator-associated infection: the role for inhaled antibiotics. Curr Opin Pulm Med 2015;21:239–49.

---

aerosolized antibiotics for ventilated patients was primarily driven by the negative results of an investigation of topical antibiotics used not for treatment but for the prevention of pneumonia in critically ill patients in 1975. It is worth reviewing this investigation because it shows how critical antibiotic delivery and choice of patients are.[30] All the patients in the ICU were treated for their entire intensive care unit admission with atomized polymyxin B and, if intubated, they also received instilled polymyxin B.

Table 1
Toxicity related to aerosolized antibiotics

Drug	Adverse Events
Aminoglycosides	Bronchial Constriction Renal toxicity[a] Tinnitus, vestibular Toxicity, hoarseness
Colistin	Nephrotoxicity[b] Bronchospasm[b] Neurologic toxicity
Aztreonam lysine	Cough, bronchoconstriction
Vancomycin	Not well described
Cefotaxime/ceftazidime	Not well described

[a] Renal toxicity rarely seen with tobramycin (Tobi, PARI Pharma GmbH, Weilheim, Germany.
[b] Nephrotoxicity and bronchospasm more severe than with aminoglycosides.

This protocol of (1) universal administration, (2) non--time-limited regimen, and (3) atomization to the oropharynx led to polymyxin B–resistant organisms and pneumonia with a 64% mortality. The investigators called the topical treatment a dangerous form of therapy and this led to what to what is now called the 40 years of fear of inhaled antibiotics.

RATIONALE FOR AEROSOLIZED ANTIBIOTIC THERAPY IN VENTILATED PATIENTS

Now that the treatment of multidrug-resistant organisms (MDRO) has become increasingly problematic, more sophisticated targeted therapy delivered directly to the lung is being revisited. The theoretic reasons for using targeted antimicrobial therapy in mechanically ventilated patients include:

- Direct delivery to the site of infection
- Concentrations in the lung that would not be tolerated if given intravenously
- The microflora of the gut are not altered, thus reducing the emergence of MDRO
- May shorten the duration of systemic antibiotics

Of these 4 rationales, the first 2 are well proved. It has been shown in multiple studies that antibiotic concentrations achieved in the lung in secretions as well as bronchoalveolar lavage (BAL) with targeted therapy far exceed the minimum inhibitory concentration (MIC) of pathogens with very low or nondetectable levels in the serum.[31–34] These high concentrations in secretions result in a large ratio of maximum concentration/MIC.[35] This index has been shown to be important for eradication of organisms in the milieu of thick purulent secretions, biofilm, and diminished mucociliary clearance of patients with cystic fibrosis.[35] The success of inhaled antibiotics in patients with cystic fibrosis is promising because ventilated patients also have injured and inflamed airway epithelium from instrumentation of the airway, poor mucociliary clearance, and endotracheal tube biofilm.[36,37]

Biofilm is a slow-growing community of bacteria that live in an extracellular polymeric matrix that consists of polysaccharide, DNA, and proteins.[37,38] It may be present in ventilated patients' airways as well as in their endotracheal tubes (**Fig. 1**). If only IV therapy is used and concentrations are not bactericidal, biofilm formation may be induced, making the infections even harder to eradicate.[39]

The data on effects of inhaled therapy on gut flora have not been measured directly. There are data suggesting a decrease in respiratory MDRO after treatment even when patients are on concomitant systemic therapy.[40,41] These investigations are discussed later, as are potential effects on systemic antibiotic use.

Inhaled Antibiotics Therapy for Prevention of Ventilator-associated Pneumonia

The use of inhaled antibiotics as prophylaxis for VAP is not well supported at this time. The polymyxin B data from the 1970s have been discussed previously. A meta-analysis by Falagas and colleagues[42] reviewed the literature from 1950 to 2005. Of the 12 prophylactic trials, there were only 8 investigations that were either RCTs or prospective comparative trials. Aerosolized gentamicin was used in 3 trials, polymyxin in 2, tobramycin in 1, and ceftazidime in 1. There were 1877 patients included in the meta-analysis. Primary outcomes were incidence of VAP and mortality. Secondary outcome was colonization with *P aeruginosa*. Analysis of the 5 RCTs showed a reduction in VAP in the treated patients with an odds ratio (OR) of 0.49 (95% CI, 0.32–0.76). However, there was no effect on mortality, and there were insufficient data to assess the effect on bacterial colonization. Addition of the 2 nonrandomized trials to their meta-analysis yielded similar results for VAP; however, in

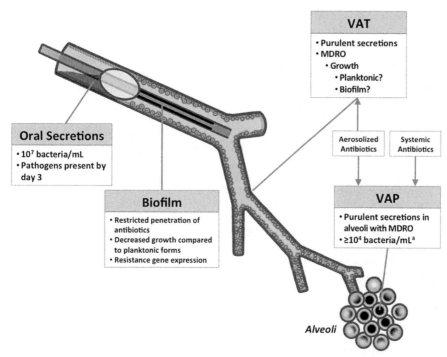

Fig. 1. The multifactorial process that leads to VAT and VAP. Subglottic secretions, disturbed mucociliary clearance, damaged mucosa, and bacterial biofilm may all play a role in the pathogenesis of proximal and distal infection. Within a few days of ICU admission, the bacteria are frequently MDRO. [a]The 10[4] CFU/mL cutoff for the microbiologic diagnosis of VAP may not pertain to patients with prolonged mechanical ventilation. (*Modified from* Aerosolized antibiotics for ventilator associated infections. Chapter 10.4. In: Dhand R, editor: Textbook of aerosol medicine. Knowville TN: International Society of Aerosols in Medicine; 2015. p.1–28.)

this analysis, there was a reduction in VAP in patients colonized with *P aeruginosa* in the group that received prophylaxis compared with the group that received no prophylaxis (OR, 0.51; 95% CI, 0.30–0.86). Although these data are of interest, current guidelines from both the Centers for Disease Control and Prevention and the ATS do not recommend this therapy.[3] These older prophylactic studies used a variety of delivery devices, often have no data on concentrations of the antibiotic in the lung, and represent pathogens that have since evolved to be more resistant. RCTs with standardized delivery methods; appropriate new end points, such as ventilator-free days; reduction in the use of systemic antibiotics; and effects on bacterial resistance are needed.

EVIDENCE FOR TREATING VENTILATOR-ASSOCIATED TRACHEOBRONCHITIS AND/OR VENTILATOR-ASSOCIATED PNEUMONIA: META-ANALYSES OF TREATMENT EFFECTS

The early evidence supporting the use of inhaled antimicrobials in ventilated patients was analyzed by Ioannidou and colleagues[43] in a meta-analysis of small RCTs done from 1950 to 2007.[44] The clinical efficacy of topical administration (aerosolization or instillation) with or without concurrent usage of systemic antibiotics for treatment of

VAP was examined. Of 685 potential relevant articles there were only 5 RCTs with a combined total of 176 patients suitable for analysis.[26,27,44–46] Antibiotics used included tobramycin, sisomicin, and gentamicin. In 4 of the 5 trials the aerosolized antibiotic was adjunctive to IV therapy.[26,27,44–46] This meta-analysis showed that patients receiving aerosolized or instilled antibiotics had higher rates of resolution of signs and symptoms of VAP (clinical diagnosis), (intention-to-treat fixed effect model OR 2.39, 95% CI 1.29–4.44; random effect model OR 2.75, 95% CI 1.06–7.17), and when analyzed for clinically evaluable patients had an OR = 3.14 and 95% CI = 1.48 to 6.70, and in a random effects model OR = 3.07 and 95% CI = 1.15 to 8.19. There were no statistically significant differences between therapeutic regimens for mortality or toxicity.

There have been 2 more recent meta-analyses.[47,48] Zampieri and colleagues[47] analyzed the results of RCTs or matched observational studies that compared nebulized antibiotics with or without IV antibiotics with IV antibiotics alone for VAP treatment. The primary outcome was clinical cure and secondary outcomes were microbiological cure, ICU and hospital mortality, duration of mechanical ventilation, and ICU length of stay. For the main outcome analysis, 812 patients were included. Inhaled antibiotics had higher rates of clinical cure (risk ratio [RR] = 1.23; 95% CI, 1.05–1.43). There was no difference in microbiological cure (RR = 1.24; 95% CI, 0.95–1.62), mortality (RR = 0.90; CI 95%, 0.76–1.08), duration of mechanical ventilation (standardized mean difference = −0.10 days; 95% CI, −1.22–1.00; 96.5%), ICU length of stay (standardized mean difference [SMD] = 0.14 days; 95% CI, −0.46–0.73; 89.2%), or renal toxicity (RR = 1.05; 95% CI, 0.70–1.57). The investigators noted that the number of patients included was less than the information size required for a definitive conclusion by trial sequential analysis but that nebulized antibiotics seemed to be associated with higher rates of clinical cure in the treatment of VAP.

Valachis and colleagues[48] conducted a meta-analysis of adjunctive colistin versus IV colistin alone. Sixteen studies fulfilled the inclusion criteria: 8 were comparing adjunctive aerosolized versus IV colistin (7 observational cohort or case-control studies and 1 randomized trial) and underwent meta-analysis. Eight were single arm and were therefore only systematically reviewed. The clinical response meta-analysis showed that the addition of inhaled colistin to IV treatment had an OR of 1.57 (95% CI, 1.14–2.15; P = .006) microbiological eradication OR of 1.61 (95% CI, 1.11–2.35; P = .01), and for infection-related mortality OR was 0.58 (95% CI, 0.34–0.96; P = .04). The overall mortality was not significantly affected, nor were nephrotoxicity or nephrotoxicity.

Rationale for Inhaled Colistin for Ventilator-associated Pneumonia

Many of the studies mentioned earlier used colistin (polymyxin E) and antibiotics from the 1970s. Highly resistant P aeruginosa and Acinetobacter have led to the reintroduction of this antibiotic in an aerosolized form as well as a prodrug, colistimethate sodium (CMS).[49,50] The mechanism of colistin's bactericidal activity is destabilization of the lipopolysaccharide (LPS) of the outer membrane, and in addition it neutralizes the LPS thereby decreasing antiendotoxin activity.[50] Its IV use was discontinued for about 40 years because of its neurologic and renal toxicity when used parenterally and the advent of less toxic antibiotics.[51,52]

There have been multiple small nonrandomized clinical trials, 1 RCT, 1 review, and 1 meta-analysis focused on inhaled and IV colistin treatment of MDR gram-negative species, in particular Acinetobacter and Pseudomonas.[13,14,19,20,22,23,49,53–56] These bacteria both produce extended-spectrum β-lactamases as well as metallolactamases. *Acinetobacter* is often sensitive only to polymyxin B or colistin (polymyxin E) and there are now reports of colistin resistance as well.[19,56]

Included in the review of the literature by Ioannidou and colleagues[43] mentioned earlier were 2 nonrandomized prospective trials of aerosolized colistin that included patients with these organisms.[43,54,57] Kwa and colleagues[54] treated 21 patients with respiratory tract infections with *Acinetobacter* and *Pseudomonas* species. Patients who received systemic antibiotics and aerosolized colistin had a good clinical response with a reduction in signs/symptoms of infection. Hamer[57] treated MDR *Pseudomonas* with aerosolized colistin in a small case series of 3 mechanically ventilated patients with VAP who also showed an improvement in signs of infection.

In an open-label, noncontrolled, prospective investigation, Michalopoulos and colleagues[22] treated 60 critically ill patients with a mean Acute Physiology and Chronic Health Evaluation II (APACHE II) score of 16.7. Patients received aerosolized colistin for the treatment of VAP caused by MDR pathogens. *A baumannii* was present in 37 of 60 patients, *P aeruginosa* in 12, and *Klebsiella pneumoniae* in 11 of the 60 patients. Half of these pathogens were susceptible only to colistin. Fifty-seven of the 60 patients received concomitant IV treatment with colistin or other antimicrobial agents. Bacteriologic and clinical response of VAP was observed in 83% of the patients.

Berlana and colleagues[14] described the microbiologic outcomes in an investigation including 71 courses of aerosolized colistin used to treat 60 respiratory infections with *A baumannii* and 11 with *P aeruginosa*. The mean duration of therapy was 12 ± 8 days. The *Acinetobacter* were eradicated in all the end-of-treatment cultures that were available; however, *Pseudomonas* was eradicated only in 57%.

Kofteridis and colleagues,[18] in a retrospective matched case-control study, compared the effect of IV colistin alone with IV colistin and aerosolized colistin. Each group had 43 patients. *A baumannii* was the most common pathogen (77% of isolates), followed by *K pneumoniae* (14%)and *P aeruginosa* (9.3%). The patients in the group with aerosolized and IV colistin had a higher rate of clinical cure than did patients in the IV colistin group (23 [54%] of 43 patients versus 14 [32.5%] of 43 patients) but it did not meet clinical significance ($P = .05$). No significant differences in eradication of pathogens ($P = .679$) or mortality ($P = .289$) between the 2 groups were observed. Overall, the mortality in the ICU was 42% (18 of 43 patients) in the IV colistin group, compared with 24% (10 of 43 patients) in the aerosol and IV colistin group ($P = .066$). This study, unlike all others described, found IV therapy to be no different from IV and aerosolized colistin in bacterial eradication. There is no description of the method of aerosolization so it is possible that the negative findings may be related to the method of delivery.

Korbila and colleagues,[19] in a similar retrospective cohort study, compared IV colistin alone (43 patients) with IV colistin plus aerosolized colistin (78 patients) and showed a significant improvement in clinical outcome (resolution of signs and symptoms of infection) in 62 out of 78 (79.5%) of the patients who received IV plus inhaled colistin versus 26 out of 43 (60.5%) patients who received IV colistin alone ($P<.025$). The use of inhaled colistin was independently associated with the cure of VAP in a multivariable analysis (OR = 2.53; 95% CI, 1.11–5.76). No significant differences were observed in the 2 groups, inhaled colistin plus IV colistin and IV colistin respectively, for all-cause ICU mortality (28 out of 78 patients [35.9%]vs 17 out of 43 [39.5%], respectively; $P = .92$) or all-cause in-hospital mortality (31 out of 78 patients [39.7%] vs 19 out of 43 [44.2%]; $P = .63$).

In a retrospective cohort study, Arnold and colleagues[17] assessed treatment of VAP caused by *P aeruginosa* and *A baumannii* VAP. Patients with only IV therapy (n = 74) were compared with those who received inhaled colistin (n = 19) and with those who received aerosolized tobramycin (n = 10) in a retrospective study and the cohort group was not well matched to the experimental groups. Patients treated with inhaled antibiotics had more MDRO (52.6% vs 14.9%; *P* = .001) and higher APACHE II scores (21.4 ± 5.7 vs 17.5 ± 5.3; *P* = .004) Despite these differences, Kaplan-Meier curves for the probability of 30-day survival from VAP onset showed that patients receiving aerosolized antibiotics had statistically greater survival (*P* = .030 by the log rank test).

RANDOMIZED CONTROLLED TRIALS OF AEROSOLIZED ANTIBIOTICS FOR VENTILATOR-ASSOCIATED TRACHEOBRONCHITIS OR VENTILATOR-ASSOCIATED PNEUMONIA

There have only been 5 randomized placebo controlled studies of inhaled adjunctive antibiotics for VAT and VAP since 2005.[31,40,41,58,59] In a double-blind, placebo-controlled phase 2 study, aerosolized amikacin delivered via vibrating mesh technology was given as adjunctive therapy to 67 ventilated patients with gram-negative pneumonia.[31] Systemic antibiotic therapy was given by the responsible clinician following ATS guidelines.[60] Randomization was to aerosolized amikacin 400 mg daily with placebo (normal saline) 12 hours later, or 400 mg twice daily or placebo twice daily. The mean number of IV antibiotics at the end of the study (mean 7 days) were 2 times greater with placebo than with twice-daily amikacin (*P*<.02).[31]

Palmer and colleagues[40], in a double-blind placebo-controlled trial, randomized 43 critically ill intubated patients with VAT (defined as the production of purulent secretions ≥2.0 mL over 4 hours) and organisms on Gram stain to aerosolized (Aero-Tech II nebulizer, Biodex Medical Systems, Shirley, NY) [31] gentamicin (80 mg every 8 hours) and/or vancomycin treatment (120 mg every 8 hours) dictated by Gram stain at the time of randomization.[40] Systemic antibiotics were administered by the clinician responsible for the patient. Both placebo and active treatment groups received similar amounts of appropriate systemic antibiotics at randomization. Treatment with aerosolized antibiotics resulted in decreased signs and symptoms of VAP and decreased clinical pulmonary infection score (CPIS), and facilitated weaning and reduction in the use of systemic antibiotics compared with the placebo patients. Patients treated with aerosolized antibiotics had marked reduction in bacterial growth. Gram stains of cultures with zero growth revealed that, in the aerosolized antibiotic group, 7 of 12 cultures (58%) during week 1 and 6 of 8 (75%) during week 2 had no organisms on Gram stain. In placebo, only 3 of 14 cultures (21%) during week 1 and 4 of 18 (22%) during week 2 had Gram stains with no organisms.

The investigation by Palmer and colleagues[40] also provided preliminary data for the treatment of methicillin-resistant *S aureus* (MRSA) via aerosolized vancomycin in ventilated patients. Three placebo patients who had VAT secondary to MRSA as well as VAP at the time of randomization had no improvement during the study despite being on appropriate systemic antibiotics. Three patients with MRSA and VAT received aerosolized vancomycin. Two of these did not have VAP at randomization and remained free of VAP at the end of treatment. The 1 patient who had MRSA and had VAP had clinical resolution at the end of aerosolized vancomycin treatment as well as eradication of the MRSA.

A recent randomized controlled study compared the effects of placebo (normal saline) plus IV antibiotics with aerosolized CMS and IV antibiotics. CMS is a prodrug that must be converted in the lung to active colistin.[58] All patients were on systemic antibiotics chosen by the responsible physicians. The baseline characteristics of the patients were similar and mean APACHE II score of both groups were 18.5 and 19.1, for placebo and CMS respectively. Conventional systemic antibiotic therapy for VAP in both groups were comparable. Most of the cases of VAP were caused by MDR, *A baumannii*, and/or *P aeruginosa*. All isolates of gram-negative bacteria were susceptible to colistin. Favorable clinical outcome was 51.0% in the aerosol CMS plus systemic antibiotic group and 53.1% in the placebo plus systemic antibiotic group (P = .84). Patients in the CMS group had significantly more favorable microbiological outcome (defined as eradication or presumed eradication) compared with patients in the control group (60.9% vs 38.2%; P = .03). This investigation differs from all others described because CMS was used, which is thought to be less potent than colistin. The concentration of active drug in the lung is not as predictable as in those studies using colistin and this may explain the less favorable clinical outcome compared with the other RCTs. Also, jet nebulizers and ultrasonic nebulizers were used so the equivalence of deposition site and concentration is unknown.

Most recently, in a double-blind placebo-controlled study, critically ill intubated patients with prolonged mechanical ventilation were randomized if they showed signs of respiratory infection (purulent secretions and CPIS >6).[41] Using a well-characterized aerosol delivery system, inhaled antibiotic or saline placebo was given for 14 days or until extubation. The responsible clinician determined administration of systemic antibiotics for VAP and any other infection. Compared with placebo, inhaled antibiotic significantly reduced CPIS (mean ± standard error of the mean, 9.3 ± 2.7 to 5.3 ± 2.6 vs 8.0 ± 23 to 8.6 ± 2.10; P = .0008). The effects on bacterial growth are shown in **Fig. 2**.

The most recent RCT, conducted by Kollef and colleagues[59] in 2016, administered a combination of amikacin and fosfomycin to ventilated patients with gram-negative VAP. All patients received IV meropenem or imipenem (dosed for gram-negative coverage for 7 days, and longer if clinically indicated). There were 143 patients randomized, 71 to amikacin fosfomycin inhalation system (AFIS), and 72 to placebo. CPIS change from baseline between treatment groups was not different (P = .70). The secondary end point of mortality and clinical cure at day 14 or earlier was also not significant (P = .68), nor was the end point of no mortality and ventilator-free days (P = .06). Mortality was 17 (24%) in AFIS, and 12 (17%) in placebo (P = .32). The AFIS group had significantly fewer positive tracheal cultures on days 3 and 7 compared with placebo. These results differ from most of the earlier RCTs. This trial used the same vibrating mesh nebulizer through the entire trial. It is not clear from the literature whether efficiency and delivery deteriorate over time using a single vibrating plate.

HOW DO AEROSOLIZED ANTIBIOTICS AFFECT EMERGENCE OF BACTERIAL RESISTANCE COMPARED WITH SYSTEMIC ANTIBIOTICS?

Increased bacterial resistance in the ICU has been shown to have a direct relationship to the amount of systemic antibiotic prescribed. However, there have been very few data in the literature analyzing the impact of aerosolized antibiotics on the emergence of resistance. The meta-analysis by Ioannidou and colleagues[43] mentioned previously described a 6.5% (3 out of 46) incidence of new resistance at the end of treatment in the 5 RCTs included.

Seven trials report data on the emergence of resistance.[14,18,21,40,41,59,61] No new resistance to drug administered was detected. Included are 5 RCTs with resistance data. Koftederis and colleagues[18] described no new resistance in the group that

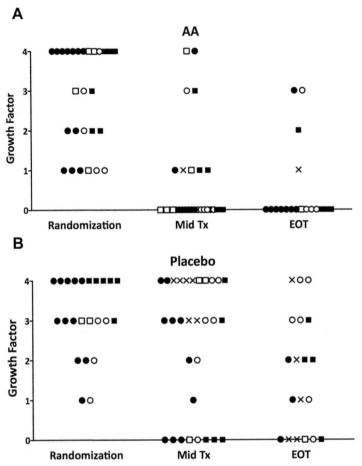

Fig. 2. Bacterial growth from tracheal aspirates obtained at time of randomization, mid-treatment (Mid Tx), and at end of treatment (EOT) for (*A*) aerosolized antibiotics (AA) and (*B*) placebo. Growth is quantified using a graded scale of 0 to 4 from semiquantitative cultures: multidrug-resistant gram-negative organisms (*filled circles*), nonresistant gram-negative organisms (*open circles*), resistant gram-positive organisms (*filled squares*), nonresistant gram-positive organisms (*open squares*), and newly resistant organisms on treatment (*x*). Some patients had multiple isolates. At Mid Tx all the isolates with zero growth represent organisms detected at randomization that did not grow in isolates sampled at Mid Tx. At EOT the isolates with zero growth represent organisms detected at randomization and Mid Tx that did not grow in samples obtained at EOT. There was a clear difference in pattern of bacterial growth between AA and placebo. Two AA isolates showed persistent growth at EOT: 1 methicillin-resistant *S aureus* (*filled square*) that was not eradicated by AA but had no gram-positive cocci on Gram stain, and 1 persistent *Acinetobacter* (*filled circle*) with organisms present on Gram stain. More newly resistant organisms were seen in the placebo group. (*Reprinted from* Palmer LB, Smaldone GC. Reduction of bacterial resistance with inhaled antibiotics. Am J Respir Crit Care Med 2014;189(10):1230; with permission of the American Thoracic Society, 2014.)

received aerosol but there were no data provided for the patients who received only systemic antibiotics. Palmer and colleagues[40] showed that 8 of 24 participants receiving placebo inhaled antibiotic and systemic antibiotics acquired resistant organisms during treatment compared with zero of 19 aerosolized antibiotic patients ($P = .0056$). In the placebo group receiving only systemic antibiotics, 4 participants with sensitive bacteria (3 *P aeruginosa* and 1 *K pneumoniae*) developed resistance on treatment. Two participants acquired a resistant *Acinetobacter* and 2 acquired MRSA. One of 19 aerosolized antibiotic participants transiently acquired a resistant organism, a resistant *Acinetobacter* that resolved during therapy. All patients who acquired resistant organisms received systemic antibiotics. Lu and colleagues'[61] randomized trial of IV versus inhaled antibiotics (as exclusive treatment) again showed the emergence of resistance only in the comparator group that received systemic antibiotics. In another investigation with more chronically ventilated patients, aerosolized antibiotics eradicated 26 of 27 organisms present at randomization compared with 2 of 23 organisms in the placebo group ($P = .0001$) despite both groups being on similar amounts of appropriate systemic antibiotics. Inhaled antibiotics eradicated the original resistant organism on culture and Gram stain at end of treatment in 14 out of 16 patients compared with 1 of 11 for placebo ($P = .001$). Resistance to systemic antibiotics significantly increased in placebo patients receiving only systemic antibiotics ($P = .03$). In chronically intubated critically ill patients, inhaled antibiotics successfully eradicated existing MDRO organisms and reduced the pressure from systemic agents for new microbial resistance. Note that most of the data described earlier are for the effects of centrally deposited drugs on pathogens in the large airways. Data on drug concentrations in the parenchyma and resistance in the alveolar space in those cases are well described. In 2 studies with more peripheral deposition using vibrating mesh with delivery to the distal lung, resistance was higher in the group on placebo compared with those patients receiving inhaled antibioitics.[59,61]

FUTURE RESEARCH

Well-designed multisite studies are needed to confirm the data summarized in this article. These protocols will need objective criteria for diagnosing respiratory infection. **Box 2** shows important end points that need to be included. If the emergence of resistance in the ICU continues to escalate, the prescribers of systemic antibiotics will be responsible for the evolution of MDRO. Future investigations are needed to determine the role of inhaled antibiotics in mechanically ventilated patients and their overall effect on MDRO. Contrary to the data on topical therapy from the 1970s,[32] it is now worth exploring whether targeted therapy may become one of the new tools combating antimicrobial resistance.

Box 2
Outcomes of interest in future multisite trials of inhaled antibiotics

- Systemic antibiotic days during mechanical ventilation
- MDRO in respiratory tract and nonrespiratory sites
- Ventilator-free days
- Recurrence of respiratory infection
- Incidence of *Clostridium difficile*

SUMMARY

- There is a growing body of data that suggest that inhaled antibiotics may have a role in the treatment of respiratory infection in the ICU.
- Three of 5 recent RCTs have shown positive clinical outcomes with reduction in CPIS score, facilitation of weaning and/or a reduction in the use of systemic antibiotics when aerosolized inhaled antibiotics were used as adjunctive therapy for VAT and/or VAP.[45,46,61]
- A decrease in the MDRO after inhaled treatment has been seen in single-site RCTs in patients treated with inhaled antibiotics compared with IV therapy alone.[45,46]
- In view of the threat of increasingly resistant organisms present in the ICU, including both MDR gram-negatives and MRSA, large multicenter trials targeting antimicrobial therapy to the lung are needed. Trials targeting early respiratory infection could determine whether inhaled therapy causes a significant reduction in the use of systemic antibiotics.
- Clinical trials must be designed to assess not only clinical end points such as resolution of signs and symptoms of respiratory infection but data should also be acquired for new primary outcomes, such as effects on the amounts and duration of systemic antibiotic used. Trials should also document antimicrobial resistance in the ICU and incidence of nosocomial infections such as C difficile.

ACKNOWLEDGMENTS

The author thanks Lorraine Morra for her expert technical assistance.

REFERENCES

1. Peleg AY, Hooper DC. Hospital-acquired infections due to gram-negative bacteria. N Engl J Med 2010;362(19):1804–13.
2. Kalanuria AA, Ziai W, Mirski M. Ventilator-associated pneumonia in the ICU. Crit Care 2014;18(2):208.
3. Kalil AC, Metersky ML, Klompas M, et al. Management of adults with hospital-acquired and ventilator-associated pneumonia: 2016 clinical practice guidelines by the Infectious Diseases Society of America and the American Thoracic Society. Clin Infect Dis 2016;63(5):e61–111.
4. Browne E, Hellyer TP, Baudouin SV, et al. A national survey of the diagnosis and management of suspected ventilator-associated pneumonia. BMJ Open Respir Res 2014;1(1):e000066.
5. Vincent JL, Rello J, Marshall J, et al. International study of the prevalence and outcomes of infection in intensive care units. JAMA 2009;302(21):2323–9.
6. Metersky ML, Wang Y, Klompas M, et al. Trend in ventilator-associated pneumonia rates between 2005 and 2013. JAMA 2016;316(22):2427–9.
7. Safdar N, Dezfulian C, Collard HR, et al. Clinical and economic consequences of ventilator-associated pneumonia: a systematic review. Crit Care Med 2005; 33(10):2184–93.
8. Lambert ML, Suetens C, Savey A, et al. Clinical outcomes of health-care-associated infections and antimicrobial resistance in patients admitted to European intensive-care units: a cohort study. Lancet Infect Dis 2011;11(1):30–8.
9. Masterton RG, Galloway A, French G, et al. Guidelines for the management of hospital-acquired pneumonia in the UK: report of the Working Party on Hospital-acquired Pneumonia of the British Society for Antimicrobial Chemotherapy. J Antimicrob Chemother 2008;62(1):5–34.

10. Chastre J, Luyt CE. Optimising the duration of antibiotic therapy for ventilator-associated pneumonia. Eur Respir Rev 2007;16(103):40–4.

11. Boucher HW, Talbot GH, Bradley JS, et al. Bad bugs, no drugs: no ESKAPE! an update from the infectious diseases society of America. Clin Infect Dis 2009; 48(1):1–12.

12. Arias CA, Murray BE. Antibiotic-resistant bugs in the 21st century–a clinical super-challenge. N Engl J Med 2009;360(5):439–43.

13. Falagas ME, Kasiakou SK. Colistin: the revival of polymyxins for the management of multidrug-resistant gram-negative bacterial infections. Clin Infect Dis 2005; 40(9):1333–41.

14. Berlana D, Llop JM, Fort E, et al. Use of colistin in the treatment of multiple-drug-resistant gram-negative infections. Am J Health Syst Pharm 2005;62(1):39–47.

15. Athanassa ZE, Myrianthefs PM, Boutzouka EG, et al. Monotherapy with inhaled colistin for the treatment of patients with ventilator-associated tracheobronchitis due to polymyxin-only-susceptible Gram-negative bacteria. J Hosp Infect 2011; 78(4):335–6.

16. Athanassa ZE, Markantonis SL, Fousteri MZ, et al. Pharmacokinetics of inhaled colistimethate sodium (CMS) in mechanically ventilated critically ill patients. Intensive Care Med 2012;38(11):1779–86.

17. Arnold HM, Sawyer AM, Kollef MH. Use of adjunctive aerosolized antimicrobial therapy in the treatment of *Pseudomonas aeruginosa* and *Acinetobacter baumannii* ventilator-associated pneumonia. Respir Care 2012;57(8):1226–33.

18. Kofteridis DP, Alexopoulou C, Valachis A, et al. Aerosolized plus intravenous colistin versus intravenous colistin alone for the treatment of ventilator-associated pneumonia: a matched case-control study. Clin Infect Dis 2010;51(11):1238–44.

19. Korbila IP, Michalopoulos A, Rafailidis PI, et al. Inhaled colistin as adjunctive therapy to intravenous colistin for the treatment of microbiologically documented ventilator-associated pneumonia: a comparative cohort study. Clin Microbiol Infect 2010;16(8):1230–6.

20. Li J, Nation RL, Milne RW, et al. Evaluation of colistin as an agent against multi-resistant gram-negative bacteria. Int J Antimicrob Agents 2005;25(1):11–25.

21. Lu Q, Luo R, Bodin L, et al. Efficacy of high-dose nebulized colistin in ventilator-associated pneumonia caused by multidrug-resistant *Pseudomonas aeruginosa* and *Acinetobacter baumannii*. Anesthesiology 2012;117(6):1335–47.

22. Michalopoulos A, Kasiakou SK, Mastora Z, et al. Aerosolized colistin for the treatment of nosocomial pneumonia due to multidrug-resistant Gram-negative bacteria in patients without cystic fibrosis. Crit Care 2005;9(1):R53–9.

23. Michalopoulos A, Fotakis D, Virtzili S, et al. Aerosolized colistin as adjunctive treatment of ventilator-associated pneumonia due to multidrug-resistant Gram-negative bacteria: a prospective study. Respir Med 2008;102(3):407–12.

24. Pereira GH, Muller PR, Levin AS. Salvage treatment of pneumonia and initial treatment of tracheobronchitis caused by multidrug-resistant Gram-negative bacilli with inhaled polymyxin B. Diagn Microbiol Infect Dis 2007;58(2):235–40.

25. Perez-Pedrero MJ, Sanchez-Casado M, Rodriguez-Villar S. Nebulized colistin treatment of multi-resistant *Acinetobacter baumannii* pulmonary infection in critical ill patients. Med Intensiva 2011;35(4):226–31 [in Spanish].

26. Klastersky J, Carpentier-Meunier F, Kahan-Coppens L, et al. Endotracheally administered antibiotics for gram-negative bronchopneumonia. Chest 1979; 75(5):586–91.

27. Klastersky J, Geuning C, Mouawad E, et al. Endotracheal gentamicin in bronchial infections in patients with tracheostomy. Chest 1972;61(2):117–20.

28. Klastersky J, Huysmans E, Weerts D, et al. Endotracheally administered gentamicin for the prevention of infections of the respiratory tract in patients with tracheostomy: a double-blind study. Chest 1974;65(6):650–4.
29. Pines A, Raafat H, Plucinski K. Gentamicin and colistin in chronic purulent bronchial infections. Br Med J 1967;2(5551):543–5.
30. Feeley TW, Du Moulin GC, Hedley-Whyte J, et al. Aerosol polymyxin and pneumonia in seriously ill patients. N Engl J Med 1975;293(10):471–5.
31. Luyt CE, Clavel M, Guntupalli K, et al. Pharmacokinetics and lung delivery of PDDS-aerosolized amikacin (NKTR-061) in intubated and mechanically ventilated patients with nosocomial pneumonia. Crit Care 2009;13(6):R200.
32. Miller DD, Amin MM, Palmer LB, et al. Aerosol delivery and modern mechanical ventilation: in vitro/in vivo evaluation. Am J Respir Crit Care Med 2003;168(10):1205–9.
33. Niederman M, Sanchez M, Corkery K. Amikacin aerosol achieves high tracheal aspirate concentrations in intubated mechanically ventilated patients with Gram-negative pneumonia: a pharmacokinetic study. Am J Respir Crit Care Med 2007;175:A326.
34. Palmer LB. Ventilator-associated infection: the role for inhaled antibiotics. Curr Opin Pulm Med 2015;21(3):239–49.
35. Mendelman PM, Smith AL, Levy J, et al. Aminoglycoside penetration, inactivation, and efficacy in cystic fibrosis sputum. Am Rev Respir Dis 1985;132(4):761–5.
36. Gil-Perotin S, Ramirez P, Marti V, et al. Implications of endotracheal tube biofilm in ventilator-associated pneumonia response: a state of concept. Crit Care 2012;16(3):R93.
37. Inglis TJ, Lim TM, Ng ML, et al. Structural features of tracheal tube biofilm formed during prolonged mechanical ventilation. Chest 1995;108(4):1049–52.
38. Costerton JW, Stewart PS, Greenberg EP. Bacterial biofilms: a common cause of persistent infections. Science 1999;284(5418):1318–22.
39. Marr AK, Overhage J, Bains M, et al. The Lon protease of *Pseudomonas aeruginosa* is induced by aminoglycosides and is involved in biofilm formation and motility. Microbiology 2007;153(Pt 2):474–82.
40. Palmer LB, Smaldone GC, Chen JJ, et al. Aerosolized antibiotics and ventilator-associated tracheobronchitis in the intensive care unit. Crit Care Med 2008;36(7):2008–13.
41. Palmer LB, Smaldone GC. Reduction of bacterial resistance with inhaled antibiotics in the intensive care unit. Am J Respir Crit Care Med 2014;189(10):1225–33.
42. Falagas ME, Siempos II, Bliziotis IA, et al. Administration of antibiotics via the respiratory tract for the prevention of ICU-acquired pneumonia: a meta-analysis of comparative trials. Crit Care 2006;10(4):R123.
43. Ioannidou E, Siempos II, Falagas ME. Administration of antimicrobials via the respiratory tract for the treatment of patients with nosocomial pneumonia: a meta-analysis. J Antimicrob Chemother 2007;60(6):1216–26.
44. Hallal A, Cohn SM, Namias N, et al. Aerosolized tobramycin in the treatment of ventilator-associated pneumonia: a pilot study. Surg Infect (Larchmt) 2007;8(1):73–82.
45. Le Conte P, Potel G, Clementi E, et al. Administration of tobramycin aerosols in patients with nosocomial pneumonia: a preliminary study. Presse Med 2000;29(2):76–8 [in French].
46. Brown RB, Kruse JA, Counts GW, et al. Double-blind study of endotracheal tobramycin in the treatment of gram-negative bacterial pneumonia. The Endotracheal Tobramycin Study Group. Antimicrob Agents Chemother 1990;34(2):269–72.

47. Zampieri FG, Nassar AP Jr, Gusmao-Flores D, et al. Nebulized antibiotics for ventilator-associated pneumonia: a systematic review and meta-analysis. Crit Care 2015;19:150.
48. Valachis A, Samonis G, Kofteridis DP. The role of aerosolized colistin in the treatment of ventilator-associated pneumonia: a systematic review and metaanalysis. Crit Care Med 2015;43(3):527–33.
49. Florescu DF, Qiu F, McCartan MA, et al. What is the efficacy and safety of colistin for the treatment of ventilator-associated pneumonia? A systematic review and meta-regression. Clin Infect Dis 2012;54(5):670–80.
50. Nation RL, Li J. Colistin in the 21st century. Curr Opin Infect Dis 2009;22(6): 535–43.
51. Elwood CM, Lucas GD, Muehrcke RC. Acute renal failure associated with sodium colistimethate treatment. Arch Intern Med 1966;118(4):326–34.
52. Duncan DA. Colistin toxicity. Neuromuscular and renal manifestations. Two cases treated by hemodialysis. Minn Med 1973;56(1):31–5.
53. Falagas ME, Kasiakou SK, Tsiodras S, et al. The use of intravenous and aerosolized polymyxins for the treatment of infections in critically ill patients: a review of the recent literature. Clin Med Res 2006;4(2):138–46.
54. Kwa AL, Loh C, Low JG, et al. Nebulized colistin in the treatment of pneumonia due to multidrug-resistant *Acinetobacter baumannii* and *Pseudomonas aeruginosa*. Clin Infect Dis 2005;41(5):754–7.
55. Rios FG, Luna CM, Maskin B, et al. Ventilator-associated pneumonia due to colistin susceptible-only microorganisms. Eur Respir J 2007;30(2):307–13.
56. Munoz-Price LS, Weinstein RA. Acinetobacter infection. N Engl J Med 2008; 358(12):1271–81.
57. Hamer DH. Treatment of nosocomial pneumonia and tracheobronchitis caused by multidrug-resistant *Pseudomonas aeruginosa* with aerosolized colistin. Am J Respir Crit Care Med 2000;162(1):328–30.
58. Rattanaumpawan P, Lorsutthitham J, Ungprasert P, et al. Randomized controlled trial of nebulized colistimethate sodium as adjunctive therapy of ventilator-associated pneumonia caused by Gram-negative bacteria. J Antimicrob Chemother 2010;65(12):2645–9.
59. Kollef MH, Ricard JD, Roux D, et al. A randomized trial of the amikacin fosfomycin inhalation system for the adjunctive therapy of Gram-negative ventilator-associated pneumonia: IASIS Trial. Chest 2016;151(6):1239–46.
60. American Thoracic Society, Infectious Diseases Society of America. Guidelines for the management of adults with hospital-acquired, ventilator-associated, and healthcare-associated pneumonia. Am J Respir Crit Care Med 2005;171(4): 388–416.
61. Lu Q, Yang J, Liu Z, et al. Nebulized ceftazidime and amikacin in ventilator-associated pneumonia caused by *Pseudomonas aeruginosa*. Am J Respir Crit Care Med 2011;184(1):106–15.

Moving?

Make sure your subscription moves with you!

To notify us of your new address, find your **Clinics Account Number** (located on your mailing label above your name), and contact customer service at:

Email: journalscustomerservice-usa@elsevier.com

800-654-2452 (subscribers in the U.S. & Canada)
314-447-8871 (subscribers outside of the U.S. & Canada)

Fax number: 314-447-8029

Elsevier Health Sciences Division
Subscription Customer Service
3251 Riverport Lane
Maryland Heights, MO 63043

*To ensure uninterrupted delivery of your subscription, please notify us at least 4 weeks in advance of move.

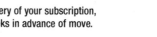

Printed and bound by CPI Group (UK) Ltd, Croydon, CR0 4YY

08/05/2025

01864703-0010